WOMEN'S HEALTH FOR LIFE

MEDICAL ADVICE YOU CAN TRUST
SYMPTOMS · TREATMENT · PREVENTION

EDITOR-IN-CHIEF **DR SARAH JARVIS** MA, BM BCH, DRCOG, FRCGP
& A TEAM OF WORLD-CLASS WOMEN DOCTORS

LONDON, NEW YORK, MELBOURNE,
MUNICH AND DELHI

Project Editor Hilary Mandleberg
Senior Editor Jennifer Latham
Senior Art Editor Isabel de Cordova
Designers Kenny Grant, John Round
Editors Ann Baggaley, Debbie Beckerman,
Claire Cross, Jo Godfrey-Wood, Mary Lindsay,
Cathy Meeus, Pip Morgan, Martyn Page,
Nikki Sims, Susannah Steel, Kathy Steer,
Diana Vowles
Managing Editor Dawn Henderson
Managing Art Editor Christine Keilty
Senior Production Editor Jenny Woodcock
Senior Jacket Creative Nicola Powling
Picture Research Liz Moore, Jenny Baskaya
Creative Technical Support Sonia Charbonnier
Senior Production Controller Wendy Penn

First published in Great Britain in 2009 by
Dorling Kindersley Limited, 80 Strand, London
WC2R 0RL
A Penguin Company

First paperback edition published in 2010 by
Dorling Kindersley Limited

2 4 6 8 10 9 7 5 3 1

Copyright © 2009, 2010 Dorling Kindersley
Limited, London
Text copyright © 2009, 2010 Sarah Jarvis pages
8–9, 12–23, and 318–331

Note to readers: *Women's Health for Life*
provides general information on a wide
range of health and medical topics. The book
is not a substitute for medical diagnosis,
however, and you are advised always to consult
your doctor for specific information on personal
health matters. The Publisher cannot accept any
liability or responsibility for any loss or damage
allegedly arising from any information
or suggestion in this book.

All rights reserved. No part of this publication may
be reproduced, stored in a retrieval system, or
transmitted in any form by any means, electronic,
mechanical, photocopying, recording or otherwise,
without the prior written permission of the
copyright owner.

A CIP catalogue record for this book
is available from the British Library

ISBN 978-1-4053-5378-6

Colour reproduced by MDP, UK
Printed and bound in Portugal
by Printer Portuguesa

Discover more at
www.dk.com

The Authors

EDITOR-IN-CHIEF

DR SARAH JARVIS, **MA, BM BCH, DRCOG, FRCGP,** has been a GP for 19 years and has moonlighted as a medical writer and broadcaster for most of that time. She is passionate about empowering people to make their own health decisions, and has published four previous books and over 800 patient information leaflets. Sarah is the doctor for BBC Radio 2 and for BBC 1's "The One Show". She also works with numerous charities to help raise awareness about heart disease, diabetes, and women's health.

DR ANNE BALLINGER MD, FRCP is a Consultant Gastroenterologist and General Physician at Queen Elizabeth the Queen Mother Hospital, Margate, Kent. She qualified at University College London School of Medicine and completed her postgraduate training in London.

DR LISA DAVIES BM BCH, BA (OXON), FRCP, FRCP(E) trained at Oxford University and is now a Consultant Respiratory Physician at University Hospital Aintree and an Honorary Senior Lecturer at the University of Liverpool.

DR CHARLOTTE FEINMANN MD, MSC, FRCPSYCH, FDS (HON) is a Liaison Psychiatrist with 30 years' clinical and academic experience in women's health and long-term conditions.

MISS TAMSIN GREENWELL MD, FRCS (UROL) is a Consultant Urological Surgeon and Honorary Senior Lecturer in Female and Reconstructive Urology at UCLH/ UCL and London Bridge Hospitals. She is also Urology Tutor at The Royal College of Surgeons of England.

DR DAWN HARPER MBBS, MRCP, DCH, DFFP is a GP and runs clinics on women's health and weight management. She presents "Embarrassing Bodies" on Channel 4, is a regular on BBC Radio 1, and writes columns for several women's magazines.

DR PATRICIA MACNAIR MB CHB, MA, DA (FARCS) is a Hospital Physician working part-time in Medicine for the Elderly. She also works as a freelance medical journalist and broadcaster, primarily for the BBC.

DR FIONA MACNEILL MBBS, FRCS, MD is Consultant Breast and Oncoplastic Reconstructive Surgeon at Royal Marsden Hospital, London. She is also Breast Tutor at the Royal College of Surgeons of England.

R85

Please return / renew by date shown.
You can renew at: **norlink.norfolk.gov.uk**
or by telephone: **0344 800 8006**
Please have you library card & PIN ready

7/3/13

NORFOLK LIBRARY
AND INFORMATION SERVICE
NORFOLK ITEM

30129 060 936 946

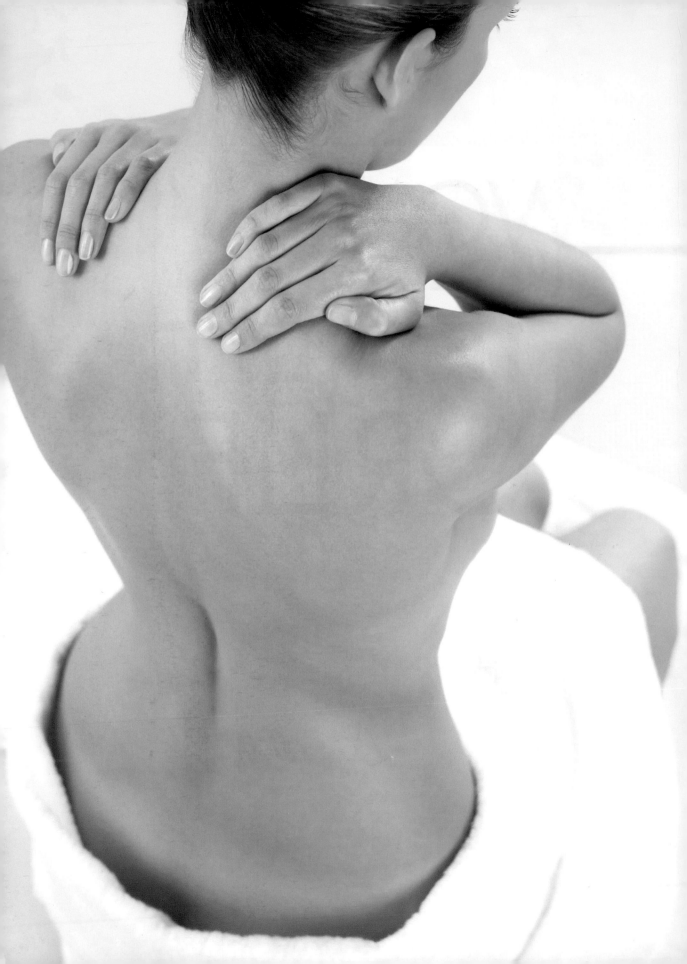

DR GHADA MIKHAIL BSC, MBBS, MD, FRCP is a Consultant Cardiologist and Honorary Senior Lecturer at the Imperial College Healthcare NHS Trust, London.

PROFESSOR KAREN MORRISON MA (CANTAB), BMBCH (OXON), DPHIL, FRCP is Bloomer Professor of Neurology, and Head of Department of Clinical Neurosciences at Birmingham University. She is also Honorary Consultant Neurologist, University Hospitals Birmingham NHS Foundation Trust.

DR NERYS ROBERTS MD, FRCP, MRCPCH, BSC is a Consultant Dermatologist at a London University teaching hospital, specializing in the diagnosis and treatment of both children and adults. She is also a Trustee of the skin research charity, START.

DR NINA SALOOJA DM, MSC (ED), FRCP, FRCPATH is a Consultant Haematologist at The Hammersmith and Charing Cross Hospitals, London, which form part of the Imperial Academic Health Science Centre.

DR NURHAN SUTCLIFFE MD, FRCP is a Consultant Rheumatologist at the Barts and The London NHS Trusts. She treats patients with all rheumatological conditions and has research and clinical interests in Sjögren's Syndrome.

DR MELANIE TIPPLES MRCOG, FRCSED is a Consultant Obstetrician and Gynaecologist at St Richards Hospital, Chichester. Her special interests are gynaecological scanning, gynaecological cancers, and colposcopy.

The Contributors

DR CATHERINE A. BIRNDORF MD Clinical Associate Professor of Psychiatry and Obstetrics and Gynecology, New York Presbyterian Hospital, Weill Cornell Medical Center, New York, USA

DR BETH B. DUPREE MD, FACS is a breast surgeon in Bensalem, Pennsylvania, USA.

DR CORDELIA GRIMM MD, MPH Consultant to the Internal Medicine Residency Program, Good Samaritan Hospital of Baltimore, Baltimore, and an Assistant Professor of Clincial Medicine at John Hopkins University of School of Medicine, Baltimore, USA.

DR DEBRA JALIMAN MD Assistant Clinical Professor, Department of Dermatology, Mount Sinai School of Medicine, New York, USA.

PROFESSOR MARY JANE MINKIN MD, FACOG Clinical Professor, Department of Obstetrics and Gynecology, Yale University School of Medicine, New Haven, Connecticut, USA.

DR DONNICA L. MOORE MD President of the Sapphire Women's Health Group in the USA, and host of DrDonnica.com, a women's health information website.

DR ALEXANDRA C. SACKS MD Resident in Adult Psychiatry, New York Presbyterian Hospital, Weill Cornell Medical Center, New York, USA.

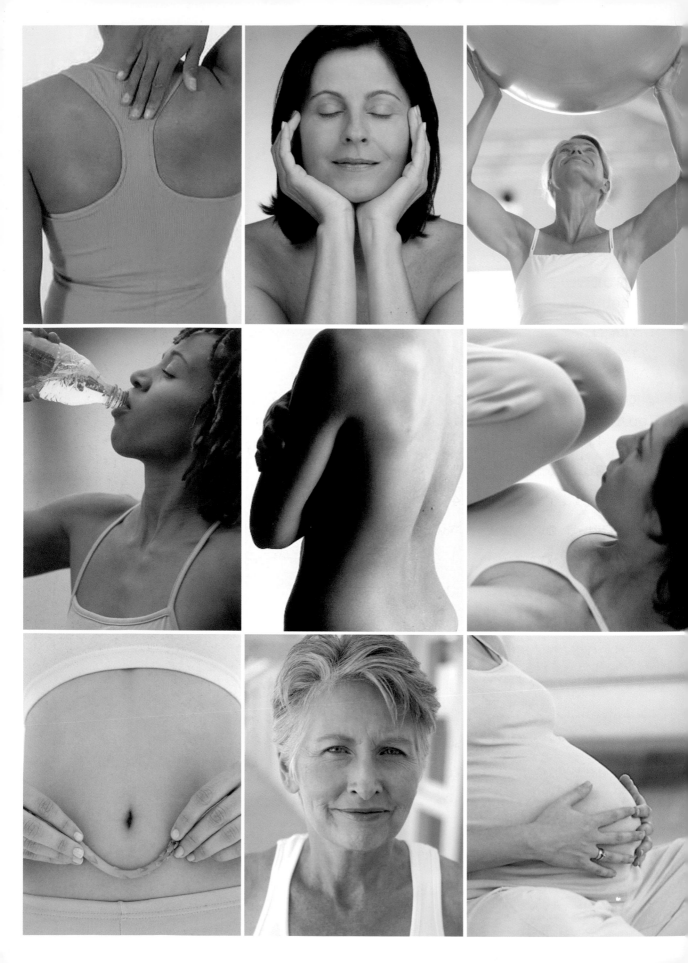

Contents

Message from the Editor-in-Chief

Our health is the most precious commodity we have, and we women are usually very good at making the most of it, which is important not just for our own sakes, but for the sake of those around us – our partners and husbands, our children, and our ageing relatives – who may all depend on our staying healthy.

Women's Health for Life is a celebration of the thousands of miracles that keep women's delicate bodies in the healthy balance that's needed. It explains, in easy-to-understand terms, the miracle of all our body systems, whether it's our bones and joints, our brain and nerves, our digestive system, or our heart and blood. It also explains the very special changes that we women undergo during the course of our reproductive lives, such as menstruation, pregnancy, perimenopause, and menopause.

But of course, there's more. Sometimes things go wrong and we need to seek medical advice. But medicine – like our bodies – is hugely complicated. It's also, like us, ever-changing, so it's not surprising that, despite our best efforts, we sometimes find the medical advice we're given bewildering and hard to understand.

Women's Health for Life helps you navigate your way through these complexities and provides you with plenty of practical advice and useful tips. For instance, it deals with a huge variety of common and important medical conditions – both physical and mental – giving you a checklist of symptoms for each so you can recognize the warning signs or discover that it's OK to relax. It also tells you what you might have in the way of tests and examinations that will help your doctor diagnose a condition, and it then explains the treatment you can expect to receive once a diagnosis has been reached. In many instances, there are things you can do to help yourself, too. *Women's Health for Life* gives you all the latest information on the self-help measures you need to continue to live life to the full, even if you're coping with a long-term condition.

Women's Health for Life has been written by several of the most credible, respected and trusted authorities in women's health. Some, like me, are working GPs, who deal with many of the health-related concerns that affect us all, and with the anxiety that symptoms can cause. Others are top specialists, whose contribution has been to provide a comprehensive outline of the possible causes of the conditions they treat each and every day, and of the latest medical advances in their specialist fields.

Uniquely, *Women's Health for Life* is designed to be easy to navigate, with a simple structure and clear, understandable illustrations, graphs and charts. It will provide you with all the information you require, whichever way you want to approach it, whether that's by reading it from cover to cover – it's divided into neat, bite-sized chunks that make doing this easy – or by dipping in and out according to your needs and interests.

If you start at the beginning, you'll find an answer to the question of whether men really do have an "excuse" for their different behaviour. Chapter 1, entitled "We're Different", explains how we differ from men in not just our anatomy and response to disease, but even in our behaviour and intelligence. Perhaps you're more interested in why your body seems to have changed over the years, and what you can expect in decades to come. Chapter 2, "Understanding the Changes", will tell you everything you need to know. Carry on to Chapter 3, "Staying Well", and you'll learn how to stay in tip-top shape and how adopting a healthy lifestyle can help to keep many diseases at bay, while Chapter 4, "Know the Signs", helps you pinpoint on your body the signs and symptoms that may indicate you have a medical condition. Handy cross-references from this chapter to the other chapters in the book will lead you to the more detailed health information you need in order to be really well informed.

After that come the chapters on the body systems, all with plenty of cross-references to other areas of health that may be connected to your personal query. Finally, turn to our Resources, where each of our team of authors offers a list of the organisations that they think are the most useful sources of information for the public within their speciality.

We're sure you'll find *Women's Health for Life* interesting and informative. We're confident that you'll want to keep it as a reference tool. Above all, we hope you have as much fun using it as we did writing it!

Dr Sarah Jarvis

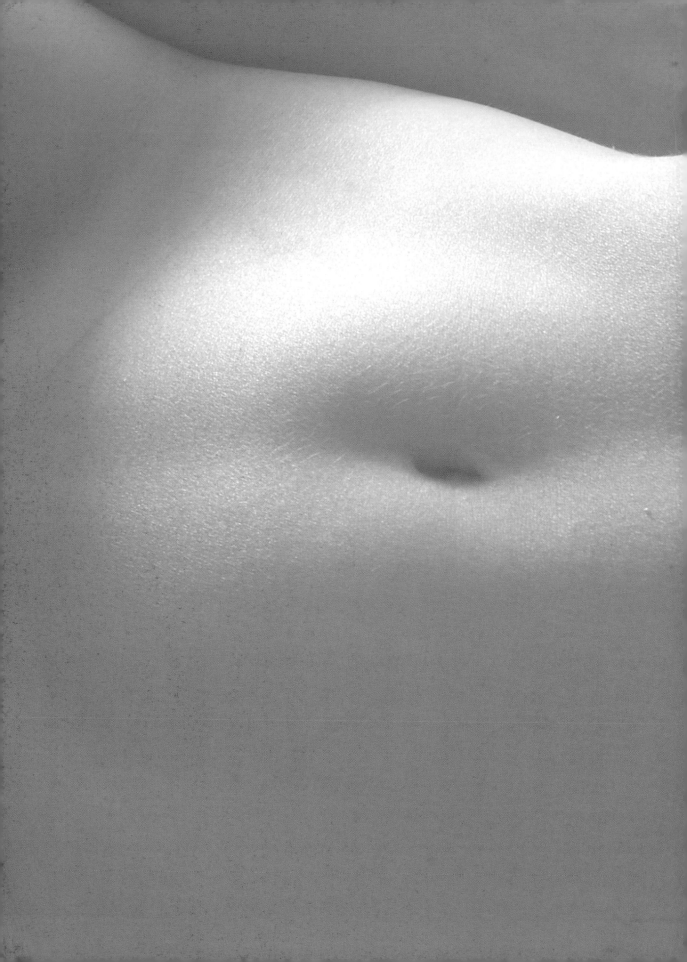

We're different

Dr Sarah Jarvis MA BM BCH DRCOG FRCGP

Girls and boys: what are the differences?

Until puberty there are very few visible differences between boys and girls, apart from the obvious difference – the presence, or otherwise, of a penis – and the fact that boys have a slightly different build. At puberty, though, the differences – both internal and external – become much more apparent.

AN EXTRA X MAKES A BIG DIFFERENCE

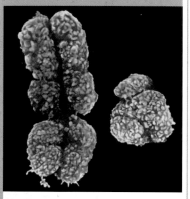

X and Y chromosomes
The X chromosome (left) is much larger than the relatively puny Y chromosome (right).

Men have one X and one Y chromosome (XY), while women have two X chromosomes (XX). Women can only pass on an X chromosome, but a man can pass on an X or a Y. When it comes to the sex of your baby, your partner's sperm has the final say! If a baby develops from your egg and a sperm with an X chromosome, it will be a girl (XX), but if it is fertilized by a sperm with a Y chromosome, it will turn out to be a boy (XY).

Women's bodies are designed to give birth and to nurture babies and men's are designed to father them. Puberty is when we reach sexual maturity, when, physically, we become capable of fulfilling these functions. It is, therefore, a time of enormous change, both physical and emotional.

THE START OF PUBERTY

The age at which their puberty starts is something that many children worry about. Although it varies from child to child and is influenced by a number of factors, including heredity, puberty begins between the ages of eight and thirteen in a girl, and between ten and fifteen in a boy.

One of the factors that influences the onset of puberty is nutrition; poor nutrition can cause a delay. As nutrition improved in the developed world between the late 19th and the mid-20th centuries, the average age when puberty started went down by well over a year. In today's developed world, malnutrition is rare and as a result, especially in the USA over the last 50 years or so, there seems to be a continuing trend towards an even lower average age of puberty. The evidence is stronger in girls than in boys, and is even more marked among African-American girls. In fact, in 1999 in the USA, new guidelines were produced, which suggested that puberty should only be considered abnormally early ("precocious puberty") if breast or pubic hair development starts before the age of seven in white girls and six in black girls.

In the UK, the changes have been less marked; there has probably only been a reduction of six months or so in the average age of puberty in the last few decades. In the UK, puberty in girls is considered to be precocious if it starts before the age of eight.

HOW GIRLS CHANGE AT PUBERTY

The dominant female hormone is oestrogen. At puberty it is produced in greater amounts and is crucial to a girl's sexual development. Its main physical effects are on:
The skeleton A girl's hips and pelvis widen, making her well suited anatomically for giving birth.

The face Girls develop jaw and facial features that are much finer and more delicate than boys'.

Body hair Girls develop pubic hair and hair under their arms.

The skin and sweat glands Girls start to suffer from body odour and acne.

Body fat Girls begin to get more body fat on their hips, thighs, and buttocks, as well as on their breasts. Most women are designed to have more body fat than men.

The breasts Soon after their body hair starts to appear, the breasts increase in size. Girls' nipples also change during puberty, becoming darker and more prominent and better designed for breastfeeding.

The ovaries and uterus The reproductive organs grow and mature. Girls begin their periods; the average age in the UK is 12 and a half.

HOW BOYS CHANGE AT PUBERTY

Testosterone is the main hormone that comes into play in boys at puberty. It has amazingly wide-ranging effects that last throughout life. At puberty, its main physical effects are on:

The skeleton A boy's shoulders start to widen so that by the time he is a man, he will have shoulders that are wider than his hips.

The muscles A boy's muscles become bigger and heavier. Those of his upper body in particular develop more than a girl's.

The vocal cords and the larynx (also known as the voice box) A boy's voice "breaks" and he develops a typically deeper voice.

The face Changes in a boy's bones and muscles result in the development of a heavier jaw.

Body hair Boys develop pubic and underarm hair and, depending on inherited characteristics, hair on the face, neck, chest, and back.

The skin and sweat glands Boys start to suffer from body odour and acne.

The genitals A boy's penis grows, his testicles descend and get larger, and he is able to ejaculate.

THE CHANGING BODY OF A GIRL

As a young girl grows from childhood into puberty and becomes a woman, her body changes. She gradually develops breasts, pubic hair, and an hourglass figure with a well-defined waist and broadened hips.

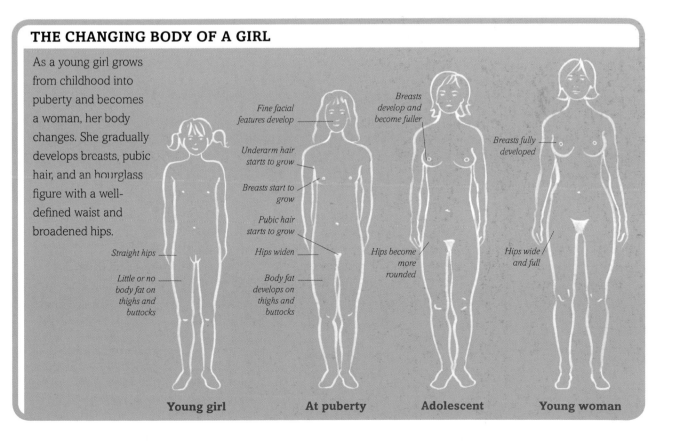

Fine facial features develop

Underarm hair starts to grow

Breasts start to grow

Pubic hair starts to grow

Breasts develop and become fuller

Breasts fully developed

Straight hips

Little or no body fat on thighs and buttocks

Hips widen

Body fat develops on thighs and buttocks

Hips become more rounded

Hips wide and full

Young girl **At puberty** **Adolescent** **Young woman**

The adult woman

By the time we reach adulthood, women are, on average, 20 per cent shorter, and 30 per cent weaker physically, than men. There are also differences in the amount of fat and muscle on our bodies, the basic rate of our metabolism, and the structure of some of our bones and joints.

Hair Women have, on the whole, less body hair than men, although it doesn't stop many of us feeling we've still got too much. Our facial hair and other body hair are usually very light, although this can become darker and coarser in later life. Our pubic hair forms a straight line at the top. Fortunately, the hair on our heads is rather longer lasting than the average man's. Although it becomes thinner as we age, and a little sparser, we can expect to end our lives with almost as much as we started with (unless you suffer from a condition such as alopecia, see p370).

Skeleton Most women have more delicate facial features than men. Generally, we also have smaller heads, shorter necks, smaller, narrower chests, and more rounded shoulders, as well as smaller hands and feet, and shorter legs and arms.

In terms of evolution, being big was an advantage for a man if he was facing a sabre-toothed tiger or another, perhaps hostile, man. Women's priorities centred around childrearing, so we relied on those big burly menfolk to fend off predators while we protected our young. Women also have a broader, shallower pelvis than a man, which is essential for giving birth.

Body fat The extra fat we gain at puberty over the hips, thighs, and buttocks, in combination with our wider hips and pelvis, gives women their traditional "hourglass" shape. Contrast this with a man's trunk, which is more like an upside-down triangle, with broader shoulders and narrower hips. Our excess body fat is probably another trick of evolution, allowing women to

MALE AND FEMALE BODIES

At puberty, male and female bodies become different shapes. Women have an "hourglass" shape with wider hips, while a man has broader shoulders that give his torso an inverted triangle shape.

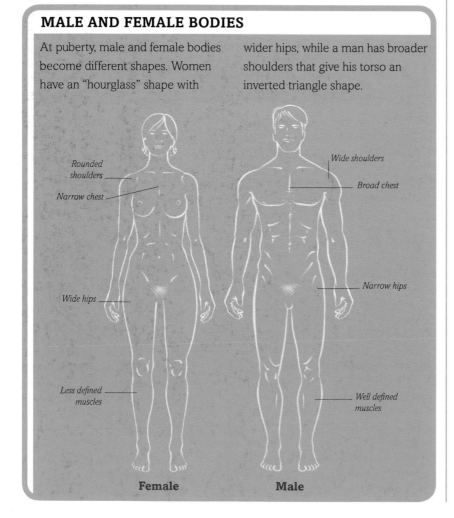

Rounded shoulders

Narrow chest

Wide hips

Less defined muscles

Wide shoulders

Broad chest

Narrow hips

Well defined muscles

Female　　　　**Male**

draw on their stores of fat to feed their young in times of famine. But the fact that we have more body fat and less body water than men also makes us more prone to the effects of alcohol (see p65).

Muscles Women naturally have smaller, less well-defined muscles than men and they are also less visible because of their covering of fat. Back in the mists of time, men needed more muscle to hunt than women did to raise young.

Breasts Our breasts usually begin to develop shortly after our body hair starts to appear. By the time puberty is complete, the breasts are sufficiently developed physically to produce milk, although this doesn't usually happen until we are well into pregnancy.

Genitals Unlike men, most of our reproductive equipment is on the inside. The only part that can be seen is the entrance to the vagina, with its two sets of lips, labia (outer and inner), framing the tiny clitoris at the front where they join.

The reproductive system

Inside her ovaries a newborn girl has many thousands of immature eggs. When her ovaries start to ovulate, they release mature eggs (the average woman produces one a month during most of the time she has periods) and she can start to reproduce.

A man can stay fertile for the rest of his life (the oldest recorded man to father a child was an Australian aged 93), but a woman can't get pregnant naturally after the menopause, and often not for

A WOMAN'S PELVIS COMPARED TO A MAN'S

The human pelvis consists of two large hip bones that join the sacrum at the base of the spine and meet in front at the pubic symphysis where they form the pubic arch. They create a space called the pelvic inlet that protects the bladder and, in a woman, the ovaries and womb. A woman's pelvis makes childbirth easier and is generally wider, shallower, and more delicate than a man's. Her inlet is larger and more circular, her sacrum is shorter and less curved, and the pubic arch is wider and less angular. During pregnancy the pubic symphysis joint softens and becomes more flexible, allowing the baby to pass through the birth canal during delivery. Our unique pelvis is the secret of our success in the delivery room.

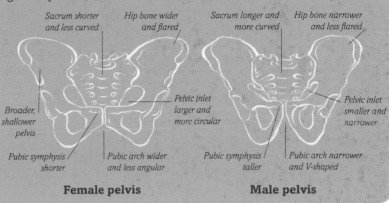

Sacrum shorter and less curved · *Hip bone wider and flared* · *Sacrum longer and more curved* · *Hip bone narrower and less flared*

Broader, shallower pelvis · *Pelvic inlet larger and more circular* · *Pelvic inlet smaller and narrower*

Pubic symphysis shorter · *Pubic arch wider and less angular* · *Pubic symphysis taller* · *Pubic arch narrower and V-shaped*

Female pelvis   **Male pelvis**

several years before it. What's more, we often only begin ovulating regularly a year or two after we start having periods.

Metabolism This is a term that describes how much energy the body uses. Our basal metabolic rate is equivalent to the amount of calories we burn just to stay alive without doing anything else. That includes breathing, keeping our heart, liver, and other organs going, and using our brains.

Amazingly, about 70 per cent of the energy we burn is just to keep us alive. For the average woman, another 20 per cent is used in physical activity and 10 per cent is for digestion and creating heat to keep ourselves warm.

On average, women naturally have a lower basal metabolic rate than men, partly because we're usually smaller – and, not surprisingly, it takes more energy to keep a bigger body going.

However, even compared to a man of the same size, a woman's body has a lower metabolic rate because she naturally has a higher proportion of fat combined with a lower proportion of muscle. This also means that when the average woman eats exactly as much as the average man, she is more likely to put on weight.

Sickness and disease

Since women differ from men so much physically, it's not surprising that we differ in our susceptibility to illness, too. The good news for us is that women in the Western world live, on average, five years longer than men. But that doesn't necessarily mean we have fewer diseases.

WHAT DISEASES DO WOMEN GET?

While women are slightly less likely to suffer from the biggest killers – heart disease and cancer – than men we're more likely to get other diseases.

Mental health problems

Women tend to have more in the way of mental health problems, such as depression (see pp210–11), anxiety (see pp204–5), and eating disorders (see pp216–17). These can seriously affect our quality of life and that of our loved ones, too.

We also suffer from Alzheimer's disease (see pp184–5) more than men, though this may be because we live longer and Alzheimer's disease gets more common with age. Again, this distressing condition affects our quality of life and that of our carers.

Bony conditions When it comes to bony conditions, we women are much more prone than men to osteoporosis, or thinning of the bones (see pp260–2).

Similarly with osteoarthritis (see pp263–5) – another bony condition that affects more women than men. Like osteoporosis and Alzheimer's, it's largely a condition that develops because of old age. But the truth of the matter is that many of the conditions that women get more commonly than men are clearly debilitating but kill only slowly, if at all. Osteoarthritis and osteoporosis cause crippling pain, and can make it very difficult to live independently, but you don't die as a direct result of them.

DRUGS TESTED MAINLY ON MEN

Drugs treatments have made great strides in modern times – for example, the development of statins for reducing high cholesterol levels in the blood. However, many drugs are tested on men, leaving women wondering whether the drugs are suitable for them. It is increasingly clear that women respond to some drugs differently, may need a different dose, or may experience different side-effects. What seems to be needed in medical research and clinical drug trials is a more representative profile of participants – one that includes women of all kinds.

Cancer Men are more likely to die from cancer than we are, due largely to smoking-related lung cancer. We, of course, are afflicted by cancers of our own, especially breast cancer (see pp152–7) and cervical cancer (see p107).

Heart disease and stroke More men than women die from heart disease (see pp160–75) and stroke (see p196), although, once we're past the menopause, the heart-protective effect of our oestrogen wanes and our risk increases sharply. Interestingly, some people who die from heart disease never even know they have it: over a third die from a heart attack without ever having had a diagnosis of heart disease.

Smoking, drinking, and taking drugs Overall, men are more likely than we are to smoke, drink too much alcohol, and take illegal drugs. This means that they're more likely to suffer (and sometimes die) from diseases linked to these unhealthy habits.

Sadly, the gap between us has been closing in recent years. This is because men are more health-conscious, but also because women are now more likely to smoke, drink, and use drugs (see pp22–3).

DOMINANT AND RECESSIVE GENES

We all have two of most genes – one of each of a pair of chromosomes (see p12) – inherited from our parents. A gene is a code for a particular characteristic. Some genes are "dominant", others are "recessive". If you inherit a dominant gene you will develop the characteristic associated with it. For example, the gene for brown eyes is dominant, so you will have brown eyes if you inherit a brown-eyed gene from one parent, even though you inherit a blue-eyed gene (recessive) from the other. You'll only have blue eyes if you inherit a blue-eyed gene from both parents and you'll have brown eyes if you inherit a brown-eyed gene from both.

Diseases can also be passed on via our genes. The genes for some, such as colour blindness and haemophilia (a condition in which the blood does not clot properly because an essential clotting factor is either partly or completely missing), are recessive and are carried only on X chromosomes (see p12). Men have only one X chromosome, so if they inherit an affected one, they'll get the disease. A woman has two, so can inherit the affected X chromosome from one parent, but the normal dominant gene from the other. She won't get the disease, but can pass on the affected X chromosome to a child, making her a "carrier".

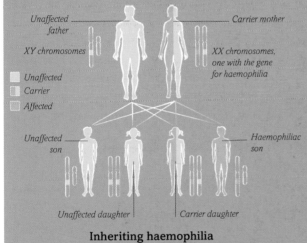

Unaffected father
XY chromosomes
Unaffected
Carrier
Affected
Unaffected son
Unaffected daughter
Carrier mother
XX chromosomes, one with the gene for haemophilia
Haemophiliac son
Carrier daughter

Inheriting haemophilia
The diagram shows how diseases such as haemophilia are passed on. It is extremely rare for a woman to get haemophilia.

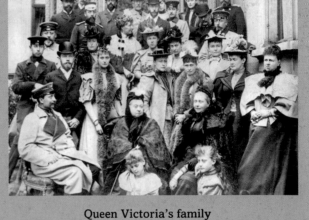

Queen Victoria's family
Queen Victoria was a carrier of haemophilia and the disease spread to other royal houses because of this.

ILLNESS AND CHANGING HORMONES

Several medical conditions tend to be more or less problematic during pregnancy or the menstrual cycle when female hormones change rapidly. They include:

Asthma During pregnancy, some women report their asthma gets better, although women with severe asthma are more likely to find their symptoms becoming worse.

Rheumatoid arthritis During pregnancy rheumatoid arthritis symptoms improve in up to three-quarters of sufferers. Unfortunately, a similar proportion experience a flare-up once pregnancy is over.

Migraine About two-thirds of sufferers have fewer attacks or less severe migraines during pregnancy, especially in the last six months. In up to 1 in 12, migraines get worse. See also menstrual migraine, p182.

Depression About 1 in 5 women get depression during pregnancy; in about 50 per cent it is clinically significant. Many women with depression find their symptoms become worse in the days leading up to their period; these women are more prone to depression around the menopause. Depression and mood changes are a risk of hormonal contraception, hormone infertility treatment, and HRT.

Venus and Mars: the brain and intelligence

Are women better then men at multitasking but not as good at reading a map? There's no doubt that men and women have differences in behaviour. Here we'll look at some of those differences and discuss the theories surrounding them. A good place to start is with the brain.

The human brain contains some 10,000–15,000 million nerve cells, called neurons, and one million billion synapses (the connections between nerve cells). But the way in which the brain functions is still, to an extent, a medical mystery, so we can't say with certainty how much the physical differences between people's brains affect or contribute to their behaviour.

The hemispheres It is believed that these two halves of the brain probably work differently. The left side helps us think analytically, while the right side helps us look at things as a whole, involving value judgements and emotion. Men are more likely to be "left-brain dominant" while women are thought to use both hemispheres more equally.

The corpus callosum transfers information between both halves of the brain. Women have a bigger corpus callosum than men, which may account for the fact that women score better on tests of thought fluency and speech.

The limbic system affects our emotions and is, on the whole, bigger in women. Together with

THE BRAIN – WHERE WOMEN ARE DIFFERENT

Women have slightly smaller brains than men (they weigh about 100g less) but, as we know, size isn't everything. Elephants, for instance, have much larger brains than humans, but nobody believes they have more intellect. And though women's brains are smaller than men's, they both have a very similar ratio of brain weight to body weight. Women also have 4 per cent fewer brain cells than men, but this doesn't mean they use them less! There are other male/female differences too!

The frontal lobe of the brain plays a major part in making judgements, planning future actions, and in language. Women have far more cells here than men.

HOW OUR BRAINS ARE DIFFERENT

There are numerous anatomical differences between female and male brains; some of the key ones are highlighted here.

Left hemisphere helps us think analytically; men are more likely to be left-brain dominant

Right hemisphere involves judgements and emotions; women are thought to use both hemispheres more equally

Overhead view

Grey matter processes information and is larger in men

White matter connects the different parts of the brain and is larger in women

Segment overhead view

Corpus callosum links the two hemispheres and is larger in women

Frontal lobe helps make decisions and solve problems, and is larger in women

Hypothalamus, part of the limbic system, links the brain to the hormone system and is smaller in women

Limbic system regulates emotion and is larger in women

Side view

a female brain's greater ability to transfer information between its two sides, these facts may help account for women's greater emotional sensitivity. The bigger limbic system may also mean that women feel negative emotions more keenly, laying them open to a greater risk of depression.

Grey matter and white matter

Processing information goes on in the grey matter, while white matter connects the different parts of our brain, enabling us to carry out various tasks. Women tend to have far more white matter than men, while men are endowed with far more grey matter. Could any or all of these differences above be an explanation for the popular theory that women are better at "multi-tasking" than men?

The hypothalamus controls the endocrine system that produces many of the hormones in the body. The functions it regulates include sexual function, sleep, water content, and body temperature. In men the hypothalamus is about twice as big and contains twice as many cells as it does in women.

MEASURING INTELLIGENCE

Despite the physical differences between the male and female brain, there seems to be little, if any, difference between them as far as overall intelligence is concerned. The average IQ (intelligence quotient) score for men and for women is very similar, but that doesn't mean we're all the same. In fact, far more men than women

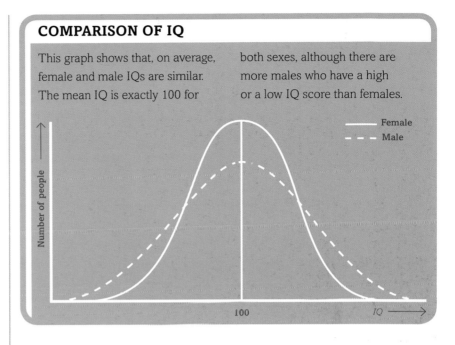

COMPARISON OF IQ

This graph shows that, on average, female and male IQs are similar. The mean IQ is exactly 100 for both sexes, although there are more males who have a high or a low IQ score than females.

Female
Male

Number of people

100 IQ

get very high or very low scores. That means there are probably more very clever men around than there are very clever women, but probably there are also more men than women at the bottom of the class.

Another problem is, though, that while "average" scores tell us about the average ability of men and women in a whole population, they can't tell us how well individuals do, or the range of their results.

Nor is measuring intelligence that straightforward. The most common tests include the IQ test and the SAT test. There has been huge debate as to whether such tests disadvantage women by using situations that men (or boys) are more familiar with than girls. For example, a question that asks about the relative speeds of two cars might be easier for a man to answer than a woman.

HORSES FOR COURSES?

Research has shown that, on the whole, men perform better than women at visual-spatial tests, so they are good at understanding the things we see and putting them in context – for instance, the way a car engine is put together. Men also tend to be better at tests involving maths.

Women do better at tests involving language and words, as well as verbal reasoning. They also score better on some memory tests.

It's not surprising then that men greatly outnumber women in top academic posts in the sciences, but there's little or no difference between the numbers of men and women reaching the top in the arts and humanities.

Venus and Mars: personality

Do the physical differences between the male and female brain account for the personality differences between men and women? Those who believe the "nature" theory argue that they do. Others believe that "nurture", or the way we're brought up, is what makes women so different from men.

In psychology, there is reasonable consensus that personality can be described by dividing it into five broad factors or dimensions. These so-called "big five" are Openness, Conscientiousness, Extraversion, Agreeableness, and Neuroticism. This psychological model is often referred to as OCEAN. Each of the five factors includes several personality traits:

Openness Imagination, curiosity, a sense of adventure, and an appreciation of new ideas.

Conscientiousness A sense of duty, self-discipline, a tendency to plan ahead rather than acting on the spur of the moment, and the need for achievement.

Extraversion A tendency to seek the company of others, exuberance, energetic approach to life, looking at the positive, and assertiveness.

Agreeableness Co-operation, peacemaking, compassion, helpfulness, and a tendency to fall in with the wishes of others rather than create conflict.

Neuroticism A sensitivity to anxiety, depression, or other negative emotions, moodiness, and a tendency to "blow problems out of proportion" and to see obstacles as insurmountable.

NATURE OR NURTURE?

In psychological tests, women consistently score higher in the areas of Agreeableness and Neuroticism. Perhaps surprisingly, such differences are greater in cultures where "traditional" models of the roles of the two genders have become less widespread. Thus the difference between the genders seems to be greater in Europe and the USA than it is in more traditional cultures.

Nature theorists Scientists who believe in the "nature" theory argue that we're "hard-wired" for either a male or female personality. They point to the differences in a woman's limbic system and the better connections between a woman's brain hemispheres (see p18) as the reason for the higher scores in the psychological tests. They also believe that, because the structure of a woman's brain is different from a man's, that accounts entirely for the way in which women process information. This, in turn, determines which particular skills in IQ tests (see p19) women will find more or less easy than men, and why women tend to look at the bigger picture when making decisions.

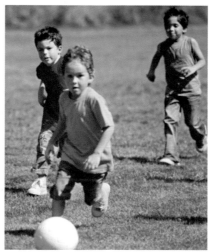

Differences between girls and boys

As every parent knows, girls are more likely to talk with each other as they sit together in the playground, whereas boys very often choose to play a physical game such as football.

Nurture theorists Another group of scientists argues vigorously that women are born with the capacity to have the same type of personality and intellectual skills as men. The differences are due to socialization – this is the way certain "female" personality traits are imposed on us by society and become deeply ingrained. These theorists believe that once physical strength was no longer needed for survival, men imposed other ways of subjugating women – for example, by claiming they were less intelligent or over-emotional and by relegating them to a secondary role in society.

Nature and nurture A third group argues that some innate differences exist between men and women, which society reinforces. Moreover, some think that the differences between men and women's brains are no more marked than the differences that exist between individual men or individual women. The truth is that behaviour is incredibly complicated and is almost certainly influenced profoundly by both our genetic make-up and our upbringing.

PERSONALITY, GENDER, AND PROFESSION

We have looked at the differences between men and women with respect to areas of intelligence (see p19). But how much of an influence does our personality have on how we get on in our profession, and what part do gender differences in personality play? It's possible that personality may have an impact on job performance. For instance, in one study, higher job performance was linked with higher levels of Openness and Extraversion and lower performance with rising levels of Neuroticism.

However, there are many other models of personality than the five OCEAN categories, and critics of the "big five" say they do not take into account other personality traits such as Sense of Humour, Motivation, and Identity. It's possible that these characteristics may also show differences between men and women, and may have a significant effect on job performance.

Personality tests also depend on completely honest replies. Many people will be tempted to adjust their answers to give the results they think their potential employers will want. For instance, applicants for teacher training might consider exaggerating their enjoyment of being the centre of attention to increase their Extraversion score.

It would therefore be unwise to come to any sweeping conclusions about likely job performance based on assessment of personality. Sadly, this means that determining your future career purely on the basis of personality testing would also be highly risky.

"Behaviour is influenced profoundly by both our genetic make-up and our upbringing."

ONLINE AND KEEPING IN TOUCH

The internet is one of the great phenomena of our time. Given how much we rely on it today, it's amazing to think that it only went public for the first time in 1991. Overall, men have taken to computer use more readily than we women – which accords with their dominance in visual-spatial intelligence tests.

By 2005, however, men and women were making use of the internet in almost equal numbers. Nevertheless, research shows that men are still more likely to hog the computer: around 68 per cent of men are "in charge of" the computer in their home, compared to around 45 per cent of women.

There are also differences between what men and women do with the internet when they are online. Women tend to use it to search for health and medical information, maps, and religious information, but also to find support groups. Men, on the other hand, rely on it more for weather reports, sports results, news, and to rate goods they're considering buying.

According to statistics from the USA, women also use email for different purposes than men. They are more likely to use it to maintain social ties, while men use email more to keep in touch with organizations.

The stresses and strains of modern life

Most women have the chance to be as well educated as our male peers and we generally have the same opportunities. But the downside is we're probably juggling a career and family life. No wonder, then, that women suffer from the same ills as men, but also from "modern life".

It was not so long ago that women were taught to aspire to nothing more in life than making a good marriage. And as recently as the late 19th century – and still true in some parts of the world – a woman was regarded as her husband's possession, to be beaten with impunity if he wished.

It's remarkable that many of the changes that liberated women are relatively recent. The Suffragettes, for example, began their struggle in the early 20th century. Their battle was finally won in America in 1920 when women were granted the vote on the same terms as men. Britain followed suit in 1928.

It was only as recently as World War II that women were encouraged to look for jobs outside the home, and that was to take the place of men who were enlisted in the armed forces.

But perhaps the most significant breakthrough for the liberation of women came as recently as 1960, when the contraceptive pill was launched in the USA. Within two years, more than a million American women were enjoying their sexual freedom by using the pill.

BEING ONE OF THE BOYS – AT WORK AND AT PLAY

Over many decades, women have been pushing extremely hard to be accepted as equals by their male peers. But achieving acceptance in the workplace often involves becoming "one of the boys" in the social arena – and that means drinking and smoking.

Increased drinking Women, as we will discover (see p65), aren't designed to drink as much alcohol as men. Not only do they come to harm at lower levels of drinking, but they also appear to damage their bodies in a shorter space of time than men.

In the UK, there has been an astonishing 38 per cent increase in the average weekly consumption of alcohol by women in the ten years since 1998. During the same period, alcohol consumption among men has increased by a much more modest 9 per cent.

By 2003, 33 per cent of women aged 20 to 25, and 19 per cent of women aged 25 to 44 were drinking at "hazardous" levels,

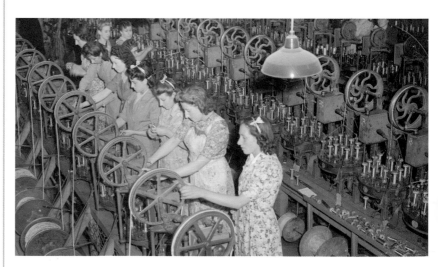

Women working in industry in World War II
These women working in a factory during World War II are typical of the thousands who started working outside the home for the first time. They were needed for the war effort.

compared to the 16 per cent and 14 per cent respectively in the same age groups in 1989.

Nor is this change in drinking patterns confined to any particular social group of women. In fact, recent research suggests that the women in their thirties who are most likely to drink to excess are the most successful, professional women with high-pressure jobs that place them under huge stress.

Increased smoking In the past, too, women were much less likely than men to smoke. Nowadays, the gap is narrowing dramatically – possibly as young women continue to smoke or take up smoking as part of a misguided attempt to keep their weight down.

EATING DISORDERS

Anorexia nervosa (sometimes referred to "the dieter's disease") is around ten times more common among females than males. Bulimia nervosa – in which people overeat, then purge themselves by vomiting or taking laxatives – is a largely female preserve, too. These two eating disorders are psychological conditions, but they can have serious physical consequences as well as causing a great deal of family stress. For more detail, see pp216–17.

Both anorexia and bulimia have shown dramatic increases in recent decades, and it seems that the stresses and strains of modern life are mostly to blame. The "typical" woman most at risk of such eating disorders is young, attractive, and high-achieving. Young women who excel at sports or occupations in which physical conditioning is paramount – ballet and athletics as well as modelling and acting – are particularly vulnerable. Often, though, these women describe their eating disorders as a kind of "coping mechanism" for the high expectations placed on them.

OUR AGEING SOCIETY

Further stress on women comes from our ageing society. As average life expectancy continues to rise, so does the proportion of the elderly in the population. Women are much more likely than men to act as carers for elderly relatives, particularly their parents. As more and more women work full time, this adds to the pressures on them.

What is more, although death rates from many serious medical conditions (such as heart disease and diabetes) are going down, the number of people debilitated by such illnesses is still going up. So as women delay having children, they are more likely to find themselves in the difficult position of having to care for both children and parents at the same time.

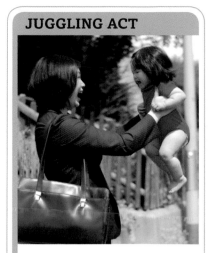

JUGGLING ACT

Busy mothers
A common sight at the nursery or school gate is a busy mother collecting her child at the end of the working day.

Women are increasingly going out to work without reducing their domestic commitments. Working women still act as the primary home-maker and care-giver for children. In a 1990s survey of doctors in their thirties, the stress of juggling domestic and professional commitments was the most common barrier to career fulfilment for women. Not one man in this survey even mentioned the problem!

Ample evidence suggests that women can't "switch off" from other problems as easily as men – perhaps because of differences in their brains (see pp18–19) or social conditioning. Whatever the cause, most women juggle more tasks than men. And while this is an achievement we should all be celebrating, it can also be a recipe for stress-related illness.

"Perhaps the most significant breakthrough for the liberation of women came in 1960 with the launch of the contraceptive pill."

Understanding the changes

Dr Patricia Macnair MBChB MA DA(FARCS)

Through the decades

Women today are living longer than their mothers and much longer than their grandmothers. Our overall quality of life is better, too: we are healthier, more active, and more independent than ever before. Much of this state of affairs is due to medical advances and public health measures, but we also know how to look after ourselves more proactively. This chapter summarizes the stages we go through as our lives unfold through the decades and reminds us of the common-sense rules of health that many of us are liable to forget.

The moment you are conceived, the stage is set for a life of individuality. The genes you inherit from your parents distinguish you from everybody else on the planet, unless you're an identical twin! These genes contribute to who you are, what you look like, what your constitution is, and what diseases you may inherit.

At the same time, your changing environment – everything from your time as a developing fetus in your mother's womb and as a newborn infant in the cradle, to the hormonal merry-go-round of your adolescence – contributes not only to your health but also to the kind of illnesses from which you may suffer. These two influences – genes and environment – make up the two components of the "nature versus nurture" discussion. Together, they determine the essence of your mental and physical wellbeing. This is also the melting pot from which psychologists draw the biopsychosocial model to explain the workings of mental health. But while we know that genes and environment are extremely important, both can be influenced tremendously – both positively or negatively – by the crucial lifestyle choices that we make.

TOP 10 GOOD HABITS FOR LIFE

Get into as many good habits as possible when you are young, preferably by your 20s. This will help to lay the foundations for enjoying your life right through the decades that come after.

1 Eat a balanced diet Include five servings of fruit and vegetables a day (see pp52–5).

2 Maintain a healthy weight See pp58–9 for how to calculate your body mass index (BMI) and why.

3 If you smoke, stop If you need help, join a support group or talk to your doctor (see also p64).

4 Moderate your drinking Limit your alcoholic intake to fewer than 2 units per day (see p65).

5 Drive carefully Accidents, including road accidents, are a leading cause of death.

6 Get a good night's sleep Sleep deprivation affects your mood, productivity, relationships, and safety.

7 Practise responsible sexual behaviour If you don't want to get pregnant or contract an STI.

8 Brush and floss your teeth routinely Good oral hygiene protects your overall health, not just your teeth.

9 Drink 2–2.5 litres (3½–4 pints) of fluid per day This includes coffee and tea in moderation as well as water.

10 Protect yourself from the sun Always wear protective clothing and sunscreen (see p66).

AS TIME GOES BY

Women differ from men in many ways, but one of the most distinctive is the way we age. Women go through unique stages in life and experience particular changes, not only based upon our reproductive and hormonal status, but also the kind of health problems associated with the various decades of our lives. On average, women in the United Kingdom live five years longer than men. Yet, as time goes by, we also tend to suffer from more chronic illnesses and take more medication.

Usually, when you read or hear the term "the change" in conjunction with women's health, you think about the menopause. Yet there are many other age-related transitions that women experience, such as reaching the "magic" age of 35 (see p30). These changes are not always dictated by age as such, but by when or whether you start a family. As this chapter shows, these transitions are also linked to the development of any acute or chronic medical problems you may have. These problems may affect your risk of developing other illnesses in the future, your need for additional preventive measures, or your need for further diagnostic or health-screening surveillance checks.

PREVENTION IS BETTER THAN CURE

Age inevitably causes a physical decline and your risk of developing certain diseases, such as cancer, heart disease, and osteoporosis, increases. Using a decade-by-decade approach, this chapter looks at the typical changes in women's bodies as we age, the health risk factors associated with each decade, and our changing nutritional needs. However, not all diseases have risks that depend on age, so the chapter offers many tips and tests for prevention and for looking after your health.

Recommended check-ups and screening tests begin in your 20s and should continue throughout your life. If the list of what you need appears to mount up from your 30s onwards, don't be dismayed! These are just precautions. You may feel healthy now, but many medical conditions can be prevented or treated more effectively if they are caught early. There are also some suggested questions to ask your doctor as you start each decade.

Whatever your age and whatever your circumstances, the best way to minimize any health risks and prevent many problems from developing is to adopt healthy habits (see box, left). And remember two things: first, even taking small steps towards improving your health is better than doing nothing at all; and second, it's never too late to start improving your health.

FEMALE LIFE EXPECTANCY

The figures below show the estimated life expectancy at birth for females in a selection of different countries. Male life expectancy at birth in many countries is consistently five to seven years less.

Country	Life expectancy
Andorra	86.23
Japan	85.56
France	84
Canada	83.86
Switzerland	83.63
Australia	83.59
Spain	83.32
Norway	83.32
Italy	83.07
Sweden	83
Iceland	82.62
Finland	82.31
Germany	82.11
New Zealand	82.08
Greece	82.06
Netherlands	81.82
Portugal	81.36
UK	81.3
USA	80.97
Ireland	80.7
Denmark	80.41
South Korea	80.10
Poland	79.44
Mexico	78.56
Saudi Arabia	78.02
Venezuela	76.48
Brazil	76.38
Turkey	75.46
China	74.82
Russia	73.03
India	71.17
Pakistan	64.83
Nigeria	48.07
South Africa	41.66

Your 20s

This decade is exciting; you are brimming with youth and vitality and unless you become a mother, you will have plenty of time to develop a career and interests. Use personal time well by looking after yourself and setting good health habits for life, standing you in good stead for a long, healthy future. The earlier you start caring for yourself, the more you will benefit as you age.

FERTILITY AND SEXUAL HEALTH

Your 20s are a time when you are generally fertile and sexually active. The average age of a first pregnancy in the UK is now 27. Since so many women become pregnant for the first time – either intentionally or unintentionally – during their 20s, family planning and preconception counselling are especially important during this decade.

We think of the importance of antenatal care as mostly benefiting the baby, but pregnancy-related complications are significant risks for the mother as well: in some countries pregnancy-related complications are high on the list of causes of death for women in their 20s.

You may have contracted a sexually transmitted infection (STI) during your adolescence. HIV/AIDS is the most worrying, though death from it for this age group is less and less common these days. But there are also other STIs, and many of these can have a devastating effect on your long-term health and fertility. You should always practise safe sex and have appropriate screening tests as recommended.

MENTAL HEALTH

Mental health is important at every age, but the 20s can be a time of particular strain due to what are often major changes in your life and in your role in society. As a result, depression is common and suicide/self-harm is the second-most common cause of death in this decade. The good news is that depression is treatable, both with medical therapy and "talk therapy" (see pp210–11).

ADDICTIVE BEHAVIOURS

Unfortunately, for many women, the 20s may be characterized by bad habits started in the teens as risk-taking behaviour. If you do have addictive behaviours, such as smoking (see p64), alcoholism (see p220), substance abuse (see p221), or eating disorders (see pp216–17), try to kick them fast. Help is available if you need it.

Drive carefully, too, because accidents, including motor vehicle accidents, are the single most important cause of death in women in their 20s in the UK.

CANCER

It is rare for women in their 20s to be affected by cancer. However, you're never too young to be vigilant and to take precautions, especially concerning melanoma, the most aggressive form of skin

QUESTIONS TO ASK YOUR DOCTOR IN YOUR 20s

The following are just some of the questions you can ask your doctor at the start of your 20s:

- Are there any vaccines I need?
- Should I be taking any vitamins or supplements?
- Do I need to think about having any additional screening or diagnostic tests?
- Are there any behavioural or lifestyle changes I should make for optimal health?

"Take time to look after yourself and it will stand you in good stead for the future."

TESTS RECOMMENDED IN YOUR 20s

These are the tests and check-ups that are useful to have during your 20s. Some of the routine check-ups, such as the breast awareness (including self-examination), you can and should do yourself on a regular basis. You can ask your doctor, dentist, and optician about which tests are appropriate for you. These are the medical recommendations.

Routine check-ups

✔ Practise breast awareness regularly (see p154)

✔ Have regular cervical smear tests: the NHS offers this every 3 years for women from the age of 20 in Wales, Scotland, and Northern Ireland, and from the age of 25 in England

✔ Have your eyes tested at least every 2 years (some people qualify for free tests on the NHS)

✔ Go for a twice-yearly dental check-up and cleaning

Additional screening tests

✔ If you are thinking of getting pregnant, see your doctor for preconception advice. You may also need screening tests and a cervical smear test (see p107) before you conceive.

---

cancer (see p360). Make sure you protect yourself properly from the harmful effects of the sun and see your doctor if you find that any moles have changed appearance.

VITAMIN AND MINERAL SUPPLEMENTS IN YOUR 20s

Most women who are not planning to get pregnant do not need vitamin or mineral supplements, but some exceptions apply:

Multivitamins If you have heavy periods, have been anaemic, or are vegan, you may benefit from a daily multivitamin with iron.

Folic acid If you are thinking of starting a family, take a folic acid supplement (400mcg a day) from before you conceive until you are 12 weeks pregnant.

Calcium and vitamin D If you are a vegan or do not eat dairy products, you may need calcium and vitamin D supplements (see also p262).

VACCINES FOR YOUR 20s

Consider having the following vaccines during your 20s.

HPV This vaccine prevents the two most important cancer-causing strains of human papilloma virus (HPV), responsible for around 70 per cent of cervical cancers. One HPV vaccine also targets HPV strains responsible for the majority of genital warts. While it is ideally given before a woman becomes sexually active, ask your doctor if it is right for you.

Flu Many groups of people are on the list of who "should" receive a flu jab annually, so if you want to reduce your risk of catching flu ask your doctor about having a jab.

Tetanus You will need a tetanus booster every ten years.

Catch-up vaccines Ask your doctor if you need any boosters or vaccinations missed in childhood. You may have missed rubella vaccine (catching rubella during the first trimester of pregnancy can cause major fetal abnormalities).

LEADING CAUSES OF DEATH FOR WOMEN IN THEIR 20s

Statistical research in the United Kingdom shows that the leading causes of death among women aged 15–34 are:

1 Accidents	4 Addiction/substance abuse
2 Suicide and injury	5 Homicide
3 Cancer	6 Cirrhosis/liver diseases
	7 Epilepsy
	8 Ischaemic heart disease
	9 Cerebrovascular diseases
	10 Congenital malformations

Your 30s

The 30s are generally considered a time of robust health for most women, but this decade can also be a transitional time in terms of your physical and emotional wellbeing. One of the biggest physical and psychological health issues may be learning to take care of your own health needs, despite the competing demands of caring for others or focusing on your career and relationships.

35 – A "MAGIC" NUMBER

Fertility is not the only physiological factor which declines in your 30s. Ironically, 35 is a "magic" number of sorts in women's health. You may notice the beginning of age-related visual changes after 35 and many women may notice changes in their hair colour and in their skin. It's also a turning point because the risk of a number of medical problems and concerns begins to rise significantly, including:

- Miscarriage
- Birth defects (notably Down's Syndrome; see chart, opposite)
- Depression
- Breast cancer
- The beginning of bone loss
- Slower metabolism, which may make it more difficult for you to lose weight
- Fibroids
- High blood pressure
- Auto-immune diseases.

FERTILITY AND SEXUAL HEALTH

For many women, their 30s (and increasingly their 40s) are a time when they face fertility concerns.

A growing percentage of women delay pregnancy until their 30s. While this is a relatively small proportion, a woman over 35 not only has a greater risk of infertility but is also considered to be of "advanced maternal age", which carries medical risks for the mother.

The older a woman is, the more likely she is to suffer complications during pregnancy, such as high blood pressure, pre-eclampsia and eclampsia, diabetes, and haemorrhage during the birth.

Years ago, women over 35 weren't allowed to take the contraceptive pill. We now know that it is safe for healthy, non-smoking women over 35 to continue taking low-dose oral contraceptives as long as they have no other contraindications.

While the average age of the menopause is 51, many women enter it earlier, either naturally, surgically (through removal of the uterus or the ovaries), or as a result of chemotherapy or radiotherapy in the treatment of cancer. This can happen as early as the 30s.

Then there is a condition called premature ovarian failure (POF), which is estimated to have caused the menopause to start by the age of 39 in 1 in 100 women. In fact, women can be affected with POF at any age, even during their teens.

BONE HEALTH

The 30s is an important time for you to think about the health of your bones. While we think that our bones stop growing once we stop growing in height, they are actually continually remodelling. Women continue to build bone mass until the age of 30.

Bone mass generally remains stable until the menopause. Then it declines relatively quickly unless you make changes in your lifestyle and medication.

The most important steps that you can take in this decade to prevent bone density loss include: **Developing good exercise habits** (see pp56–7) and focusing on weight-bearing exercise. This includes walking, running, dancing, or aerobics, and strength-training **Getting sufficient calcium** and vitamin D in your diet (see pp54–5, and p262).

TESTS RECOMMENDED IN YOUR 30s

The routine check-ups and screening tests that are recommended during your 30s are similar to those in your 20s and you should carry on the good habits, such as breast self-awareness and good eating and sleeping habits, which you established during that decade. Ask your doctor if there are any particular tests that are appropriate for you.

Routine check-ups

✔ Practise breast awareness (including self-examination) regularly (see p154)

✔ Have a cervical smear test (see p107) according to your doctor's recommendations: the NHS offers this every 3 years for women in their 30s

✔ Have your eyes tested at least every two years (some people qualify for free tests on the NHS)

✔ Go for a twice-yearly dental check-up and cleaning

✔ Have your weight and height measured every year: this will help to measure any bone loss later on

✔ Have your blood pressure taken every 3–5 years, or yearly if you are at high risk of heart disease or high blood pressure

✔ If you have a family history of heart disease at a young age or inherited disorders of blood lipids, you may want to ask your doctor to check your cholesterol and triglyceride levels

✔ Check your skin regularly for any moles or suspicious abnormalities or changes (see pp358–60).

Additional screening tests

✔ If you are thinking of getting pregnant, see your doctor for preconception advice. You may also need screening tests and a cervical smear test (see p107) before you conceive

✔ If there is a history of bowel cancer in your family you may want to ask your doctor about screening tests such as faecal occult blood testing or colonoscopy (see p308).

HEART HEALTH

Your 30s is the time when risk factors for heart disease begin to increase. In this decade, it's important to maintain a healthy weight (pp58–9), address risky habits (pp64–5), and correct any abnormalities in blood pressure and levels of sugar, cholesterol, or triglycerides in your blood (see pp162–3). Doing regular aerobic exercise (see pp56–7) is vital for maintaining a healthy heart.

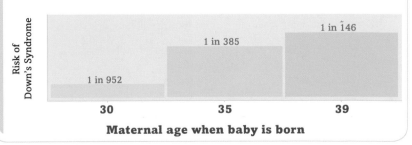

RISK OF DOWN'S SYNDROME

The risk of a baby having a chromosomal abnormality, the most common of which is Down's Syndrome (see the chart below), increases sharply if the mother is in her mid to late 30s when the baby is born.

Risk of Down's Syndrome		
1 in 952	1 in 385	1 in 146
30	**35**	**39**

Maternal age when baby is born

WEIGHT ISSUES

Try to keep your weight under control as best you can. If you are overweight or obese you are at increased risk of:

- Heart disease, heart attack, stroke, and type 2 diabetes
- Metabolic syndrome
- Endometrial cancer
- Gallstones
- Stress incontinence
- Polycystic ovary syndrome
- Obstetric problems, including miscarriage, pre-eclampsia, gestational diabetes, and needing a caesarean section
- Postmenopausal breast cancer: 30 per cent of these cancers are associated with weight gained after the menopause.

"Between her 30s and 50s, the average woman loses 0.5 per cent of bone density each year."

EXERCISE

We all know that exercise is good for us and there's no such thing as being too old for it – especially when you are still only in your 30s! The benefits of taking plenty of exercise include:

- Easier weight management
- An increase in HDL ("good") cholesterol and a decrease in triglycerides and LDL ("bad") cholesterol in the blood
- Decreased blood pressure
- Slower resting heart rate
- Increased bone density and a reduced risk of osteoporosis

- Decreased risk of colon cancer, kidney stones, breast cancer, and depression
- Decreased stress and anxiety
- Improvement in self-esteem and overall mental health
- Improvement in sleep patterns and overally sleep quality.

VITAMIN AND MINERAL SUPPLEMENTS IN YOUR 30s

Most healthy women don't routinely need supplements of vitamins and minerals in their 30s – the ideal is to get all you need from a balanced diet (see pp52–5). But if you have very heavy periods or a restricted diet, such as vegan or fructarian, you may need supplements. Remember some vitamin supplements can interact harmfully with some medicines or with the absorption of other nutrients, so always check with your doctor.

Folic acid/omega-3 fatty acids
If you are breast-feeding, pregnant,

QUESTIONS TO ASK YOUR DOCTOR IN YOUR 30s

The following are just some of the questions you can ask your doctor at the start of your 30s:

- Should I be taking any vitamins or supplements?
- Are there any additional

screening or diagnostic tests that I need to take?

- Are there any behavioural or lifestyle changes I should be making in order to increase my optimal health?

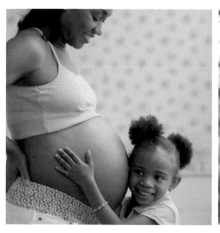

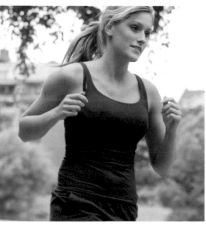

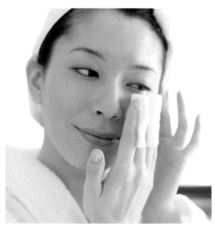

or are thinking of starting a family, take a folic acid supplement (400 micrograms a day) – and possibly an omega-3 fatty acid supplement (200mg a day) as well – from before you conceive until you are about 12 weeks pregnant.

Calcium Your bone density starts to drop now, especially if you're a smoker, take long-term steroids, or have suffered from anorexia (see osteoporosis pp260–2).

To help protect your bones you need 800mg a day of calcium, which you can get by eating three servings of dairy foods a day. If your diet is not giving you enough, you may want to take a daily calcium supplement.

Vitamin D This essential vitamin aids calcium absorption and bone health. The recommended daily intake for women under 65 is 5mcg a day (10mcg if you are pregnant or breast-feeding). While vitamin D is found in foods such as oily fish, eggs and butter, it is also manufactured in the skin in response to exposure to sunlight. In the UK, you should get enough

vitamin D from 15–20 minutes of daily sunlight between April and September, at peak sun time and without using sunblock, but be careful not to stay out in the sun long enough to burn, as this will increase your risk of developing skin cancer (pp358–60).

VACCINES FOR YOUR 30s

You may think that you don't need any more vaccines, unless you are travelling to an exotic destination. However, you may want to consider having the following vaccines during your 30s.

Flu If you are worried about catching flu talk to your doctor.

If you are at risk you should be offered a flu vaccination, but most healthy people in their 30s will not be offered it routinely and will have to pay privately if they want it.

Rubella (German measles) If there's a chance that you may become pregnant, make sure you are immune to rubella. A rubella infection during the first trimester of pregnancy can cause major fetal abnormalities.

Tetanus, diphtheria, pertussis (TDP/tDap) Ask your doctor when you had your last TDP/tDap jab. You will need a tetanus booster every 10 years.

Catch-up vaccines See p29.

LEADING CAUSES OF DEATH FOR WOMEN IN THEIR 30s

The leading causes of death among women aged 15–34 in the UK are:

1 Accidents
2 Suicide and injury
3 Cancer
4 Addiction/substance abuse
5 Homicide

The leading causes of death among women aged 35–54 in the UK are:

1 Cancer
2 Cirrhosis/other liver diseases
3 Ischaemic heart disease
4 Heart disease
5 Suicide and injury

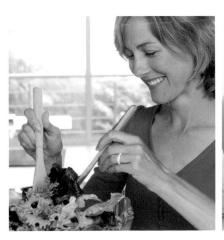

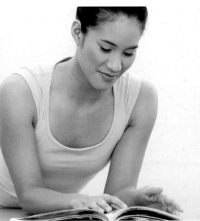

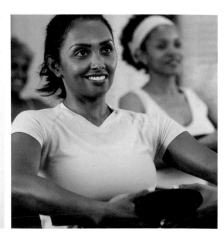

Your 40s

The 40s can be a wonderfully settling decade for women. Many describe this decade as a time when they can appreciate their accumulated life's wisdom, their professional lives have had time to develop, their family lives are often established, and, even though they are beginning to show a few more signs of ageing, they are still enjoying good health.

FERTILITY AND SEXUAL HEALTH

An increasing number of women choose to become pregnant in their 40s, yet face realistic concerns about decreasing fertility. Ironically, many women in this decade are unsure about which contraceptive methods are safe for them. If they have irregular periods, they often mistakenly think that they no longer have to be worried about getting pregnant. As a result, women in their 40s have the second-highest rate of unintended pregnancy (after the teens).

If you are heterosexually active, haven't yet reached the menopause, and are not using reliable contraception, you can still become pregnant. The good news is that if you are a healthy, non-smoking woman in your 40s, it is no longer considered unsafe for you to take the contraceptive pill or use the contraceptive patch, as long as you don't have any contraindications; many very low-dose alternatives are now available.

The age at which women reach the menopause is, on average, 51. However, many women begin it earlier, either naturally or because of surgery – after hysterectomy or ovary removal – or as a result of treatments for cancer (chemotherapy or radiotherapy). The average age of a surgical menopause is 42.

LIBIDO

Many women have reported that they experience a decreased libido during their 40s, even before they reach menopause. It is unclear whether this is driven by hormones, psychology, or social forces, but it is probably a combination of all three. If you are feeling that your libido has decreased, the best thing to do would be to discuss it with both your partner and your doctor. Many women are not aware, for example, that decreased libido is a potential side effect of many

PERIMENOPAUSE

The hormonal hallmark of this decade is the perimenopause. This is the period that lasts for between two and ten years preceding your menopause (see Chapter 5). Your ovaries start to produce less oestrogen, causing inevitable reduction in your fertility. While you may still have regular periods during this time, falling oestrogen levels may cause, for example, early bone loss. You may also notice one or more of the following symptoms:

- Changes in your menstrual flow or frequency
- Increased premenstrual symptoms
- Increased acne
- Increased moodiness or irritability
- Sleep disturbances.

You may also begin to notice menopausal symptoms such as:

- Hot flushes
- Night sweats
- Vaginal dryness

If such symptoms are bothering you, there are several over-the-counter or prescription remedies available. However, you should also consult your doctor to be sure that your symptoms are due to normal, age-related hormonal changes and that they are not caused by another medical problem.

TESTS RECOMMENDED IN YOUR 40s

The routine check-ups and additional screening tests that are recommended in your 40s are almost the same as those in your 30s. However, it is important to talk to your doctor if you are worried about annoying perimenopausal symptoms. And since it may be 10 years before you are offered NHS breast screening, you should also continue your breast self-awareness.

Routine check-ups

✔ Practise breast self-awareness (including self-examination) regularly (see p154)

✔ Have a cervical smear test (see p107) according to your doctor's recommendations: the NHS offers this every 3 years for women in their 40s up to the age of 49

✔ Have your eyes tested at least every 2 years (some people qualify for free tests on the NHS)

✔ Go for a twice-yearly dental check-up and cleaning

✔ Everyone over the age of 40 should have a regular cardiovascular health risk assessment, which can be done by your doctor. This includes a blood test to check cholesterol and triglyceride levels, measurement of weight and blood pressure, and assessment of smoking habits. If your risk score is high you may need treatment or regular monitoring

✔ See your doctor if you are experiencing any perimenopausal symptoms which bother you

✔ Check your skin regularly for moles or suspicious abnormalities or changes (see pp358–60).

Additional screening tests

✔ If you are thinking of getting pregnant, see your doctor for preconception advice. You may also need screening tests and a cervical smear test (see p107) before you conceive.

✔ If there is a history of bowel cancer in your family you may want to ask your doctor about screening tests such as faecal occult blood testing or colonoscopy (see p308)

✔ Ask your GP or practice nurse about a cardiovascular risk assessment, including a cholesterol check if you've never had one or if you have any risk factors (see p163)

✔ If you have a family history of type 2 diabetes, and especially if you are overweight, you may want to ask your doctor to check your blood glucose levels occasionally to screen for diabetes

✔ If you have risk factors for osteoporosis (see pp261), talk to your GP about the possibility of a DEXA scan to measure your bone density.

---

medicines, including birth control pills and some antidepressants (which are increasingly prescribed to women in this age group).

OTHER MENSTRUAL CHANGES

Not all menstrual irregularities are due to perimenopausal changes (see box, left). Fibroids increase during the 40s and may be found in more than 60 per cent of women over 45, although only about half have symptoms. Fibroids are three times more common among women of Afro-Caribbean origin. Both endometriosis and endometrial hyperplasia may become a problem, too. All these conditions may contribute to heavy menstrual cramps (dysmenorrhoea) and heavy menstrual bleeding (menorrhagia).

BREAST HEALTH

Breast cancer is the commonest cause of cancer deaths among women in their 40s and the number-one killer in this age group, causing around 2,000 deaths a year in the UK. But the incidence rises with age and NHS screening doesn't start until 50. Most of these younger deaths are among women with a strong family history of the disease who may have inherited genes putting them at particular risk. If this applies to you, ask your doctor whether a mammogram or other screening (such as genetic tests) is appropriate. If you discover a breast lump, a lump changes, and/or you have a strong family history of the disease, discuss this immediately with your doctor.

"Women in their 40s have the second-highest percentage of unplanned pregnancies."

OTHER PHYSICAL CHANGES

"Female, fertile, fat, and 40" is an old medical expression describing the classic risk factors for a number of medical problems, from type 2 diabetes to gallstones. Changes in your metabolism seem to make it suddenly more difficult to lose weight and much easier to put it on, especially around the abdomen.

Perhaps the condition of greatest concern is one that is only just being understood: during this decade you are at a much greater risk of developing metabolic syndrome. While the definition of this syndrome varies, the consensus is that it includes a constellation of conditions that create a high risk for coronary artery disease. These conditions include type 2 diabetes, obesity, increased LDL ("bad" cholesterol), low HDL ("good" cholesterol), high blood pressure, elevated triglycerides, and insulin resistance.

Other changes may include:
- Visual changes (especially the need for reading glasses)
- Hair becoming greyer
- Some hair loss (or growth in the wrong places)
- Urinary incontinence (this may begin now or worsen)
- Early bone loss, especially if you are at risk of osteoporosis.

MENTAL HEALTH

The majority of women in their 40s enjoy good mental health, but up to 10 per cent of them (twice as many as men) may experience significant clinical depression (see pp210–11). Obvious risk factors for depression include separation, divorce, bereavement, financial problems, and lack of social support. But there may be other causes, too, such as a history of PMS, illness, being a certain personality, and having a family history of depression.

VITAMIN AND MINERAL SUPPLEMENTS IN YOUR 40s

Most healthy women don't routinely need supplements of vitamins and minerals in their 30s – the ideal is to get all you need from a balanced diet (see pp52–5). But if you have very heavy periods or a restricted diet, such as vegan or fructarian, you may need supplements. Some

---

QUESTIONS TO ASK YOUR DOCTOR IN YOUR 40s

The following are just some of the questions you can ask your doctor at the start of your 40s:
- Should I be taking any vitamins or supplements?
- Are there additional screening or diagnostic tests that I need?
- Are there any lifestyle changes I should make for optimal health?
- If I am at risk for heart disease, should I take a junior aspirin once a day?

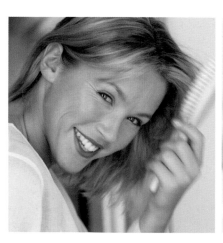
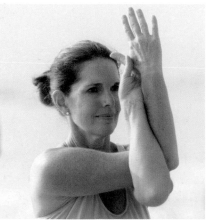
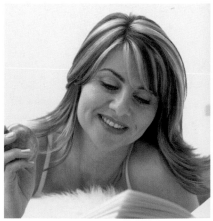

vitamin supplements can interact harmfully with some medicines or the absorption of other nutrients, so always check with your doctor.

Folic acid/omega-3 fatty acids If you are breast-feeding, pregnant, or are thinking of starting a family, take a folic acid supplement (400 micrograms a day) – and possibly an omega-3 fatty acid supplement (200mg a day) as well – from before you conceive until you are about 12 weeks pregnant.

Calcium Your bone density continues to drop, especially if you're a smoker, take long-term steroids, or have suffered from anorexia (see osteoporosis pp260–2). If your diet is not giving you enough calcium (800mg a day – for this you need to eat three servings daily of dairy foods), you may want to take a daily calcium supplement to make up the difference. However, speak to your doctor before you do so.

Vitamin D The recommended daily intake for women under 65 is 5mcg a day (10mcg if you are pregnant or breast-feeding) You

LEADING CAUSES OF DEATH FOR WOMEN AGED IN THEIR 40s

Statistical research in the United Kingdom shows that the leading causes of death among women aged 35–54 are:

1 Cancer (all types)
2 Cirrhosis/other liver diseases
3 Ischaemic heart diseases
4 Cerebrovascular diseases
5 Suicide and injury
6 Accidents
7 Chronic lower respiratory diseases
8 Flu and pneumonia
9 Epilepsy
10 Diabetes

can find it in many foods, but your skin also makes it in response to exposure to sunlight (see p33).

VACCINES FOR YOUR 40s

You might need one or two vaccines during your 40s, such as:

Flu If you are worried about catching flu talk to your doctor. Those at high risk should be offered flu vaccination, but most healthy people in their 40s won't be offered it and will have to pay privately if they want it.

Rubella (German measles) In case you become pregnant, make sure you're rubella-immune. If you catch rubella in the first trimester of pregnancy, your baby can develop major abnormalities.

Tetanus, diphtheria, pertussis (TDP/tDap) Ask your doctor when you had your last TDP/tDap jab. You'll need a tetanus booster every 10 years.

Catch-up vaccines Ask if you need any boosters or vaccinations missed in childhood (see p29).

> "Early bone loss can start in your 40s, so make sure your diet is rich in calcium and vitamin D."

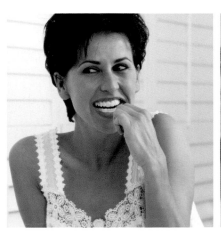

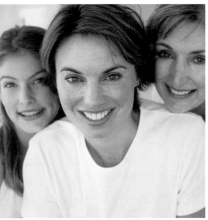

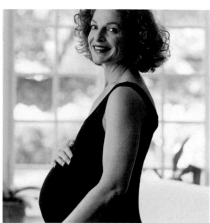

Your 50s

Most women go through the menopause in their 50s. For many, the years following the menopause are a cause for celebration, leading to renewed energy in the "third act" of their lives. Women no longer have to worry about contraception or unplanned pregnancy, and can now enjoy the increased independence that comes with children (if they have them) leaving the nest.

SEXUAL HEALTH

For many women, one advantage of the menopause is no longer worrying about contraception. Consequently, women in this age group often forego condom usage with a new partner. This may be partly why the incidence of sexually transmitted diseases (STIs) in women in their 50s has increased. Other reasons include higher divorce rates, better social networking and changing attitudes to sex in middle life. Research has pinpointed increases in genital warts, herpes, gonorrhoea, and syphilis. If you are sexually active and not in a mutually monogamous relationship, you are at the same risk of getting STIs as younger women unless you practise safe sex.

BONE HEALTH

Many other subtle changes within the body result from the decline of oestrogen production occurring with the menopause. Bone loss is the most dramatic: 20 per cent of your lifetime-expected bone loss occurs during the first five years of menopause, after which it continues to decrease more slowly. The National Osteoporosis Society recommends that women who are at risk of osteoporosis talk to their doctor about having a bone-density scan (see pp260-1).

BOWEL HEALTH

After the age of 50, digestive health and bowel problems become far more common. Levels of "friendly bacteria" in the gut fall and conditions such as indigestion, constipation, diverticulitis, and even bowel cancer start to increase (bowel cancer is the third most common cause of cancer deaths in this age group).

The NHS bowel cancer screening programme doesn't start until the age of 60, but there is plenty that you can do to look after your bowel health, such as following a healthy diet with plenty of fibre and taking prebiotic and probiotic supplements. You should also be vigilant for changes in your bowel habit – for example, if you need to open your bowels more often, if you become very constipated, or if you pass blood or mucus, you should seek urgent advice from your doctor (see also pp306–9 for more information).

OTHER PHYSICAL CHANGES

The following changes may also occur during your 50s:

- You may need reading glasses for some close-work tasks
- Your hearing starts to fade
- A continued decrease in your metabolism accounts for persistent weight gain, even though your calorie intake is the

LEADING CAUSES OF DEATH FOR WOMEN IN THEIR 50s

The leading causes of death among women aged 35–54 in the UK are:	The leading causes of death among women aged 55–74 in the UK are:
1 Cancer (all types)	1 Cancer (all types)
2 Cirrhosis/other liver diseases	2 Ischaemic heart disease
3 Ischaemic heart diseases	3 Cerebrovascular disease (stroke)
4 Cerebrovascular diseases	4 Chronic lower respiratory diseases
5 Suicide and injury	5 Flu and pneumonia

TESTS RECOMMENDED IN YOUR 50s

The tests and check-ups that you began in your 30s and 40s continue into your 50s, with the exception of preconception advice, which you are no longer likely to need. Now is the time to discuss menopausal concerns and bone-density issues with your doctor. In addition, ask your doctor if there are any particular tests that are appropriate for you.

Routine check-ups

✔ Practise monthly breast awareness (including self-examination) regularly (see p154)

✔ Have a mammogram every three years (see p155)

✔ Have regular cervical smear tests (see p107): the NHS offers this test every 5 years for women in their 50s in England and Northern Ireland and every 3 years in Scotland and Wales

✔ Have your eyes tested at least every 2 years (some people qualify for free tests on the NHS)

✔ Go for a twice-yearly dental check-up and cleaning

✔ Everyone after 40 should have a regular cardiovascular health risk assessment and your doctor can do this. This includes a blood test to check cholesterol and triglyceride levels, measurement of weight and blood pressure, and assessment of smoking habits.

✔ Check your skin regularly for any moles or suspicious abnormalities or changes (see pp358–60)

✔ Ask if you should have a bone-density test (see p260).

Additional screening tests

✔ The NHS is introducing national screening programmes for bowel cancer, using faecal occult blood testing. In Scotland and Wales, you will invited if you're over 50, and in England once you reach 60

✔ Have your haemoglobin and haematocrit checked (anaemia is common in menstruating women and now that fibroids are an increased risk). However, this wouldn't be done routinely unless indicated by symptoms or other risks

✔ If you have a family history of type 2 diabetes, and especially if you are overweight, you may want to ask your doctor to check your blood glucose levels occasionally to screen for diabetes

✔ If you have risk factors for osteoporosis (see p261), talk to your GP about the possibility of a DEXA scan to measure your bone density.

---

same as before and you take as much exercise. It seems that the weight is simply harder to lose

● Fat deposits around your middle are more likely to build up and be more persistent. This is an increased risk factor for heart disease and leads to an increase in blood triglyceride levels.

● Skin changes become more obvious, with increased facial wrinkles, liver spots, skin tags, and overall dryness

● While increased forgetfulness is common during this decade, discuss significant changes in memory with your doctor.

SLEEPING PROBLEMS
Some experts attribute forgetfulness to sleep disturbances that are associated with the menopause.

Many surveys of menopausal women report that women find sleep disturbances to be the most disruptive menopausal symptom of all. In addition to hormonally mediated sleep disturbances such as these, a snoring disorder in a bed partner can also disrupt a woman's sleep!

Whatever the reason for sleep disturbances and deprivation, they can be upsetting, cause an excess amount of daytime drowsiness, and interfere with cognitive or skilled functions. (See pp60–1 for advice on sleeping well.)

> "Approximately 30 per cent of women will not experience any disruptive menopausal symptoms."

MENTAL HEALTH

More good news: myths about the "empty nest" syndrome leading to depression in menopausal women have been proved to be unfounded for the majority of women.

Depression is not associated with the menopause except for those with specific risk factors. These include women who:

- Have previously suffered from major depression
- Experienced moderate premenstrual syndrome (PMS)
- Experienced post-partum depression
- Have experienced a major bereavement, such as the death of a spouse or a child
- Smoke
- Have a young child still at home.

EARLY-ONSET ALZHEIMER'S

You may worry that increased forgetfulness is a sign of early dementia. Dementia affects about 700,000 British people and the most common form is Alzheimer's disease. Most of those with dementia are over the age of 65

QUESTIONS TO ASK YOUR DOCTOR IN YOUR 50s

Some questions you can ask your doctor at the start of your 50s:

- Should I be taking any vitamins or supplements?
- Are there additional screening or diagnostic tests that I need?
- When should I have my next mammogram?
- Do I need a bone-density test?
- Are there any lifestyle changes I should make to achieve optimal health?
- If I'm at risk of heart disease, should I take a daily junior aspirin?
- Do I need any changes in my medications?

(in fact, most are over 80, when 1 in 5 people are affected). However, about 1 in 1400 people between the ages of 40 and 65 have a condition called "early-onset Alzheimer's", and overall there's an estimated 15,000 people with early-onset dementia in the UK, many of whom are only in their 50s. Early-onset Alzheimer's often results from a genetic defect inherited through the chromosomes. So if you have a family history of early-onset dementia, discuss this with your doctor. Experts are at present concerned that this condition is underreported and many may be missing out on effective treatments. (See pp184–5 for more information on the early signs of Alzheimer's.)

VITAMIN AND MINERAL SUPPLEMENTS IN YOUR 50s

The following vitamin and mineral supplements can help you get the most out of life. However, some single-dose vitamin supplements can interact harmfully with some medicines or with the absorption of other nutrients, so check with your doctor before taking them.

Multivitamins Unless your doctor tells you otherwise, you probably no longer need iron in your multivitamin supplements.

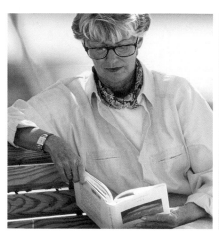
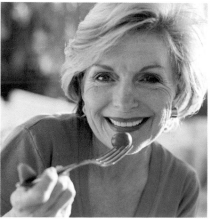
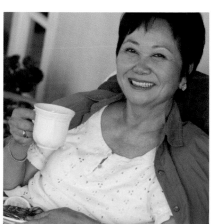

Calcium If your diet does not give you enough calcium (800mg a day, gained by eating three servings of dairy foods), you may need a daily supplement, but be sure to speak to your doctor before you take one.
Vitamin D This vitamin helps your body to absorb calcium. Most multivitamins contain vitamin D, but check the dosage – the recommended daily intake for women under the age of 65 is 5mcg a day (10mcg if you are pregnant or breast-feeding). Vitamin D is contained in many foods, but your skin also makes it from sunlight (see p33).

VACCINES FOR YOUR 50s
You may need the following:
Flu People at high risk, such as those with heart or respiratory conditions, should be offered flu vaccination. However, most healthy women in their 50s won't be offered it routinely and will have to pay privately if they want it.
Tetanus, diphtheria, pertussis (TDP or tDap) You will need a tetanus booster every 10 years.

THE MENOPAUSE

The average age of the menopause among women in the UK is 51. For most women, the menopause not only signifies the end of menstruation; when it's over, it also brings about a feeling that has been described as "post-menopausal zest" (see p137).

It is a myth that all women experience menopausal symptoms. In fact, approximately 30 per cent of British women will not experience any disruptive menopausal symptoms. However, this means that approximately 70 per cent will. While menopausal symptoms vary significantly in terms of the age of onset, severity, frequency, and duration, classic menopausal symptoms include hot flushes, night sweats, vaginal dryness (leading to irritation and painful sexual intercourse), mood swings, irritability, and sleep disturbances (see Menopause, pp136–41).

HORMONE REPLACEMENT THERAPY
One of the biggest health questions for menopausal women who have moderate to severe menopausal symptoms is whether or not to use hormone replacement therapy (see p138). One major concern is whether this therapy may or may not increase a woman's risk of serious health consequences, notably breast or endometrial cancer.

Among the huge amount of information available is a confusing study from the Women's Health Initiative (WHI), the largest-ever study of menopausal women. This study confirms only one thing: that each woman must consider her own individual circumstances, symptoms, risks, and benefits in consultation with her doctor. Women in their 50s should be reassured by the 2006 reanalysis of the WHI data, which showed that there was no increase in the risk of heart disease among those women aged 50 to 59 who were taking oestrogen.

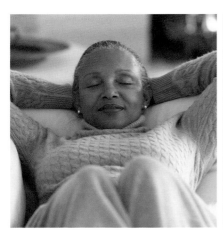
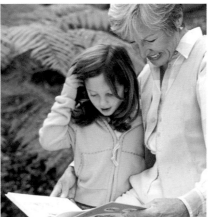
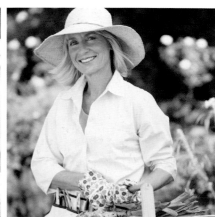

Your 60s

Women in their 60s are more active than ever before. Many continue to work beyond the usual retirement age, take up new activities, and embark on fresh relationships. In fact, the average, healthy, 60-year-old woman can expect to live another 24 years and for 18 of those, she should be in good, very good, or excellent perceived health – and she won't have given up on her sex life, either.

> "Walking, swimming, and low-impact aerobics reduce cardiac risk and maintain overall fitness and endurance."

EXERCISE

Try to keep active: if you enjoy a specific activity, continue with it, but if you're not active it's never too late to start. Consider the following physical activities:

- Walking, swimming, and low-impact aerobics reduce cardiac risk and maintain endurance and overall fitness
- Weight-bearing exercises, such as tennis, are particularly good for preventing osteoporosis
- Weight-building exercises, such as light weight training, build and maintain muscle mass and bone strength
- Exercises, such as yoga and Pilates, maintain flexibility and balance and help prevent falls.

PHYSICAL CHANGES

Physical signs of ageing are now becoming more apparent. Sight and hearing continue to decline, with 30 per cent of the over-65s experiencing significantly impaired hearing. Urinary incontinence is also an increasing problem and 10 per cent of women are affected. In addition, bladder, vision, and hearing problems, as well as decreased physical activity, may contribute to social isolation.

DISEASES OF THE 60s

Women with osteoporosis may start to develop a slight hunch and lose height. Arthritis may be come a problem that disfigures fingers and makes other joints stiff.

Heart disease is a close second to cancer as the main killer of women in their 60s. There is also an increased incidence of other diseases, such as Parkinson's and brain tumours.

MENTAL HEALTH

The impression that women in this age group suffer depression and isolation is largely inaccurate. However, women with difficult physical changes to face should take special care of mental health.

VITAMIN AND MINERAL SUPPLEMENTS IN YOUR 60s

Check with your doctor before taking supplements as some single-dose vitamins can interact harmfully with medicines or with the absorption of other nutrients. **Multivitamins** You probably no longer need iron in a multivitamin, but check this with your doctor first.

QUESTIONS TO ASK YOUR DOCTOR IN YOUR 60s

The following are just some of the questions you can ask your doctor about at the start of your 60s:

- Should I be taking any vitamins or supplements?
- Are there additional screening or diagnostic tests that I need?

- Are there any lifestyle changes I should make for optimal health?
- If I am at risk for heart disease, should I take a junior aspirin once every day?
- When should I have a bone-density test?

TESTS RECOMMENDED IN YOUR 60s

In your 60s, you need to continue with a number of recommended check-ups and tests, many of which you have already experienced in previous decades. Mammograms continue to be offered as part of the NHS screening programme until the age of 70, but the cervical screening programme stops at 65, unless you have particular risk factors.

Routine check-ups

✔ Continue to practise breast awareness regularly (see p154)

✔ Have a mammogram every three years (see p155)

✔ Have a cervical smear test (see p107) according to your doctor's recommendations: the NHS offers this every 5 years for women aged 50–64 in England and Northern Ireland and every 3 years up to the age of 64 in Wales; cervical screening is not routinely offered in Scotland after the age of 60

✔ Have your eyes tested regularly for glaucoma, cataracts, and macular degenerative disease

✔ Have your hearing tested every year

✔ Go for a twice-yearly dental check-up and cleaning

✔ After 40, everyone should have a regular cardiovascular health risk assessment (see p163). This includes a blood test to check cholesterol and triglyceride levels, weight and blood pressure measurements, and assessment of smoking habits.

✔ Check your skin regularly for any moles or suspicious abnormalities or changes (pp358–60)

✔ Have a baseline bone-density test (see p260) by the age of 65.

Additional screening tests

✔ You will be offered screening for bowel cancer on the NHS screening programme from 60–74 using the faecal occult blood test

✔ If you have a family history of type 2 diabetes, and especially if you are overweight, you may want to ask your doctor to check your blood glucose levels occasionally to screen for diabetes

✔ Ask your doctor about a thyroid screening test, known as the TSH test (see p328), to check your thyroid gland once you reach 60 – they may feel this is not necessary if you have no symptoms

✔ Have urinalysis (a urine test to screen for metabolic and kidney disorders) as recommended by your doctor

✔ Have a blood test to check for anaemia, as recommended by your doctor.

Calcium and vitamin D If your diet doesn't give you enough calcium (see p33) or vitamin D (see p41; you need 10mcg after 65), you may need a supplement.

VACCINES FOR YOUR 60s

Make sure you receive vaccines for the following diseases:

Pneumonia Routinely available on the NHS after the age of 65.

Flu Once over 65 you will routinely be offered flu jabs by your doctor; complications from flu are much more severe in older people.

Tetanus You may need a tetanus booster every 10 years.

Zoster Since 2005 there has been a vaccine to prevent shingles; as it reduces your risk by 50 percent, you may consider paying for it privately.

LEADING CAUSES OF DEATH FOR WOMEN IN THEIR 60s

Statistical research in the United Kingdom shows that the leading causes of death among women in aged 55–74 are:

1 Cancer (all types)
2 Ischaemic heart disease
3 Cerebrovascular disease (stroke)
4 Chronic lower respiratory diseases
5 Flu and pneumonia
6 Cirrhosis and other liver diseases
7 Diabetes
8 Dementia and Alzheimer's
9 Aortic aneurysm and dissection
10 Diseases of the urinary system

Your 70s

An increasing number of women live active, healthy lives well into their 70s and beyond. In fact, a 70-year-old woman in the United Kingdom has, on average, almost 12 years of life to live. The challenge is to do all you can to make those years as healthy and as mobile as possible, remembering that it's never too late to take steps to improve your health.

MENTAL AND PHYSICAL WELLBEING

Mental and social health are just as important as physical health for women in their 70s. Because of longer life expectancies for women than men, and the tendency for many women to marry men who are older, most women can expect to spend some of their later years as singles. However, "single" does not need to mean "alone".

To prevent this isolation, many women in their 70s work part-time (paid or voluntary), join clubs, take classes, form exercise groups, or pursue other interests. Pets can also be great companions.

Research studies have shown that older women who become socially isolated are three times more likely to die from cancer. Depression can raise the mortality rates of other medical problems if it is left untreated.

While most women over 70 are able to maintain a healthy quality of life, the Women's Health and Aging study found that 32 per cent of women over 70 had difficulty performing – or were unable to perform – basic self-care activities. The most common causes of this

kind of disability were musculoskeletal pain, general weakness, and balance problems.

LIBIDO

Another common myth about people in their 70s and beyond is that their sex lives are over. Yet, many of them are still sexually active. However, one large-scale study revealed that about half of the men and women surveyed reported at least one sexual problem. Among women in the study, the most common problems were low desire (43 per cent), vaginal dryness (39 per cent), and an inability to climax (34 per cent).

Decreased libido and an inability to achieve orgasm are complex

sexual issues. However, vaginal dryness can be easily treated, either with an over-the-counter, water-based lubricant or with a prescription oestrogen cream.

Most older women with treatable sexual problems have not discussed symptoms with a doctor. There are various reasons for this: they think that nothing can be done or that their problem is just a part of ageing; or else they are too embarrassed to talk about it.

DIGESTIVE HEALTH

Digestion slows down after the age of around 70 due to various dental problems, a fall in gastric acid production, and the decreased movement of food through the gut.

QUESTIONS TO ASK YOUR DOCTOR IN YOUR 70s

The following are just some of the questions you can ask your doctor about at the start of your 70s:

- Should I be taking any vitamins or supplements?
- Are there additional screening or diagnostic tests that I need?
- Should I still have an annual mammogram or cervical smear?

- Have I been tested recently for diabetes or thyroid problems?
- Are there any lifestyle changes I should make for optimal health?
- If I am at risk of heart disease, should I take a junior aspirin once per day?
- Would I benefit from some form of physical therapy?

TESTS RECOMMENDED IN YOUR 70s

The lists of check-ups and tests that are recommended for you in your 70s remain similar to those in your 60s. Make sure you keep your appointments for the routine check-ups, especially the mammograms and the tests for glaucoma, cataracts, and macular degenerative disease of the eyes. Tests for blood pressure, bone density, and colon cancer are important, too.

Routine check-ups

✔ Risk of breast cancer increases. Continue to practise breast awareness (see p154)

✔ Have a mammogram (see p155) every 3 years, even though routine screening stops after 70. Ask your doctor to arrange it.

✔ Go for a twice-yearly dental check-up and cleaning

✔ Have a baseline bone-density test if you did not have it at 65

✔ Have regular eye tests for glaucoma, cataracts, and macular degenerative disease and have your hearing tested annually

✔ Continue to have a regular cardiovascular health risk assessment (see p163), including a blood test to check cholesterol and triglyceride levels, measurement of weight and blood pressure and assessment of smoking habits

✔ Check your skin regularly for moles, suspicious abnormalities or changes (see pp358–60).

Additional screening tests

✔ Ask your doctor about faecal occult blood testing for bowel cancer if you are concerned about it (the NHS screening programme ends at 74)

✔ If you have a family history of type 2 diabetes, and especially if you are overweight, you may want to ask your doctor to check your blood glucose levels occasionally to screen for diabetes

✔ Ask your doctor about a thyroid screening test, known as the TSH test (see p328), to check your thyroid gland, though they may feel this is not necessary if you have no symptoms

✔ Have urinalysis as recommended by your doctor (a urine test to screen for metabolic and kidney disorders).

The result may be constipation and indigestion. Decreased appetite can become a problem, too. It is often caused by a reduced sense of taste and smell, or by illness or muscle wasting.

If you have decreased energy, you may think that it is a "normal" sign of ageing, but it may be that you're deficient in protein, calories, iron, vitamin B12, or vitamin D. Ask your doctor about taking a daily multivitamin or whether you should consult a dietician.

Various preventive measures can help improve the health of your digestive system. These include:

● Eating small, frequent meals
● Increasing your dietary fibre

(or take a supplement)
● Taking pre- and probiotic supplements
● Increasing your daily non-alcoholic fluid intake
● Walking for about 20 to 30 minutes each day.

BONE AND TEETH HEALTH

Tooth loss is increasingly common in this decade, due to poor dental hygiene, osteoporosis of the jaw, and gum disease.

Increasingly fragile bones in women over 70 make it vital that

LEADING CAUSES OF DEATH FOR WOMEN AGED 75 AND OVER

Statistical research in the United Kingdom shows that the leading causes of death among women aged 75 and over are:

1 Heart diseases (ischaemic)
2 Cancer (all types)
3 Cerebrovascular disease (stroke)
4 Flu and pneumonia
5 Dementia and Alzheimer's
6 Chronic lower respiratory diseases
7 Heart failure/heart disease
8 Diseases of urinary system
9 Accidents
10 Aortic aneurysm and dissection

they do not fall over. Bone-density testing, osteoporosis treatment, and taking calcium and vitamin D supplements are important, too. In women over 75, the most common surgery is hip fracture repair – but 20 per cent die within one year of surgery and 25 per cent need long-term care in a nursing home.

EYE AND EAR HEALTH
Poor vision can contribute to falls as well as make daily living more challenging. Similarly, hearing may become increasingly impaired in your 70s and beyond.

Don't be shy or embarrassed about telling your doctor your hearing needs help: there are many types of hearing aid which are neither obvious nor intrusive.

SKIN HEALTH
In your 70s and beyond, your skin continues to become increasingly thin, dry, itchy, and fragile, making bruises, cuts, and infections more common. While most of the skin problems are benign, you should still be alert to changes that are

> "Various preventive measures can help improve the health of your digestive system."

potentially cancerous. People over 70 may also experience decreased sensitivity to temperature changes. Hypothermia can be serious so keep your home adequately heated.

EXERCISE
Staying physically active is one of the most important ways of staying well. Running after your grandchildren (if you have them) is a great form of exercise, but a recent study found that women aged 72–79 who exercised moderately for at least one hour per week were far less likely to have symptoms of arthritis.

It is a myth that older people should avoid doing exercise. On the contrary, it would be harmful to your health if you did none! You simply need to find a physical activity that suits you. Regular flexibility exercises such as yoga or stretching are good for you, as are swimming and supervised strength

training. Unless your doctor has told you otherwise, age itself is no reason to discontinue any activity that you have previously enjoyed. If in doubt, check with your doctor.

VITAMIN AND MINERAL SUPPLEMENTS IN YOUR 70s
The following vitamin and mineral supplements can help you get the most out of life. However, some single-dose vitamin supplements can interact harmfully with some medications or with the absorption of other nutrients, so check with your doctor before taking them.

Multivitamins Unless your doctor tells you otherwise, you probably no longer need iron in your multivitamin.

Calcium If your diet is not providing you with an adequate amount of calcium (800mg a day, gained by eating three servings of dairy foods), you could take a calcium supplement every day to

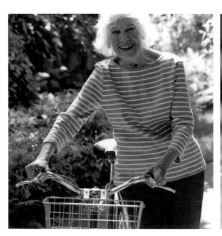

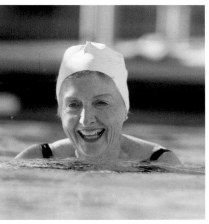

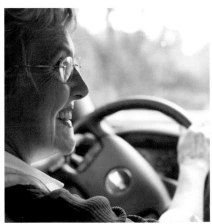

make up the difference. However, be sure to speak to your doctor before doing so and see pp52–5 and p262 for more about a healthy diet.

Vitamin D This essential vitamin aids calcium absorption and bone health. Most multivitamins contain vitamin D, but always check the dosage. Women aged above 65 need 10mcg of vitamin D each day. While it is in many foods, vitamin D is also made in the skin in response to exposure to sunlight (even if it's not a sunny day). If you don't receive 20 minutes of daily sunlight exposure, or are diligent about using total sun block, you may need to consider supplements.

VACCINES FOR YOUR 70s

You may need the following:

Flu Have a flu jab every year.

Pneumonia All adults over 65 should receive this vaccine to lower the risk of pneumonia.

Tetanus You may need a tetanus booster every 10 years.

Zoster You may want to consider vaccinating against shingles, but this jab is not available on the NHS.

DEMENTIA AND ALZHEIMER'S DISEASE

Memory problems and dementia are increasingly a cause for concern for women in their 70s. Alzheimer's disease (see pp184–5) is one of the most common forms of dementia and the average age at which it starts is 72. A significant number of people with dementia also develop signs of Parkinson's disease (p197), such as body rigidity and walking abnormalities. Certain factors increase the risk of Alzheimer's disease:

● Smokers can develop the disease 2.3 years earlier than non-smokers. Other studies estimate the increased risk of Alzheimer's and other forms of dementia with smoking is 50 per cent

● This "smoking" effect is even greater in individuals who have a genetic predisposition to develop Alzheimer's

● Those who consume two or more alcoholic drinks per day can develop Alzheimer's disease 4.8 years earlier than non-drinkers

● People with all three of the above risk factors can develop Alzheimer's disease an average of 8.5 years earlier than their risk-free counterparts.

We now know that you can reduce your risk of developing Alzheimer's disease by:

● Stopping smoking and reducing alcohol intake (see pp64–5 for advice)

● Taking regular exercise (see pp56–7 for advice). The greatest benefit of this may be in reducing the risk, or delaying the onset, of Alzheimer's. This is because neurons in the brain (particularly in the hippocampus) continue to regenerate throughout life. The process is fuelled by cerebral blood flow in the brain, which can be increased by aerobic exercise

● Taking vitamin E and omega-3 fatty acid supplements. However, their benefits have not yet been proved, nor have their effective doses been established.

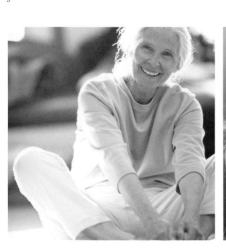

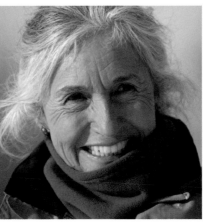

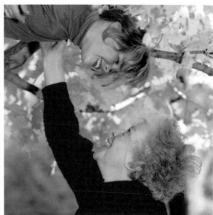

Staying well

Dr Dawn Harper MBBS MRCP DCH DFFP

Staying well

Obesity, diabetes, and heart disease seem to be the curse of the western world today. Doctors refer to these conditions as "multifactorial", which simply means that lots of different things can put us at risk of developing them. Some, like our genetics, we can't do much about, but most of the risk factors for these and lots of other conditions are entirely in our own hands. How we live our lives, what we eat and drink, and how we handle stress all play a part in how healthy we are, and even how long we will live.

We all lead increasingly busy lives, and perhaps women more so than men: more women work today than ever before, but many are still trying to juggle jobs with running the home. It is not unusual for women to start doing at 7pm what their mothers and grandmothers spent all day doing. This leaves precious little time to be proactive about health, and too many women put their own needs at the bottom of the agenda, which is a false economy for all concerned. It is easy to take good health for granted, but if you don't look after yourself you won't be able to look after anyone else. If you are lucky, your warning shot will be a gentle nudge, like one too many colds this winter because your immune system just isn't strong enough

OUR PSYCHOLOGICAL WELLBEING

It's not just our physical health that we need to maintain if we want to enjoy good health in the fullest sense – living a longer, more purposeful, and happier life is in part due to the relationships that we cultivate and enjoy.

The meaningful relationships that we have with a partner, family, friends, and wider community can help to nourish us emotionally and benefit our psychological wellbeing, as can spirituality in whatever form we best relate to it. Our sense of identity and our self-worth is inevitably grounded in these significant relationships, and being able to share our hopes, dreams, goals, and successes within a loving, intimate relationship or with a good friend is as important as being there to support each other through the conflicts, challenges, anxieties, and disappointments that we all encounter in life. Relaxing with friends and enjoying the company of others can also help us to unwind, which decreases our stress levels (see pp62–3) so that we feel revived and revitalized once again.

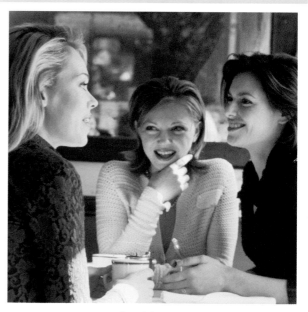

Good friends
Research studies into friendship have shown that having a good support network is vital for our wellbeing, and that feeling connected and cared for is particularly important for women.

to fight off infection. However, ignoring your own needs can have much more serious consequences. Most women don't see themselves as heart attack material, but in fact heart disease is the number one killer of women in the UK and accounts for nearly four times as many deaths as those from breast cancer. There simply aren't enough women asking their doctors about their blood pressure and cholesterol levels, and those that do are more often than not enquiring about their male relatives.

Perversely, thousands of women spend a great deal of time and money on looking good on the outside. Whether it is hairdressing, cosmetics, or freshening up our wardrobes, we are more likely to take care of our external appearance than men but, frighteningly, few of us take our internal health seriously enough. Just a few simple changes to your lifestyle could keep you feeling well for longer. Eating well, exercising regularly, and keeping stress under control will boost your immune system and keep you healthy for longer. There is nothing in this chapter that will require superhuman willpower. In fact, the exact opposite is true. Most of us can stick to a restrictive diet for a week or two or cut out alcohol for short periods, but very few of us can, or even want to, keep up that sort of lifestyle for months let alone for life.

ACHIEVABLE GOALS

If positive lifestyle changes are to have any effect on your health and longevity, they have to be achievable and sustainable, so there is no need to worry about having to begin training for a marathon. The aim of this chapter is simply to point you in the right direction to help you make relatively minor changes to your lifestyle that could make a significant impact on your health and wellbeing, leaving you and your family to enjoy your good health for longer.

> "It's easy to take good health for granted, but if you don't look after yourself you won't be able to look after anyone else."

PROTECT YOUR IMMUNE SYSTEM

Every day our bodies are exposed to literally thousands of bacteria and viruses, which could potentially cause infection. Our immune system protects us from succumbing to the vast majority of them. It is easy to take our immune system for granted, but if you get more than your fair share of the coughs and colds that go around, you probably need to be more proactive about looking after yourself:

Eat a balanced diet Healthy eating habits can boost your immune system (see pp52–5). The nutrients zinc, vitamin C (see p55), and selenium are particularly important for a healthy immune system.

Deal with your stress A little bit of stress can be good for you, making you feel more alert, but chronic stress will depress your immune system. (See pp62–3 for ways to deal with stress.)

Take time out to relax A class in yoga or pilates is a great way to unwind and exercise your body.

Don't drink too much alcohol – it will depress your immune system. The recommended limit for women is 2–3 units a day, and a maximum of 14 units a week (see also p65). Sadly, women's bodies aren't designed to cope with as much alcohol as men.

Stop smoking – smokers absorb 30 per cent less vitamin C from their diet. They also get more chest infections and upper respiratory tract infections than non-smokers, and are at increased risk of osteoporosis. (For more information on giving up smoking, see p64.)

Get enough rest How much sleep you need varies from person to person, but not getting enough sleep undoubtedly suppresses your immune system. For more information on getting a good night's sleep, see pp60–1.

Keep smiling According to research from the American Psychological Association, a positive attitude really can help protect against illness.

Wash your hands regularly Colds are passed mainly from hand to hand contact, and from there to the eyes and nose – and not via droplets in the air from other people's coughs and sneezes.

Eat a healthy diet

Eating healthily is all about ensuring that you eat a balanced diet of beneficial foods, and in the western world we are fortunate enough to have ready access to a whole variety of different foods all year round. So there really is no excuse for allowing your health to suffer as a result of a poor diet.

A good diet increases your chances of living a longer, healthier life by reducing the risk of diseases such as heart disease, stroke, and diabetes. It may even help reduce the risk of developing some cancers.

Eating healthily doesn't mean cutting out all your favourite foods and treats, but you do need to eat more of certain types of fresh foods. Eating the occasional bar of chocolate or a ready-made meal is fine, but making these foods part of your staple diet is not.

CARBS AND FIBRE

Around half of our daily calories should come from the complex carbohydrates found in all fruit, vegetables, and grains and cereals such as rice, pasta, and potatoes. Aim to eat at least five portions of fresh fruit and vegetables a day (according to the UK Foods Standards Agency, a glass of fruit juice counts as one portion). Frozen, canned, and dried fruit and vegetables also count towards your five a day. Don't fall into the trap of thinking of "carbs" as the enemy: complex carbohydrates are good for you and won't make you fat. With carbohydrates such as breads, grains, and cereals, try to choose the wholegrain, unrefined options, such as wholemeal bread and brown rice. These foods are high in fibre and help to fill you up without being high in calories. It's also important to remember that it is what you put with these foods, such as butter on bread or sugar on cereals, that adds the calories.

FOOD ALLERGIES AND INTOLERANCES

Food allergies are really quite rare; many of those who claim to be allergic to a food are probably just intolerant of it.

An allergy occurs if the body's immune system reacts to a food in a dramatic way. Symptoms include itchy skin and a rash that looks like nettle rash (urticaria). In severe cases, the lips, tongue, and throat swell, the heart rate increases, blood pressure drops, and wheezing may occur due to the narrowing of the airways. Known as anaphylaxis, this reaction is life-threatening if the obstructed airways and extreme low blood pressure are not treated quickly. An allergic reaction will often occur within an hour of contact with the allergen, and get worse with repeated exposure. Common food allergens include:
- Peanuts and tree nuts
- Cow's milk
- Hen's eggs
- Fish and shellfish
- Soya
- Wheat.

Possible triggers, identified from a patient's story, can be confirmed with blood tests or skin prick tests.

Food intolerance affects as many as 1 in 5 of us. The symptoms can be vague and include abdominal pain and bloating, nausea, constipation, or diarrhoea. The key difference is the time scale and the variability – people who are intolerant to a food develop symptoms several hours, or even days, after exposure to it, and may go through phases where they are able to tolerate it again – unlike allergy sufferers. Keep a food and symptom diary for a few weeks if you think you have an intolerance, and talk to your doctor.

The right food combinations

For a well-balanced diet, eat a range of healthy foods in the correct proportions. Complex starchy carbohydrates and proteins release energy gradually, helping you to keep going for longer, while vegetables and fruit are important sources of fibre, vitamins, minerals, and antioxidants. Protein-rich foods are also vital for building and repairing your body cells. To gauge the correct size of each food portion, use the size of the palm of your hand as a guide.

Complex starchy carbohydrates

One third of your daily energy intake should be complex carbs. Include at least 1 portion per meal.

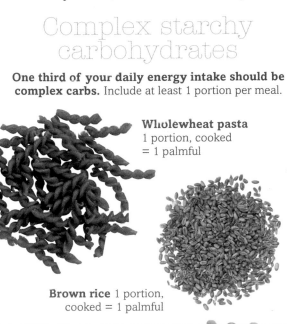

Wholewheat pasta
1 portion, cooked
= 1 palmful

Brown rice 1 portion, cooked = 1 palmful

Protein

Choose 2 portions a day. Include at least 2 portions of fish a week, 1 portion of which should be oily fish.

Salmon steak
1 portion = 1 palmful

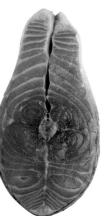

Lentils 1 portion, cooked = 1 palmful

Chicken 1 portion = 1 palmful

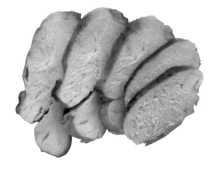

Vegetables and fruit

Eat at least 5 portions of fruit and vegetables a day. Try to choose from a wide range of different coloured fruit and vegetables.

Broccoli 1 portion = 1 palmful (e.g. 2 large spears or 4 small ones)

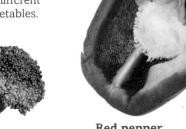

Red pepper
1 portion = ½ a pepper

Apricots
1 portion = 1 palmful
(e.g. 2 small apricots)

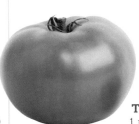

Tomato 1 portion = 1 medium-sized tomato

Dairy

Choose 2–3 portions a day. Select from cheese, milk, and yoghurt, and choose low- or reduced-fat options.

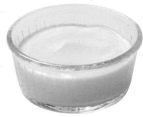

Milk
1 portion = 1 small glass (200ml/7fl oz)

Low-fat yoghurt 1 portion = 1 small pot (150ml/5fl oz)

Refined grains are known as simple carbohydrates, and the processed products made from these refined grains, such as white bread, cakes, and pastries, should be an occasional treat only.

Fruits, vegetables, wholegrains, beans, lentils, and other legumes are rich in fibre, which keeps your digestive system healthy, lowers cholesterol, and may decrease the risk of cancer. If you eat a more processed diet, you lose out on this valuable fibre, so limit the amount of processed foods you eat.

MILK AND DAIRY PRODUCTS

These foods are high in calcium, protein, and vitamins, but they can be high in fat; opt for low- or reduced-fat dairy products, such as semi-skimmed or skimmed milk. Check the labels, as some low-fat foods have added sugar to make up for the loss of flavour.

MEAT AND FISH

Lean meat, such as poultry, and fish are rich in iron, protein, vitamins, and minerals. Aim to eat at least two portions of fish a week, at least one of which should be an oily fish such as salmon, mackerel or fresh tuna, which are rich in omega-3 oils. If you can't eat this much fish, consider taking a supplement.

FATS AND SUGARS

The fats found in nuts, seeds, and oily fish provide vitamins A, D, E, and K, and essential fatty acids – which help to make healthy cell

HOW MUCH SALT CAN I HAVE?

The high salt diet that we eat in the west works against how we were ancestrally developed, and so predisposes us to salt-sensitive problems. Adults should eat no more than 6g (about 1 teaspoon) of salt a day; given that three quarters of our salt quota is included in the food we buy, it is easy to see how we exceed that amount. Check ready meal food labels for salt content, try swapping salt with herbs when you cook, and avoid adding salt to your food. Your food may taste bland at first, but in time your taste buds will acclimatize.

FIVE ESSENTIAL MINERALS

Minerals promote muscle activity, keep cells and nerves healthy, and help the body to repair itself. The recommended daily allowance (RDA) of five key minerals are given below, together with the average mineral content per 100g (4oz) of the foods listed.

ZINC
RDA: 15mg

Helps maintain a healthy immune system. Good sources include prawns (2.2mg), oysters (59mg), calves' liver (15.9mg), and wholemeal bread (1.6mg).

CALCIUM
RDA: 800mg

Crucial for strong bones and teeth. Good sources include cheddar cheese (739mg), low-fat yoghurt (162mg), semi-skimmed milk (120mg), tofu (510mg), and broccoli (40mg).

POTASSIUM
RDA: 3,500mg

Promotes muscle activity and nerve function, and prevents cramp. Found in most foods; good sources include bananas (400mg), avocados (450mg), and red kidney beans (420mg).

IRON
RDA: 14mg

Important for the manufacture of red blood cells. Lack of iron can lead to tiredness. Goods sources include red kidney beans (2mg), calves' liver (12.2mg), and dried apricots (3.4mg).

MAGNESIUM
RDA: 300mg

Necessary for a healthy nervous system. Good sources include nuts, such as almonds (270mg), steamed spinach (34mg), and wholemeal bread (66mg).

membranes. Limit these foods to a third of your daily calorific intake, as fat contains more calories per gram than any other foods. Fats can be divided into three types:

- Monounsaturated – found in olive oil, nuts, and avocados
- Polyunsaturated – found in oily fish, sunflower oil, and some spreads
- Saturated – found in sweet and savoury snacks, processed meat products, ready meals, biscuits, cakes, pastries, and some dairy. Limit these foods to a third of your total daily intake of fat. Unsaturated fats increase "good cholesterol", while saturated fats increase "bad cholesterol" (see p163).

A lot of processed foods are high in saturated fats: if you see the word "hydrogenated" on a food label, it means that some of the unsaturated fats in a food have been converted to saturated fats.

Like fat, sugar is high in calories, and provides no nutritional benefit, so limit sugary foods in your diet.

NINE ESSENTIAL VITAMINS

Small quantities of vitamins are needed by our bodies in order for them to work efficiently and resist illnesses. The recommended daily allowance (RDA) of nine key vitamins are given below, together with the average vitamin content per 100g (4oz) of the foods listed.

VITAMIN B12
RDA: 1mcg

Prevents anaemia, helps maintain a healthy nervous system, and relieves irritability. Good sources include lamb (3mcg), salmon (5mcg), cheddar cheese (2.4mcg), and eggs (2.7mcg).

VITAMIN A
RDA: 800mcg

Strengthens the immune system. Good sources include dairy foods. Beta-carotene, found in yellow and orange foods such as carrots (5,330mcg), turns into Vitamin A in the body.

VITAMIN C
RDA: 60mg

Increases the body's resistance to infection and free radicals. Good sources include oranges (54mg), red pepper (140mg), and steamed broccoli (44mg).

VITAMIN B1
RDA: 1.4mg

Necessary for converting carbohydrates into energy. Good sources include raisins (0.12mg), eggs (0.09mg), wholegrain bread (0.25mg), and branflakes (0.8mg).

VITAMIN D
RDA: 5mcg

Vital for strong, healthy bones and crucial for the absorption of calcium. Good sources include herrings (16.1mcg), mackerel (8.8mcg), salmon (7.10mcg), and eggs (1.75mcg).

VITAMIN B2
RDA: 1.6mg

Helps to keep the eyes, skin, and nervous system healthy. Good sources include rice (0.02mg, cooked), mushrooms (0.31mg), semi-skimmed milk (0.24mg), and eggs (0.45mg).

VITAMIN E
RDA: 10mg

Protects from free-radical damage and keeps skin, nerves, and muscles healthy. Good sources include sunflower seeds (37.7mg), peanuts (10mg), and almonds (23.9mg).

VITAMIN B6
RDA: 2mg

Allows the body to use and store energy from the food we eat. Good sources include chicken (0.36mg), turkey (0.49mg), cod (0.21mg), and peanuts (0.59mg).

FOLATE
RDA: 200mcg

Breaks down protein in the body and helps prevent birth defects in newborn babies. Good sources include steamed broccoli (64mcg), peas (33mcg), chickpeas (66mcg).

Exercise to stay healthy

We are leading increasingly sedentary lives and unless we make some fundamental changes, our children are likely to do even less exercise than we do. Exercising regularly will boost your energy levels, help combat stress, improve your sleep, keep you slim, and protect against weight-related illnesses.

TOP TIPS TO WALK 10,000 STEPS A DAY

Walking the equivalent of 5–7.5km (3–4½ miles) every day is easier to achieve if you try these options:

- Wear a pedometer (see below) on your waistband and measure the number of steps you take. An average pace is 50–75cm (20–30in). If you have an office-based job, you may walk as little as 2,000 paces a day, so throughout the day check your pedometer to motivate you to reach your target
- Get off the bus or tube a stop early each morning
- Use the stairs, not the lift; taking the stairs is superb exercise
- Park your car as far away from where you're going as possible
- Don't use a phone for internal calls – walk over instead.

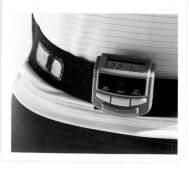

Life in the west has changed unrecognizably in a relatively short period of time. One hundred years ago, we didn't have supermarket deliveries on the internet, washing machines, or vacuum cleaners, and we didn't drive everywhere. Women used around 4,000 calories a day simply doing the chores, so they had no need for a personal trainer or gym membership. Today, we typically use a little over half of those daily calories and almost certainly take in a lot more, so it should come as no surprise that we are getting fatter. With this worrying trend comes an increased risk of a multitude of diseases, including heart disease (see pp158–74), diabetes (see pp322–5), and even depression (see pp210–11).

Women often give up formal exercise at a younger age than men. According to the British Heart Foundation, two-thirds of British women are so unfit that they cannot walk up a gradual incline at a normal pace without becoming short of breath.

HOW MUCH EXERCISE IS ENOUGH?

As a minimum, you should walk at least 10,000 paces a day (see box, left). In addition, you should aim to exercise moderately for 30 minutes five times a week, or aerobically three times a week. It doesn't matter what you do so long as it gets your heart pumping. Choose something you enjoy, such as a dance class or swimming, and if you exercise with a friend you will be more likely to keep to a routine, especially as women often put themselves at the bottom of a long agenda of family and work commitments. Be realistic about your day – it may be better to get up early and fit in your exercise at the start of the day, or

CALCULATE YOUR MAXIMUM HEART RATE (MHR)

To calculate how hard you should work your heart, subtract your age from 220. Your training range (beats per minute) is 70–85% of your MHR.

For example: if you are 40 years old, your MHR should be:

220	—	40	=	180	70–85% of 180	=	126–153 pulse rate
		Your age		MHR			Training range

follow an exercise DVD at home while the children are at school. If you can afford it, hire a personal trainer who will ensure that you stick to your plan. Set yourself targets – whether it is fitting into that little black dress for a special occasion or joining a fun run – so that you have something to help you keep motivated.

ARE YOU EXERCISING HARD ENOUGH?

If you can chat easily as you exercise, you aren't pushing yourself hard enough, but if you are gasping for breath, you are overdoing it. Somewhere in the middle is just right. To begin with, you may find just walking briskly is all you need to do to push yourself, but as you get fitter you will have to work harder to achieve the same result. Invest in a heart rate monitor and aim for a pulse rate of 70–85 per cent of your maximum heart rate (see box, opposite) as you exercise.

EXERCISE AND WEIGHT LOSS

You need to expend 3,500 calories to lose one pound of fat. It is difficult to be too dogmatic about how many calories we burn doing different activities, as the amount depends on how energetically you take part in that activity and how much you weigh: heavier women use up more calories doing exactly the same activity as their slimmer counterparts. As a rough guide, a 57kg (9 stone) woman will use up the following calories with each half hour of exercise:

Three ways to stay strong

Strength-training exercises are an important part of any fitness routine, helping to keep muscles toned and bones healthy. The exercises below work many of the major muscle groups – and they are quick and easy to do anywhere.

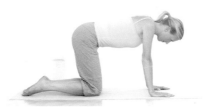

Upper body 1
A great exercise that will tone your arms, chest, and belly. Kneel on all fours, back straight, belly pulled in.

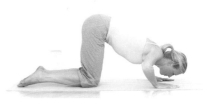

Upper body 2
Bend your elbows out the sides and slowly lower your chest to the floor. Slowly push back up; repeat 8 times.

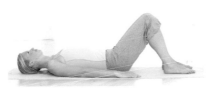

Lower body 1
This exercise will keep your spine strong, and your bottom and thighs toned. Lie with your knees raised, feet hip-width apart.

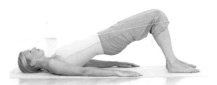

Lower body 2
Pull your belly in, squeeze your bottom, and slowly lift your hips into the raised position. Lower gently; repeat 8 times.

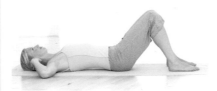

Strong core 1
For strong abdominal muscles, lie on your back, knees bent, feet hip-width apart. Rest your fingertips at the side of your head.

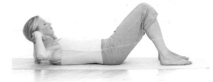

Strong core 2
Pull your belly in and curl up slowly until your shoulders are off the floor. Don't tuck your chin in. Curl down; repeat 8 times.

- Playing golf – 110 calories
- Horse riding – 120 calories
- Walking the dog – 125 calories
- Housework – 135 calories
- Gardening – 160 calories
- Gym workout – 160 calories

- Dancing – 170 calories
- Aerobics – 170 calories
- Cycling – 240 calories
- Swimming – 250 calories
- Jogging – 280 calories
- Tennis – 300 calories.

Weight issues

It is now estimated that more women than men are putting their health at risk because of weight issues. Obesity is a growing problem in many developed countries; in fact, one in three women in the UK is thought to be overweight, and 24 per cent of women are considered obese compared to 23 per cent of men.

AM I OVERWEIGHT?

You are considered overweight if you carry too much fat for your height. Doctors use a calculation called a Body Mass Index (BMI) to assess your weight in relation to your height (see box, below), although if you are an athlete or very muscular – muscle weighs more than fat – you can have a higher BMI even though you may have a healthy level of body fat and be in the peak of fitness.

Waist and hip measurements

For this reason, many doctors rely more on waist measurement as an indicator of risk for weight-related diseases, in particular diabetes and heart disease. If your waist measures more than 79cm (31in), you are at increased risk of these diseases, and the risks are very high if your waist measures more than 86cm (34in). To calculate your waist-hip ratio and measure the proportion of fat stored around your waist in comparison to your hips, measure your waist at its narrowest point, then your hips at their widest point. Divide the waist by the hip measurement to calculate your waist-hip ratio. A ratio of more than 0.8 defines you as an apple shape (see box opposite), which means that you are at risk of serious health problems.

THE RISKS OF BEING OVERWEIGHT

Being overweight will make you look and feel older, but it is how it ages you on the inside that is most important. If being overweight doesn't bother you from a cosmetic point of view, it is easier to accept your weight as normal and ignore the health warnings. But being obese can knock as much as ten years off your life. The health risks make for sobering reading:

Diabetes Being overweight is the main cause of Type 2 diabetes (see pp322–5), which predisposes you to a range of serious illnesses including heart disease, stroke, kidney disease, and blindness.

High blood pressure The heavier you are, the higher your blood pressure is likely to be (see p161), which increases your risk of heart disease and stroke.

Heart disease and stroke Obese women are 3.2 times more likely to have a heart attack (see p166), and 1.3 times more at risk of stroke (see p196).

CALCULATE YOUR BMI

To calculate your own BMI, divide your weight (in kilograms) by the square of your height (in metres).

If your BMI is:
Below 18.5 you are underweight
18.5–25 you have a healthy BMI

25–30 you are overweight
Over 30 you are clinically obese
Over 40 you are morbidly obese.

For example: if you are 1.6m (5ft 3in) and weigh 65kg (10st 3lb), your calculation would be:

1.6m (5ft 3in) Height (in metres)	**×**	1.6m (5ft 3in) Height (in metres)	**=**	2.56 Height (squared)	65kg (10st 3lb) Weight (in kilograms)	**÷**	2.56 Height (squared)	**=**	25.39 Your BMI

CALCULATE YOUR DAILY CALORIE REQUIREMENT

If you have a healthy BMI for your height, you can calculate your daily calorie requirement to maintain a healthy weight: [(0.062 x your weight in kilograms) + 2.036] x 239.
If you are aged 35–55, deduct 200–300 calories from this total. If you are aged 55 or over, deduct 400–600 calories.

Then multiply the number of calories by your activity level to reach your correct daily intake:
- no formal exercise: multiply by 1.4
- 30 minutes of moderate exercise a day: multiply by 1.5
- three or more sessions of intense aerobic activity a week: multiply by 1.6

For example: if you weigh 65kg (10st 3lb), are 41 years old, and exercise aerobically three times a week, the calculation would be:

$$\left[\ (0.062 \times 65 = 4.03) + 2.036 = 8.205\ \right] \times 239 = 1{,}449$$

Your weight (65kg) | Basic calories

$$-\ 200 = 1{,}249 \times 1.6 = 1{,}998$$

For ages 35–55 | Activity level | **Total calories per day**

High cholesterol The heavier you are, the higher your cholesterol will be. High cholesterol is linked to angina (see p164), heart attack (see p166), and stroke (see p196).
Cancer The fatter you are, the more likely you are to succumb to cancer of the breast, womb, ovary, or kidney.
Infertility Overweight women are more likely to have irregular periods, find it difficult to get pregnant, and at increased risk of complications in pregnancy (see pp124–31).
Osteoarthritis Obese women are three times more likely to suffer from arthritic knees (see p263–5), which can be hard to treat.
Depression Overweight women are more likely to suffer from depression (see pp210–11).

THE RISKS OF BEING UNDERWEIGHT

If your BMI calculation is below 18.5, your body has fallen below a critical weight and you are at risk of infertility and osteoporosis. A low body weight can be linked to depression and anxiety, and you may need professional help for these (see Chapter 9, pp200–27).

ACHIEVING A BALANCE

If you're overweight or underweight, first work out how many calories your body needs to stay healthy (see box above), and follow the advice on healthy eating (see pp52–5). If you need to lose weight, reduce your weekly allowance by 3,500 calories to lose a steady 0.5kg (1lb) a week.

APPLE SHAPED

If you are overweight and "apple shaped" (a normal apple shape is shown below), you are more at risk of developing diabetes or heart disease than if you store fat on your thighs and bottom (pear shaped). This may be because apple shapes store fat around their internal organs, making them resistant to the effects of the hormone insulin (see p324).

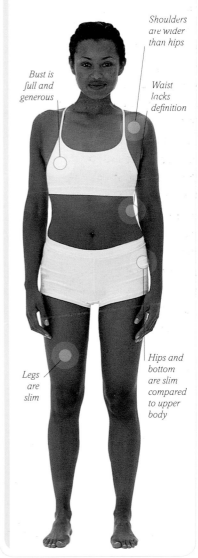

Shoulders are wider than hips

Bust is full and generous

Waist lacks definition

Legs are slim

Hips and bottom are slim compared to upper body

Sleep well

A good night's sleep is essential to our physical and emotional wellbeing. Most of us can cope with the occasional bad night, but disturbed sleep on successive nights can knock your immune system, leave you feeling irritable and less able to concentrate or make decisions, and make you prone to stress.

Although we all vary in our need for sleep – our requirements change according to our activity levels during the day, and throughout our lives as we age – experts believe that between seven and nine hours of sleep a night is probably the optimum amount. Of course, there is more to sleep than the number of hours we actually spend in bed.

NORMAL SLEEP PATTERNS
At night we oscillate between two types of sleep pattern – rapid eye movement (REM) sleep, and non-rapid eye movement (NREM) sleep. We probably spend about a quarter of the time in the lighter REM sleep (when most of our dreaming is thought to occur) and the rest in the deep, more refreshing NREM

sleep, which is divided into four stages, each stage being a little bit deeper than the last.

If we are constantly disturbed during the night, we are deprived of the NREM sleep – what could also be called "battery recharge sleep" – that we need, and we therefore wake up tired and feeling unrefreshed.

YOGA FOR RELAXING

To help you unwind at the end of the day, try this simple yoga sequence known as the hare pose. It will help you to relax your body and calm your mind ready for bed. Hold each posture for 10 seconds, turning your attention inwards. Feel a great stretch in your back, hips, and knees as you repeat the sequence three times.

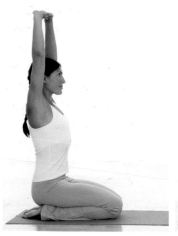

Step 1
Kneeling on a soft surface, stretch your hands towards the ceiling, fingers interlocked, palms facing upwards.

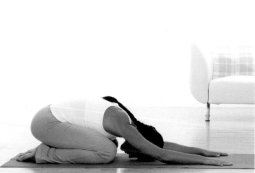

Step 2
Bend forwards and stretch your arms out in front of you. Open your knees if you need to. Rest your forehead on the floor.

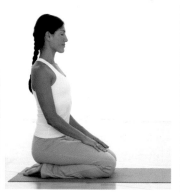

Step 3
Return to a seated position, palms on thighs. Close your eyes and breathe deeply and slowly.

INSOMNIA SUFFERERS

Persistent sleep problems are very common; your sleep pattern can easily be affected by how you are feeling. Women are twice as likely as men to suffer from insomnia, and social factors such as being unemployed or divorced seem to increase the risk of developing it. The incidence of insomnia also seems to increase the older we get, because we tend to need less sleep and sleep less deeply.

Listed here are some of the factors that may influence the quantity and quality of sleep that you get, and some suggestions as to how to resolve them so that you sleep more easily.

Stress Try to resolve any stressful problems you encounter before you go to bed. However, if your mind is still preoccupied, take a pen and paper to bed with you so that you can jot down any thoughts as you think of them. This should help you to switch off properly and get to sleep knowing that you will have an aide memoire when you wake. For more information on dealing with stress, see pp62–3.

Anger There is a lot to be said for not letting the sun go down on an argument. Try to resolve all disputes outside of the bedroom.

Depression Sufferers of depression may find that they can get off to sleep quite easily, but wake in the early hours and are unable to get to sleep again. If you suffer from low moods or depression and you repeatedly wake too early, talk to your doctor.

Hormones The hot flushes and night sweats that occur around the menopause are a common cause of sleep problems. If you are struggling to sleep, don't rule out a short course of HRT. Your doctor will explain the risks and benefits to you, but if you decide that HRT isn't for you, there are non-hormonal alternatives that may prove helpful.

Pain Few of us can get to sleep, let alone stay asleep, when we are in pain, so if you are struggling with pain, talk to your doctor about fine-tuning your treatment.

Noise Whether you have a noisy neighbour or a snoring partner, use a pair of good-quality earplugs to block out the noise.

Room temperature and light Being too hot or cold in bed can affect your ability to get to sleep, as can too much light in the room. Adjust the conditions to suit you better and help you settle quickly.

Caffeine Avoid drinks that contain caffeine – including coffee, tea, and cola – after 6pm.

Alcohol Don't rely on alcohol – it may help you get off to sleep by making you feel tired, but it interferes with your normal sleep rhythms and you won't get a proper night's sleep.

Smoking Nicotine is a stimulant. If you have to smoke, at least avoid smoking after 6pm.

Drugs If you notice a change in your sleep pattern after you have started taking medication, talk to your doctor. The new drug could be to blame and there may be a more suitable alternative.

TOP TIPS FOR A GOOD NIGHT'S SLEEP

There are several golden rules to follow if you want to be assured of a restful night.

- **Stop working** at least an hour before you go to bed to allow yourself enough time to unwind and switch off
- **Make your bedroom calm** and as comfortable as possible so that going to bed is a peaceful experience
- **Go to bed at the same time** each night and avoid catnaps during the day at all costs. A good night's sleep is all about routine
- **Be active during the day**, but avoid exercising late at night – it may boost your energy levels, which can make it harder for you to wind down in order to get to bed at your usual time
- **Don't read or watch TV in bed.** Your bedroom should be for sleeping and sex, and your brain needs to know that!
- **Once you are in bed**, don't toss and turn and fret about whether you can get to sleep. If you are not asleep within 20 minutes of going to bed, get up again, go to another room, and read until you are tired enough to try to get off to sleep again. However, choose your reading matter carefully – a thriller could leave you feeling even more awake.

Managing stress

Most of us find it impossible to live a totally stress-free life, and it's probably unlikely that we would want to; a little bit of stress can be exhilarating, and enables us to get things done. If we have too much stress to cope with, however, then something has to give – and it shouldn't be our health.

When we experience stress or feel anxious, the stress hormones that our bodies release in response to the situation cause our heart rate and blood pressure to increase and put us in what is known as "fight or flight" mode. For our ancestors, that meant being able to react quickly enough to flee from an approaching mammoth, but today's "mammoths" don't come and go in an instant; they can hang around for days, weeks, or even months.

These days it is common for most women to find themselves multitasking as they handle busy working and home lives. Many of us have become accustomed to our pressurized lifestyles and are able to cope well in crises, but if we find ourselves over-functioning with too many demands on our time, or we have deadlines piling up at work and frequent arguments at home, over time we may begin to feel consistently stressed and

anxious, or physically run down, which all takes its toll on our mental and physical wellbeing. This may help to explain, in part, why more women than men are likely to suffer from stress.

RESPONDING TO STRESS

Stress is something that is quite difficult to define or measure on a scale, as we all respond differently to potentially stressful situations. What might wind one

DEEP-BREATHING MEDITATION

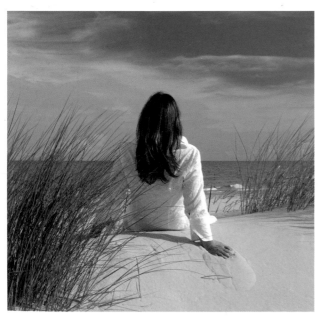

Use this simple meditation to relax and re-energize your body and mind:

1 Sit in a comfortable position, or lie flat on a bed or on the floor with your knees bent. Place one hand on your abdomen and the other on your chest. Close your eyes if you wish.

2 Quieten your body and mind. To help you relax, imagine you are on the beach, or some other favourite location; savour the sights, sounds, and smells.

3 Now slow your breathing: breathe in for a count of 5, pause for 1–2 seconds, then breathe out for a count of 5.

4 Consciously release all your tension with each out-breath. Feel your abdominal muscles push out the last of each breath, and your diaphragm expand as you inhale. Repeat as many times as you wish, even 5–10 minutes will help to you to feel calmer and centred.

person up into a frenzy can pass straight over another's head. If you've got your stress levels under control, you should feel mentally alert and vibrant, able to concentrate, make decisions, eat well, and then switch off and relax at the end of the day. If you feel anxious or tense, however, perhaps with a thumping heart or a knot in your stomach, or if you have any physical symptoms related to stress (see right), then you need to do something about your stress levels, and sooner rather than later.

WHEN STRESS AFFECTS YOUR HEALTH

Recognizing the signs of stress in yourself can go a long way to helping you know when to slow down. Common signs of stress building up include:

- Disturbed sleep and feeling tired all the time
- Depression, anxiety, panic attacks
- Frequent minor infections from a weakened immune system
- Migraine and tension headaches
- Flare-ups of skin problems, such as eczema, acne, and psoriasis
- Indigestion or symptoms of irritable bowel syndrome.

If you recognize any symptoms, the chances are that ongoing stress in your life is adversely affecting your health and you need to deal with it (see box, below). It's also important to re-learn how to relax, so practise some simple relaxation techniques or meditation (see box, opposite). If you feel that you simply don't know where to start, you are becoming overwhelmed by stress and you need to see your doctor as soon as possible.

TOP TIPS ON MANAGING STRESS

Women can get caught in the trap of wanting to be everything to everyone and then take on too much, which can put huge pressure on their time and dramatically increase their stress levels. Try these solutions:

Make lists Write down everything that you have to do in the week ahead, and then prioritize. It will help you to plan your time carefully so that the really important things get done first. If anything at the bottom of the list gets missed or time runs out on you, the chances are that it won't really matter.

Delegate No one can, or should, expect you to do everything on your own; your partner or children may not tidy up the house as well as you, but they can certainly try!

Communicate There is nothing wrong with admitting that you aren't coping with all the pressures on your time, and even the people you live with won't necessarily know how much you are juggling if you don't say. You may find that simply talking to a close family member or friend about how stressed you feel, and the reasons why, will help hugely.

Accept offers of help Whether you have a neighbour who can help with the school run, or a colleague at the office who is offering to help with your workload, the probability is that they can see that you are under pressure and want to help.

Learn to say "no" Women are slow learners here, and it is often not until we are in our mid- to late forties that most of us finally learn how to say "no". If you haven't got time to do something, say so. There are only 24 hours in a day and, try as you might, you won't find any more.

Find some "me time" It doesn't matter if it's a session at the gym or having lunch with a friend, taking some time out of your routine will help you to switch off and then be more efficient the next day, not to mention being a better mum and partner. Women are notorious for feeling guilty about doing anything for themselves, but remind yourself that there are no winners if you are stressed and your fuse is short.

Exercise regularly Regular exercise reduces stress levels and wards off depression. If you are feeling tired all the time, forcing yourself to exercise may seem like a ludicrous suggestion, but it really does work, as it leaves you feeling energized and refreshed.

Most of us can manage our stress levels by making just a few of these simple adjustments, but if you are still overwhelmed by stress and feel swamped, or if stress is making you physically unwell, you must seek help from your doctor.

Kicking bad habits

Giving up bad habits is never easy, and it requires a lot of willpower, but one thing is certain – you need to really want to give up. It is no good your partner or children urging you to stop smoking or cut out alcohol if you're ambivalent about it, but once you have made the decision, their support will be invaluable.

SMOKING

When it comes to living a long and healthy life, smoking is not an option. The truth is that half of all smokers will die from smoking-related diseases, and women are more susceptible to these diseases than men – diseases such as chronic obstructive pulmonary disease (see pp240–1), heart disease (see pp158–74), and cancers. Overall, smoking carries almost twice the risk of developing heart disease in women as it does in men, and you don't have to be a heavy smoker to be susceptible. One study of Danish women showed that those who smoked just three cigarettes a day were at almost double the risk of having a heart attack. The risk of developing other, non life-threatening, conditions, such as osteoporosis (see pp260–2), cataract (see p190), psoriasis (see pp356–7), gum disease, and tooth loss, are also higher if you are a smoker. Stopping smoking can make a big difference to your health: if you give up smoking before the age of 35, your life expectancy is only slightly less than those who have never smoked; if you give up smoking by the time you reach 50, your chances of dying from a smoking-related disease decrease by about 50 per cent.

TOP TIPS FOR GIVING UP SMOKING

Giving up smoking isn't easy, but there are several steps you can take to help to give you the determination you will need to stop:

Think of the cost Smoking 20 cigarettes a day for a year can cost approximately the same as a family holiday abroad. Stop for a moment and think what else you could spend that money on.

Write down the pros and cons of smoking Which is the longer list? Keep the list of reasons why you want to stop in your pocket so that you can read it again if your resolve begins to weaken.

Keep a diary of when you smoke Recognizing when you have your weakest moments will give you a better chance of avoiding temptation when you decide to quit.

Set a date to quit You will need all your willpower if you are going to be successful, so if you are under a lot of pressure, now may not be the best time. However, don't fall into the trap of finding endless excuses.

Make a plan of what you will do instead Giving up smoking is a life-changing event and taking up a new hobby may help to take your mind off things.

Be ready for weak moments You will have them. Ask your family and friends to help you through by focusing your attention on something else.

Think about your children If you smoke, your children will be exposed to the dangers of secondhand smoke, and are three times more likely to smoke themselves.

Stop completely You may prefer the idea of cutting back gradually, but even if you smoke fewer cigarettes, your nicotine desire will remain the same.

Get professional help Research shows that the chances of you quitting permanently are greatly improved if you have the back-up of a smoking cessation clinic. Your doctor or practice nurse will be able to advise you on this and on the various medicines, such as gums, sprays, tablets, and patches, that are available.

TOP TIPS FOR KEEPING TO RECOMMENDED ALCOHOL LIMITS

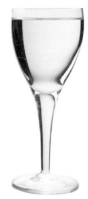

Red or white wine
small glass, 125ml (4fl oz)
12% ABV
Units: 1.5

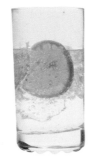

Gin and tonic
large single measure,
35ml (1fl oz)
Units: 1.4

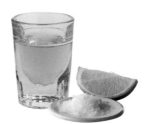

Tequila shot
large shot, 35ml (1fl oz)
Units: 1.3

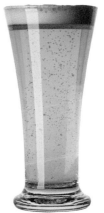

Premium beer
284 ml (½ pint)
5% ABV
Units: 1.4

Admitting that you have a drink problem is the first step towards getting better. The second is to find practical ways to cut back on the amount you drink, or give up altogether. Try these tips:

Keep a diary Make a note of every alcoholic drink you have for a week and calculate your units using the formula above. It may shock you, but don't cheat.

Only drink while you are eating.

Have at least two alcohol-free days a week.

Offer to drive if you go out, and stick to soft drinks.

Find a soft drink you like If you are serious about cutting back on the amount you drink, or stopping altogether, you need to find a substitute. If you want to have a drink or two, alternate each glass of alcohol with a soft drink – it will help to hydrate you and slow the rate at which you drink.

Think of the calories Alcoholic drinks may vary in their calorific value, but they are all fattening – and that doesn't include the nibbles that you pick at as you consume your drink and your willpower gradually fades.

ALCOHOL

In recent years there has been a marked increase in the number of women who regularly drink more than the recommended 14 units of alcohol per week. Forget the old guidelines of a glass of wine being a unit of alcohol – our glasses are getting bigger, and our wine stronger. A more accurate calculation is to look at the percentage of alcohol in your drink. That indicates the number of units in a litre of that drink. The standard size of a glass of wine is now 175ml (6fl oz), and if the wine you are drinking is 13 per cent alcohol by volume (ABV), your drink is equivalent to 2.3 units. Suddenly, exceeding the recommended limits is easy to do.

Women are more susceptible to the harmful effects of alcohol than men, and alcohol now kills more women than cervical cancer. It seems that too many of us are choosing to put our health at risk by exceeding this recommended weekly limit of alcohol.

Do you have a drink problem?

Ask yourself these questions; if you answer "yes" to two or more, you have a drink problem and need to tackle it now. Have you ever:

- Felt you should cut down on your drinking?
- Been annoyed by others criticising your drinking?
- Felt guilty about your drinking?
- Had an alcoholic drink to help you start the day?

Your doctor will be able to advise you on where to get the help you need.

Top-to-toe health care

Caring for your body and cultivating a positive self-image is all about making the most of what you have. Contrary to the media's preoccupation with surgical enhancement, there is little that the majority of us need to, or should want to, change if we are taking good care of ourselves inside and out.

Hair care

Creating a healthy head of hair is a multi-billion pound industry, but how we look after our hair on a day-to-day basis is just as important as having a haircut every few weeks.

MAINTAINING HEALTHY HAIR

Try these simple suggestions to keep your hair in optimum condition:

Wash your hair regularly Regular shampooing and conditioning will keep your hair looking and feeling healthy. Dirt accumulates in your hair as much as it does on your skin, so wash your hair as often as you wish. However, avoid using hair products containing chemical preservatives, such as parabens and sodium lauryl sulphate, as they act like detergents and strip your hair of its natural oils.

Detangle your hair first using a wide-toothed comb. Soak your hair thoroughly with warm water before shampooing it, pour the shampoo onto your hands, and rub them together before applying it to your scalp. Take at least 30 seconds to massage the shampoo into your hair. If you wash your hair every day, you should only need one application. Rinse your hair for twice as long as you think you should – dull hair is often a result of inadequate rinsing.

If you have dandruff, regular use of an anti-dandruff shampoo should keep it under control. Dandruff is not due to a dry scalp; in fact, it is more likely to be the result of an oily scalp.

Condition your hair after every wash Apply conditioner to the ends of your hair, not near the scalp.

Use the products designed for your hair type If you are not sure whether your hair is fine, medium, or coarse, ask your hairdresser.

Beware of overheating your hair Ration the use of hair dryers and straighteners. Towel your hair dry by gently patting it, and use a wide-toothed comb to comb it. If you use a hair dryer, choose one with a wide nozzle and use it about 15cm (6in) from your hair. Blow-drying already dried hair will cause hair damage, as will the over-use of hair straighteners.

Don't smoke Grey hair is largely determined by our genes, but smoking will make you prone to premature greying.

HOW MUCH SUNSCREEN DO I APPLY?

We often apply too little sunscreen when we are outside in strong sunlight. It is thought that the average adult needs about 2mg of sunscreen to protect each square centimetre of skin, which means that you need approximately 35ml (1fl oz) – about a sixth of a bottle, or a shot glass-full – to cover your body. Reapply more sunscreen at least every two hours, as sweating and being active can easily remove it.

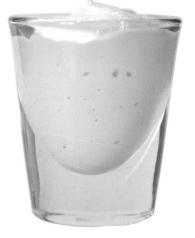

Life-size amount of suncream

Posture

Good posture is essential for the proper functioning of your muscles and joints; poor postural habits can lead to neck pain, shoulder tension, headaches, and back pain. In addition to the "Ws" exercise shown below, the exercises on p59 will also help to improve posture.

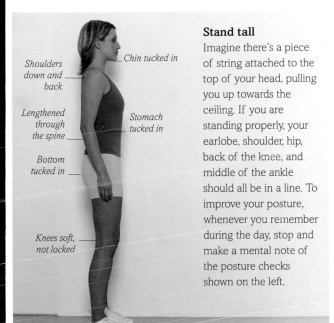

Shoulders down and back

Chin tucked in

Lengthened through the spine

Stomach tucked in

Bottom tucked in

Knees soft, not locked

Stand tall

Imagine there's a piece of string attached to the top of your head, pulling you up towards the ceiling. If you are standing properly, your earlobe, shoulder, hip, back of the knee, and middle of the ankle should all be in a line. To improve your posture, whenever you remember during the day, stop and make a mental note of the posture checks shown on the left.

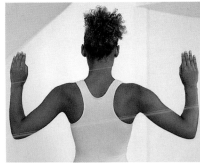

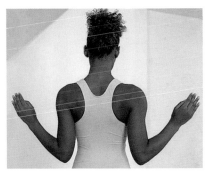

"Ws"

Step 1 You can do this exercise anywhere to strengthen the muscles in your midback. Put your arms out to your sides as shown, elbows bent.

Step 2 Draw your shoulder blades down and together as you move your elbows slowly and smoothly to your sides. Repeat the move 10 times.

Skin care

It's worth developing good skin care habits now so that your skin will be radiant and healthy for years to come.

CARING FOR YOUR SKIN

Avoid stressed, dehydrated skin by following these simple steps:

Protect yourself from the sun
A tan may make you feel and look good today, but make no mistake – prolonged exposure to the sun will irreversibly damage your skin. Protecting your skin from the sun's harmful ultraviolet rays is the best way to stay looking younger for longer (see box, opposite).

Don't smoke Smoking causes the skin to age prematurely, as it reduces the blood flow to the skin, depleting it of vital oxygen and nutrients. This damages the elastin and collagen fibres in skin. What's more, repetitive facial movements when you inhale smoke from a cigarette cause deep facial lines, especially on the upper lip and around the eyes. Tobacco smoke also contains many toxins that wreak havoc on your skin and affect its ability to repair itself.

Treat your skin gently Hot water from long showers or baths can strip the natural oils from your skin, so limit your bathing time and turn the water temperature down a notch. Other things that leave skin dry or irritated are strong soaps and certain product ingredients (see below), so avoid these. Pat your skin dry rather than rubbing to keep some of the moisture on the skin, and then use moisturizer.

Moisturize regularly Trap moisture in your skin by slathering on a moisturizer, which forms a seal over your skin and prevents water loss. Ideally, your moisturizer should contain SPF15 or higher. Avoid any products with artificial colours, fragrances, and preservatives (parfum, parabens, and sodium lauryl sulphate).

Ears

Unlike eye tests, there is no need to have routine hearing tests unless you think you have a particular problem. However, if your family complains that you are not answering them, or that you have the TV on too loud, you need to get your ears checked.

EAR MAINTENANCE

Like eyes, our ears are largely self-maintaining, but you may sometimes have an occasional problem:

Deafness from ear wax The commonest cause of deafness is earwax, which affects one in three people over the age of 50. Ear wax is made up of dead cells and a substance called cerumen produced by the gland in the lining of the ear canal. Don't be tempted to use cotton buds to try to remove the wax, as this causes irritation to the delicate lining of the ear canal, and results in further inflammation and more wax production. A five-day course of eardrops, available from pharmacies, will soften the wax and deal with the problem, but if the wax is still impacted see your doctor to ask about syringing.

Eyes

Good eyesight is crucial to our quality of life, yet many of us take it for granted. In fact, 85 per cent of what we learn is via the eyes and brain, so you should look after your eyes properly.

Eye care

Our eyes do most of their own minor maintenance work, but there are important precautions we should take to ensure good eyesight:

Attend for regular eye tests Have regular eye tests, even if you think that your vision is fine. Book an eye test every couple of years, and more often if you have eye problems (see pp189–91).

Don't smoke Tobacco smoke contains 4,000 chemicals, many of them toxic to the eyes. Smoking can cause or worsen several eye conditions, including cataracts (see p190) and age-related macular degeneration (see p191).

Protect your eyes from the sun Ultraviolet light can cause cataracts (see p190), corneal damage, and macular degeneration (see p191), one of the commonest causes of blindness in the west. Wear a wide-brimmed hat to reduce UV rays by 50 per cent and choose your sunglasses carefully. Price is no guarantee of quality – if they don't carry a label confirming that they conform to UV safety standards, don't buy them.

Eat healthily Vitamins A, C, and E are all important for healthy eyes, and a diet rich in the antioxidants lutein and zeaxanthin – found in dark-coloured fruits and vegetables – may help safeguard your vision (see p55).

Teeth, gums, and mouth

Poor dental hygiene will leave you with discoloured teeth and bad breath, which is hardly likely to make you feel your best. However, with a little bit of effort you should be able to enjoy healthy teeth well into old age.

GOOD ORAL HYGIENE

There are several simple, but vital, routines to follow if you want healthy teeth, gums, and mouth:

Attend for regular check-ups Unless they suggest otherwise, most dentists recommend check-ups every six months and a regular visit to the hygienist.

Brush your teeth well with a pea-sized blob of toothpaste containing fluoride. Brush your teeth with short, gentle strokes at least twice a day after meals for 2 to 3 minutes. You should replace your toothbrush every three months or so with a toothbrush that has soft, rounded bristles; hard bristles can hurt or damage your gums.

Floss regularly Use a piece of floss about 40cm (16in) long and wind it round the middle finger of each hand. Grip the floss between your thumb and forefinger and gently place the floss between each tooth in turn, curving it

"Gum disease may be linked to other diseases in the body, so if it persists you should speak to your doctor about it."

around the tooth and bringing it up the side of the tooth away from the gum. Repeat the process twice on each side of every tooth.

Watch your diet Sugar causes the bacteria that live naturally in your mouth to produce acid, which attacks tooth enamel and causes dental decay. Cut down on sugar in your diet and, if you have to give yourself a sweet treat, eat it in one go to reduce the number of times your teeth are under attack. Chewing sugar-free gum after meals will stimulate saliva production and will help neutralize the acid.

Don't smoke Smokers are at increased risk of stained teeth and gum disease (which results in the loosening, and then loss, of teeth).

Hands and feet

Don't forget your hands and feet in your healthcare regime – apart from your face, they are usually the most frequently exposed parts of your body, and can be a real giveaway to your age and health.

HAND AND FOOT CARE

Adopt a regular routine to care for your hands and feet:

Use a good moisturizer or barrier cream on your hands, especially in winter or after washing up. You may also want to moisturize your feet in summer to prevent the skin around your heels becoming too dry.

Remove hard skin around the soles of your feet to keep them smooth. Use a pumice stone or special foot file after a bath to remove the softened skin.

Check your nails for changes in your health. Look out for spoon-shaped nails called koilonychias (a sign of low iron levels), or nails that lift off and flake, which can be linked to thyroid disease (see p326), psoriasis (see p356), or due to a fungal infection. A horizontal ridge in the nail is often caused by a past illness: normal healthy nails grow at about 0.1mm a day, but they stop growing when we are seriously ill.

Always cut your toenails straight across and don't be tempted to shape them as you would your fingernails, since this can leave you prone to ingrowing toenails.

RESTORATIVE FOOT MASSAGE

Our feet are amazing structures, yet we rarely think about them until something goes wrong. Reduce the likelihood of problems by wearing well-fitting shoes (feet get wider as we age, so get them re-measured from time to time), and if you love high heels, wear them only for special occasions – your feet will thank you! This quick 5-minute foot massage is wonderfully relaxing, and can help to relieve mild aches and pains.

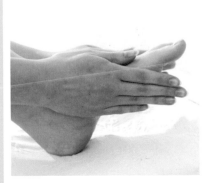

Step 1
Apply a little massage oil to one foot and use both hands to slowly and firmly stroke from toes to ankle 3–4 times.

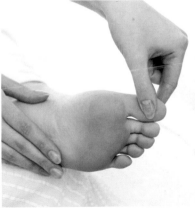

Step 2
Gently circle the ankle one way and then the other 3–4 times, then rotate and massage each toe in turn.

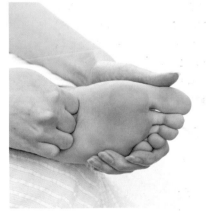

Step 3
Knead the sole of the foot with your knuckles, focusing on any tender areas, then repeat Step 1 to finish.

Knowing the signs

Dr Sarah Jarvis MA BM BCH DRCOG FRCGP

Introduction

Your body is a miraculous, highly tuned collection of muscles, nerves, blood vessels and organs, connected by an intricate network of pathways which carry messages from one part to another. It is exquisitely adapted to your needs – but it is constantly exposed to the stresses and strains of daily life, and all too often the delicate balance is disrupted. Because some of our organs have an impact on the functioning of other, often distant parts of your body, a problem in one area can produce symptoms in an unconnected part.

In this section, we give you some pointers about what symptoms in any one part of your body might mean. Sometimes the connection is clear – a burning pain in your stomach, made worse by eating, is likely to be related to your stomach. But often, the signals your body sends out don't make sense if you're not versed in the mysteries of medical science. For instance:

- Swollen ankles could mean your heart isn't pumping properly (in which case you may also find that you are breathless unless you sleep propped up on several pillows)
- Pitting of your nails could mean that you're suffering from a condition associated with skin problems
- If your doctor wants to exclude a clot on your lung, she will check you out for a painful red calf, which could be the underlying cause
- A butterfly rash on your skin could mean that you have an autoimmune condition (in which your body's defence systems turn on your own body) which can make you prone to heart and kidney problems.

IF YOU HAVE SKIN PROBLEMS

Other symptoms are found in widespread parts of the body. The skin is a particularly good example because it is often an excellent barometer of what is going on in the rest of your body. For instance:

- Dull, lifeless skin can be an indication of being run down (see Chapter 3, Staying well, pp48–69)
- Dry skin can be an indication of an underlying thyroid hormone problem

- Developing acne again later in life have can be a symptom of polycystic ovary syndrome (see p95)
- Lemon yellow tinge to the skin can be a pointer to kidney disease
- Yellow skin (and yellowing of the whites of the eyes) can be a sign of liver damage or inflammation
- Excessive bruising can suggest a problem with the blood clotting system
- Finding very mild signs of the skin condition psoriasis can indicate joint disease in some cases
- Blotchy purple bruises which don't blanche when you press on them can be a sign of meningitis or blood poisoning – get help urgently!

IF YOUR LYMPH NODES ARE SWOLLEN

The lymphatic system runs throughout your body in a complex series of interconnecting channels, which meet at junctions. Here, the lymph cells created by your body to fight off infection are stored, and congregate if there is a threat such as an infection. Sometimes a single lymph node or group of nodes becomes enlarged because of a local infection – such as tonsillitis, which can cause swollen glands in your neck. But in other conditions large numbers of lymph nodes spread all over your body can become swollen.

Many apparently innocuous signs could mean that there is a more serious underlying condition, but on the other hand, many signs that may, at first sight, seem worrying can have an innocent cause which requires nothing more than time for a full recovery.

SYMPTOM GUIDES

The symptom guides on the following pages will give you a general idea of what signs and symptoms in one part of your body may mean, and they will also point you to the relevant sections where you can find out more. These guides are, however, not a replacement for medical advice and if you are at all worried or concerned about anything then you should see or call your doctor who will be able to advise you.

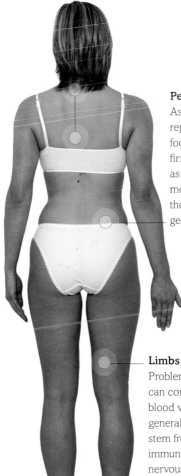

Head and face
This section covers not only pains in your head, neck and face, but conditions affecting your balance. It also offers a brief pointer to what might be at the root of changes in mood

Neck and back
The spine, stretching from the neck to the coccyx, is held in place by innumerable joints, muscles and pieces of connective tissue

Upper chest
The upper chest includes some of your most crucial organs – the lungs and heart, essential for life; and the breasts, which play such a fundamental part in marking us out as women

Pelvis
As the site of the female reproductive organs, the focus in this section is firmly on the woman. But as you can find out in the more detailed sections, there may be a more general underlying cause

Abdomen to pelvis
Most of the headings in this section relate to the digestive system. But some women-only problems can also cause abdominal symptoms

Limbs
Problems in an individual limb can come from joints, muscles, blood vessels or nerves. More generalized limb problems can stem from conditions of the immune system or the central nervous system

Head and face

You may have experienced a headache, but could you tell the difference between migraine and meningitis? The brain has a widespread impact on your body. But some parts of the nervous system can cause local symptoms affecting your eyes or ears.

Head

Headaches:
- Moderate pain worsening as the day progresses: p180
- Nausea, dislike of bright lights with severe throbbing pain: see migraine p182
- With rash, nausea, fever, and dislike of bright lights: exclude meningitis p181
- Worse on waking, nausea, impaired vision/balance: exclude brain tumours p181

Unusual changes in mood:
- With changes in menstrual pattern and libido: see menopause pp136–41
- With undue worry or panic, fatigue: see generalized anxiety disorder p204, panic disorder p205; if related to social situations: see social anxiety disorder p206
- With compulsions/obsessions: see obsessive-compulsive disorder p207
- With persistent sadness, weight loss/gain: see depression pp210–11; if seasonal: see SAD p213
- With emotional numbness, irritability, insomnia: see post-traumatic stress disorder pp208–9
- With racing thoughts, poor concentration, distractability, inflated self-esteem: see bipolar disorder p212
- During pregnancy: see perinatal depression p214
- Soon after giving birth: see postnatal depression p215
- Fear of losing or gaining weight: see anorexia nervosa p216, bulimia nervosa p217
- Personality disorders: see pp218–19
- Related to substance abuse, alcohol, and prescription drugs: see addictions pp220–1
- Lack of desire for sex: see hypoactive sexual desire disorder p222
- Lack of arousal during sex: see female arousal disorder p222, female orgasmic disorder p223
- With declining memory: exclude Alzheimer's disease pp184–5

Dizziness:
- Lightheaded, sweaty and pale: see dizzy spells and falls p192
- Sudden onset, nausea, vomiting: see vertigo/Ménière's disease p192
- With nausea, vomiting, impaired vision: see vestibular neuritis, p193, labyrinthitis p193
- Partial or total loss of consciousness with jerking or twitching limbs, abnormal sensations, detachment from reality: see epilepsy pp194–5

Skin

Rash:
- Intermittent flushed hot skin, associated with sweating: see menopause pp136–41
- Dark irregular patches: see melasma p361
- In butterfly pattern across nose and cheeks: see lupus p269

Lips:
- Tingling, blisters: see cold sores p367

Spots:
- With greasy skin and blackheads: see acne vulgaris pp362–4
- With redness and thread veins: see rosacea p364
Sore with blisters and honey-coloured crusts: see impetigo p367

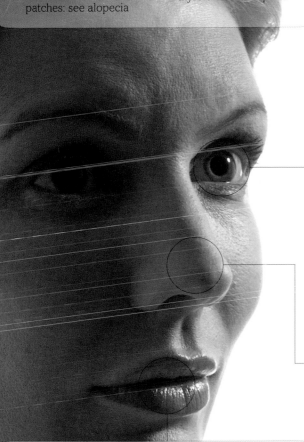

Hair

Hair loss:
- Thinning most at temples: see female pattern baldness p371
- Small round bald patches: see alopecia areata p370
- Major hairloss: see telogen effluvium p369
- Generally thinned hair with weight gain: see thyroid disorders p326

Eyes

Painful eyes:
- With redness, discharge, itching: see conjunctivitis p190
- With reduced vision, aversion to light: see acute glaucoma p191
- Dry, with dry mouth: see Sjögren's syndrome p271

Yellow eyes:
- See liver disorders pp296–9, gallstones pp294–5

Low vision:
- Long- or short-sighted: see vision disorders p189; macular degeneration p191
- Aversion to light, pain in the eyes: see glaucoma p191; with tingling in the face, numbness in limbs, unsteadiness: exclude multiple sclerosis p198

Blurred vision:
- With yellow or reddish-tinged vision, distortion: see cataracts p190

Ears, nose, and throat

Earache:
- With itchiness, pus: see otitis externa p186
- Sudden ache, reduced hearing: see otitis media p187
- Recurrent pain: see glue ear p187
- Ringing or buzzing noises: see earache p188, tinnitus p188
- Hearing loss: see p188

Blocked nose:
- With pain over forehead/cheekbones: see sinusitis p235

Neck swelling:
- Moves with swallowing: see thyroid disorders p326, goitre p329, Grave's disease p329

Sore throat:
- With sneezing and cough: see cold p232
- With fever: see flu p232
- With hoarse voice: see laryngitis p236
- With a runny nose and fever: see pharyngitis p237
- Chronic hoarseness: see vocal cord nodules p237

Mouth

Dry mouth:
- Intense thirst, frequent urination, tiredness, blurry vision: see Type 1 diabetes pp320–1
- With dry eyes: see Sjögren's syndrome p271

Difficulty swallowing:
- With chest pain: see oesophageal disorders p293

Slurred speech:
- With facial drooping, weakness, tingling in limbs, clumsiness, impaired vision: see stroke p196

Tongue
- Inflamed: see glossitis p288
- Irregular patches, smooth, red: geographical tongue p288; if black and "hairy": see tongue disorders p288
- White patches, sore, inflamed: see oral thrush p288

Upper chest

As you'll discover in Chapter 7 (Heart and circulation), women are not immune from heart disease. The chest also houses the lungs, which can be affected by long-term conditions (such as asthma) and acute ones (such as pneumonia). The heart and lungs are housed in the ribcage, with bones, joints, and muscles which can also cause symptoms.

Chest

Sharp chest pain:
- Worse on breathing with coughing up of blood and shortness of breath: see pulmonary embolism pp252–3

Central chest pain:
- With belching, acidic taste in mouth, and often related to eating: see gastro-oesophageal reflux pp290–1
- With difficulty swallowing: see oesophageal disorders p293
- Travelling to neck, jaw or left arm, brought on by cold temperature, exercise or stress and relieved by rest: see angina p164
- Heavy or squeezing, may radiate to arms, jaw, neck, back, or stomach, with sweating and nausea; shortness of breath; increasing tiredness, feeling dizzy, light-headed: exclude heart attack pp165, 166
- With breathlessness, dizzy spells, swollen ankles: see valvular heart disease p174

Palpitations:
- Heart beating too fast, too slowly, or irregularly: see palpitations, p167

Cough:
- With nasal congestion and fever: see bronchitis, p232
- Persistent cough: see chronic cough p233
- With blood in phlegm, with fever and malaise: see pneumonia p234
  And wheeze: see asthma p238
- Longstanding with gradually increasing breathlessness: see COPD p240; also with rapid weight loss, exclude lung cancer p242

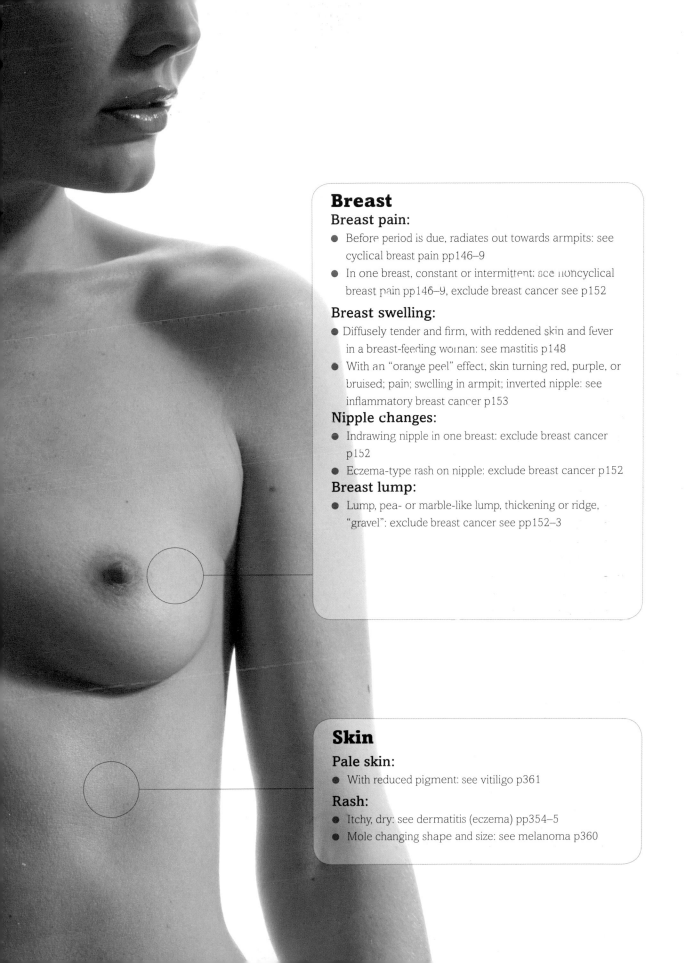

Breast

Breast pain:

- Before period is due, radiates out towards armpits: see cyclical breast pain pp146–9
- In one breast, constant or intermittent: see noncyclical breast pain pp146–9, exclude breast cancer see p152

Breast swelling:

- Diffusely tender and firm, with reddened skin and fever in a breast-feeding woman: see mastitis p148
- With an "orange peel" effect, skin turning red, purple, or bruised; pain; swelling in armpit; inverted nipple: see inflammatory breast cancer p153

Nipple changes:

- Indrawing nipple in one breast: exclude breast cancer p152
- Eczema-type rash on nipple: exclude breast cancer p152

Breast lump:

- Lump, pea- or marble-like lump, thickening or ridge, "gravel": exclude breast cancer see pp152–3

Skin

Pale skin:

- With reduced pigment: see vitiligo p361

Rash:

- Itchy, dry: see dermatitis (eczema) pp354–5
- Mole changing shape and size: see melanoma p360

Abdomen to pelvis

Many people refer to their "stomach" when what they're talking about is their abdomen. The stomach actually occupies only a small portion of your abdominal cavity. Most of the rest is taken up with your large and small bowel, with your liver at the top right hand side.

Stomach

Diarrhoea:

- Chronic: see diarrhoea p302
- With abdominal pain and fever: see gastroenteritis p300
- With blood and mucus: see inflammatory bowel disease p310
- Alternating with constipation, rectal bleeding, and weight loss: exclude colorectal cancer pp307–9

Constipation:

- Chronic: see constipation p303, diverticular disease p312
- Recent, with cramping abdominal pain: see diverticular disease p312, exclude colorectal cancer pp307–9
- With pain and bleeding when moving bowels: see haemorrhoids p314
- Tearing of opening of bowels, rectal bleeding, itching around the anus: see anal fissure p315
- With unexplained weight gain: see underactive thyroid p327; plus a loss of appetite, weight loss, muscle spasms, minor depression: see parathyroid gland disorders p330

Abdominal pain in pregnancy

- To one side, and less than 3 months pregnant: see ectopic pregnancy p125
- More than 3 months pregnant: see abruption p128
- With lots of morning sickness, sleeplessness, rapidly gaining weight in first trimester: see multiple births p131
- With high blood pressure, swollen feet, headaches, occasional nausea, vomiting: see pre-eclampsia p128
- Regular contractions. breaking of waters before week 37: see premature delivery p129
- Vaginal bleeding, cramping pains in lower abdomen, nausea/sore breasts: see miscarriage p124
- Vaginal bleeding, shoulder pain: see ectopic pregnancy p125

Upper abdomen

Upper abdominal pain:

- Nausea, bloating, belching, heartburn: see indigestion and ulcers p292
- On the right side, travelling to the right upper back, pale stools, nausea, yellowing eyes and skin: see gallstones p294
- Aches and pains around liver, mild fever, tiredness, nausea: see hepatitis B p118; with pale stools and dark urine: see hepatitis p296
- Weight loss, fever, jaundice: see alcoholic liver disease p297
- Easy bruising, jaundice, mild confusion, swollen abdomen: see cirrhosis pp298–9
- With jaundice, difficulty swallowing: exclude oesophageal cancer p306

Lower abdomen

Lower abdominal pain:

- Before menstruation: see PMS pp92–3
- Severe on one side, pressure on rectum: see ovarian cyst p94, exclude urinary tract cancer p348
- Fever, offensive vaginal discharge, severe pain: see pelvic inflammatory disease p98
- With swelling in the groin: see hernia p291
- In waves with diarrhoea: see gastroenteritis p300
- Loose, bulky greasy faeces, bloating, itchy rash: see coeliac disease p301
- Associated with alternating diarrhoea and constipation, and relieved by passing wind: see irritable bowel syndrome pp304–5
- Irregular periods, headaches, blurry vision: see pituitary gland disorders p330
- Weight gain around the abdomen, reddening in the face, increased hairiness: see adrenal gland disorders p331
- With urinary frequency: see urinary incontinence p339
- With painful urination: see urinary tract infection pp336–7, bladder pain syndrome pp343–5
- Radiating to pain in the back: see kidney stones pp346–7

Pelvis, genitals, and bladder

Only women can have children, and only women have the reproductive organs which give them that ability. From puberty, through the reproductive years to the menopause, these reproductive organs go through constant change every month.

Genitals

Vaginal discharge:

- Premenopause and postmenopause: increasingly heavy periods, and between periods and after sex, heavy, foul smelling discharge: see cervical dysplasia p106 (exclude cancer of the uterus p104)
- Unpleasant, often fishy: see vaginitis p108
- "Cottage cheese" appearance, vaginal/vulval irritation: see vaginal thrush p109
- Bloodstained, rectal pain, postcoital bleeding: exclude cancer of the vagina p111
- With burning feeling in vagina and urethra, anal irritation, bleeding in between periods: see gonorrhoea p114
- With lower abdomen pain, burning during urination: see chlamydia p115
- Green/yellowish, itchy or sore, and smells: see trichomoniasis p119

Painful vagina:

- During sex: see dyspareunia p109; with unusual bleeding and heavy, watery discharge: exclude cervical cancer p107
- With discharge: see vaginitis p108 and vulvitis p113
- Burning pain: see vulvodynia p112
- With ulcers: see genital herpes p116

Vaginal bleeding:

- Heavy periods: see menorrhagia p91
- Absent periods: see amenorrhoea p90
- Irregular: see oligomenorrhoea p90
- Irregular with hot flushes: see menopause pp136–41
- With pain: see dysmenorrhoea p91
- Irregular, noticeable facial hair and oily skin: see polycystic ovary syndrome p95
- With bleeding between periods: see endometrial polyps p100
- Heavy periods, pelvic pressure, pain, frequent urination, constipation: see fibroids p99
- With constipation, infertility: see endometriosis p101, endometrial hyperplasia p103
- With vaginal discharge, lower abdominal pain, fever: see endometritis p102
- Between periods, piercing pelvic pain: see adenomyosis p102
- Ranging from spotting to heavy bleeding, no abdominal pain, during pregnancy: see placenta praevia p130

Lumps around the vagina:

- Heaviness, protruding into the vagina: see uterine prolapse p105
- Spasms, fear of penetration, pain, loss of desire: see vaginismus p110
- With pain and swelling: see Bartholin's gland cyst p113
- With roughened surface: see genital warts p117

Skin

Rash:
- With painless sores on vulva, anus, tongue or lips: see syphilis p115

Swollen nodes:
- Blisters, headaches, fever, burning sensation when urinating: see genital herpes p116

Bladder

Painful urination:
- With increased frequency of urination: see urinary tract infection p336
- With fever and backache: see pyelonephritis p338
- With increased frequency, lower abdominal pain, blood in urine: see bladder pain syndrome pp343–5
- Passing water very frequently, intense thirst, blurry vision, lack of energy: see diabetes I p321; with recurrent skin infections: see diabetes II p322; during pregnancy: see gestational diabetes p127
- Blood in urine, frequent urination and urgency; also pain in side that won't go away: exclude urinary tract cancer pp348–9

Change in urination:
- Involuntary leakage of urine: see stress incontinence pp339–42
- Frequent, sudden urge to pass urine: see urge incontinence pp339–42

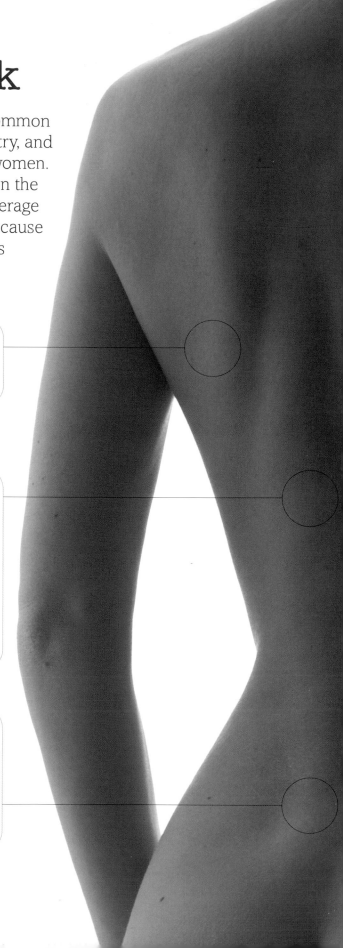

Neck and back

Low back pain is the single most common cause of time off work in this country, and neck pain is also very common in women. Not only the physical daily strains on the body, but also the stresses of the average woman's constant juggling act, can cause symptoms in the muscles and bones of the back.

Shoulder

- Pain, tenderness, loss of range of movement in joint: see painful shoulder p282

Upper back

Back pain:

- Central and associated with loss of height: see osteoporosis pp260–1

Mid back pain:

- On one side, with fever over 38°C (100°F): see pyelonephritis p338
- Pain in waves, travelling to the groin: see kidney stones pp346–7

Lower back

Lower back pain:

- Before menstruation: see PMS p92
- Travelling to buttock or thigh: see back and neck pain pp272–5
- Gradual or sudden pain, with stiffness, often recurrent: see mechanical low back pain p272

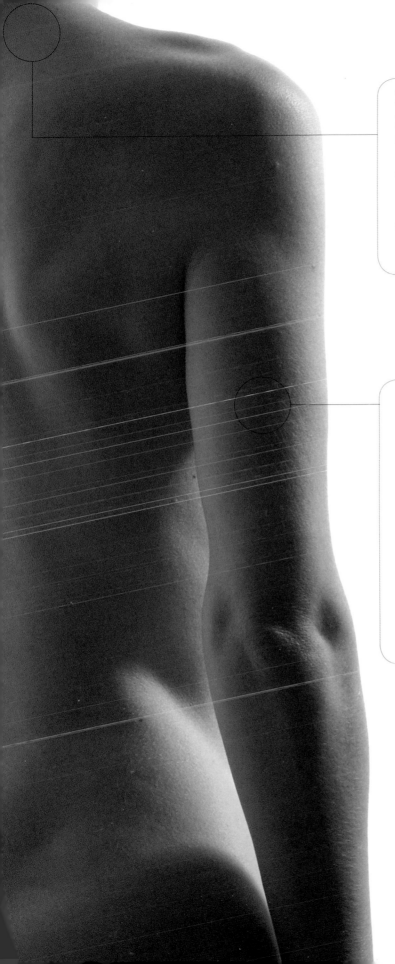

Neck

Neck pain:

- Travelling into shoulders and arms: see cervical spondylosis p272
- Associated with generalized muscle pains, swollen joints, tingling, headaches: see fibromyalgia pp276–7
- Pain, stiffness, tenderness, swelling: see repetitive strain injury p280

Skin

Rash:

- Itchy, dry; with scaling and blistering: see dermatitis pp354–5
- Scaly, raised, salmon-pink colour: see psoriasis pp356–7
- Non-healing, scaly and rough: see squamous cell carcinoma p359; with weeping scabs: see basal cell carcinoma p359
- With reduced pigment: see vitiligo p361
- Easy, spontaneous bruising, prolonged/ major bleeding: see bleeding disorders p250

Limbs

The joints and muscles of the limbs are vulnerable to sprains, strains and wear and tear. Some symptoms, however, can point to an underlying problem with the heart or circulatory system, which may need urgent medical attention.

Hands

- Pain, aching, numbness, and tingling in the hands: see carpal tunnel syndrome p283
- **Tremors:**
- Often on the same side initially, stiff limbs, slow movements: exclude Parkinson's disease p197

Joints

Joint pain:

- Painful joints, but no redness, getting gradually worse: see osteoarthritis p263
- Pain and swelling, morning stiffness: see rheumatoid arthritis p266
- Several painful hot red joints after recent infection: see reactive arthritis p267
  With swelling in big toe joint: see bunion p265
- Pain moves from joint to joint, weakness, persistent sore throat, chills: see chronic fatigue syndrome pp278–9
- With dislike of heat, thinning of hair, diarrhoea: see overactive thyroid p328

Skin

Pale skin:

- Pale skin, easy bruising, enlarged lymph glands in neck/groin: anaemia pp248–9, exclude blood cancers pp254–5

Rash:

- With reduced pigment: see vitiligo p361
- Multiple purple-coloured, like bruises, not blanching with pressure: exclude meningitis p181, clotting disorders pp250–1
- Small, yellow pimples with pus, itching: see folliculitis p366

Arms

Arm pain:

- With shoulder pain and stiffness and restricted movement: see painful shoulder p282
- Around elbow, pain and bony lump on joint: see tennis elbow p281, golfer's elbow p281
- Associated with central, heavy chest pain: see heart attack pp 165, 166
- Shooting pain in arm: see cervical spondylosis p272
- Worse after repetitive movements: see repetitive strain injury p280
- With weakness, numbness, tingling, slurred speech, impaired vision: see stroke p196

Legs

- Shooting pain in leg going to ankle: see back and neck pain pp272–5
- Aching legs with swollen veins: see varicose veins p175
- Swollen ankles with breathlessness: see heart failure p166
- Hot, red, swollen calf, pain, feeling of cramp: see deep vein thrombosis p252
- Weakness and clumsiness in the legs, with numbness or tingling: see multiple sclerosis p198
- Stiffness in the legs, with slurred speech, muscle twitching: exclude motor neurone disease p199

Feet

Toes:

- Pain, numbness, changes in skin colour: see Raynaud's phenomenon p270

Nails:

- Brittle, tingling in toes/fingers, swollen ankles: see blood deficiency problems pp248–9

Warts:

- With black spots, painful: see warts p366

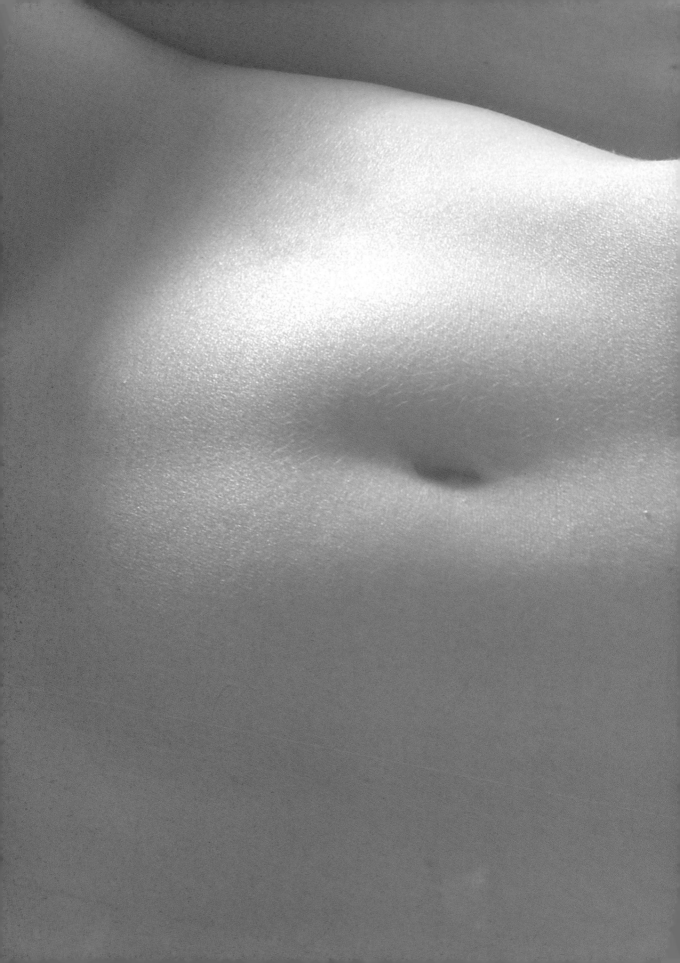

Reproductive system

Dr Melanie Tipples MRCOG FRCSEd

Reproductive system

The central role of your reproductive system is carried out by the ovaries. Even before you are born, your ovaries contain hundreds of thousands of eggs that will be released – usually one a month throughout your reproductive years – ready to be fertilized by male sperm. Unfertilized eggs are shed with the lining of the uterus during menstruation. This process is controlled by a finely balanced hormonal system, which starts to function at puberty and continues for about 40 years until your fertile phase ends at the menopause.

THE FEMALE REPRODUCTIVE SYSTEM

These diagrams show the main female reproductive organs, which are positioned low down in your abdomen, between your pelvic (hip) bones. The uterus (womb) lies just above the bladder and in front of the rectum. On either side of the uterus are the egg-bearing glands, or ovaries, which also produce the female sex hormones. Close to each ovary is a fallopian tube, a duct that carries eggs to the uterus.

The muscular walls of the uterus are capable of expanding dramatically during pregnancy to hold a developing baby. In childbirth, the cervix (the neck of the uterus) and the vagina both open out to allow the baby to pass through into the world.

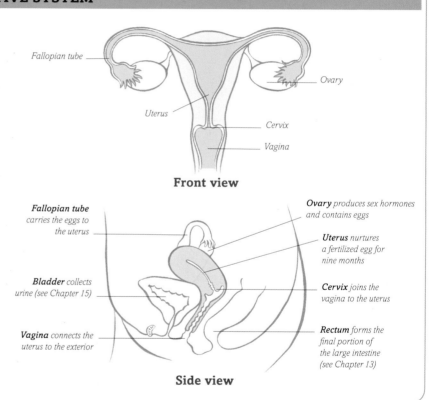

Front view

Fallopian tube

Ovary

Uterus

Cervix

Vagina

Side view

Fallopian tube carries the eggs to the uterus

Bladder collects urine (see Chapter 15)

Vagina connects the uterus to the exterior

Ovary produces sex hormones and contains eggs

Uterus nurtures a fertilized egg for nine months

Cervix joins the vagina to the uterus

Rectum forms the final portion of the large intestine (see Chapter 13)

Most of your reproductive organs are hidden deep within your pelvis. The visible parts of the system at the entrance to the vagina are known together as the vulva. These are the clitoris and the soft flaps of skin called the labia. The vagina is a flattened tube that connects with the cervix, or neck of the uterus. The uterus is a thick-walled chamber where a developing baby is nurtured during the nine months of pregnancy. A pair of ovaries (the female sex glands) lie to either side of the uterus. The fallopian tubes, which open at one end into the uterus, reach out towards the ovaries with finger-like projections. These "fingers" gather up the eggs as they are released from the ovaries (see opposite) and guide them into the tube.

Jointly, the ovaries contain about 400,000 eggs, one or more of which may be released every month. The ovaries also make the female sex hormones – oestrogen and progesterone – which are vital for sexual development, the menstrual cycle, and fertility.

YOUR MENSTRUAL CYCLE

Each month a woman's body goes through a cycle in preparation for conception and pregnancy. In the ovary an egg ripens inside a fluid-filled sac called a follicle (see right). At the same time, the lining of the uterus starts to thicken. When the fully mature egg is released from the ovary it is delivered into the fallopian tube. If it meets a male sperm in the fallopian tube, fertilization may take place. The egg takes several days to complete its journey to the uterus. If it is fertilized it may embed in the thickened lining of the uterus to start a pregnancy. If the egg is not fertilized, both it and the lining of the uterus are shed in menstrual bleeding. The cycle continues as another egg comes to maturity in the ovary.

HOW THE HORMONES ARE INVOLVED

As we have seen, the female sex hormones oestrogen and progesterone are secreted by the ovaries. The time this takes place and how much is secreted are controlled by the follicle-stimulating hormone (FSH) and the luteinizing hormone (LH), which are produced by the pituitary gland in the brain. Release of these hormones occurs in peaks and troughs during your menstrual cycle, with oestrogen and LH reaching highs just before you ovulate.

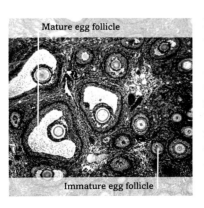

Mature egg follicle

Immature egg follicle

Developing egg follicles
Eggs within the ovary are in various stages of development, as seen in this magnified image. Usually only one egg matures and is released during each monthly cycle of ovulation.

SECTION THROUGH AN OVARY

In each of your ovaries there are many thousands of immature eggs in their follicles; other eggs are just beginning to ripen, while some are reaching full maturity. When ovulation occurs, the egg-follicle ruptures to release the mature egg. The empty follicle produces the hormone progesterone, which triggers thickening of the lining of the uterus.

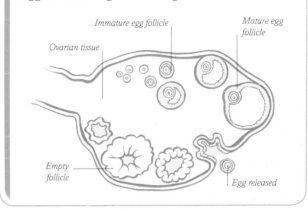

Immature egg follicle

Mature egg follicle

Ovarian tissue

Empty follicle

Egg released

LIFE AFTER CHILDBEARING

In the past, because of poorer health and nutrition – and because many women were exhausted after spending most of their fertile lives either pregnant or breastfeeding – the end of the childbearing years was often closely followed by the end of life. These days, fortunately, the situation is very different and women can expect to live upwards of 30 years after the menopause. For some women, the lack of oestrogen can have profound effects on wellbeing, both mental and physical. On the downside, at this time some of us may have "empty nest" syndrome when children leave home, problems with a partner, and frail elderly parents to care for. However, this can be a joyful time; you've got your life back after years of nurturing a family, accidental pregnancy is no longer a worry, and the stresses of your younger years have blown away.

> "Women can now expect to live upwards of 30 years after the menopause."

Menstrual problems

Menstruation is a highly complex cycle governed by your hormones. Your menstrual cycle is unique: what is regular for you might be abnormal for someone else, just as light or heavy periods vary from woman to woman. Fortunately, most menstrual problems are minor and easily treatable.

Irregular periods (oligomenorrhoea)

Your first periods are likely to be unpredictable in timing and length. After a year or so, most women settle into a regular cycle, but erratic periods often become the norm again near the menopause.

WHAT IS IT?

Many women have a menstrual cycle that varies from the 28-day average. A cycle that is routinely shorter or longer is not seen as a problem. However, irregularity may be caused by a hormone imbalance such as polycystic ovary syndrome (see p95).

WHAT NEXT?

If irregularities persist, or if you develop other problems, consult your doctor.

MY TREATMENT OPTIONS

You may be prescribed an oral contraceptive, or if you are approaching the menopause, you may be offered hormone replacement therapy (HRT).

HOW CAN I HELP MYSELF?

For two or three months, note down the dates of your periods, to see if irregularity is normal for you.

HAVE I GOT THE SYMPTOMS?

Your menstrual cycle will be considered irregular if you experience:
- Periods occurring more frequently, for example, twice monthly
- Periods occurring without there being any regular pattern.

See your doctor if you are concerned by any irregularities in your menstrual cycle, or if your periods are very frequent or very infrequent.

Absence of periods (amenorrhoea)

The most common cause of absent periods is pregnancy. Amenorrhoea can also be a side effect of illness or stress, over-exercising, or extreme weight loss.

WHAT IS IT?

Amenorrhoea is lack of periods in women who normally menstruate.

WHAT NEXT?

Once pregnancy or menopause have been ruled out, your doctor may check for hormonal disorders. You may have a blood test and an abdominal (with a full bladder) ultrasound scan, or a transvaginal (via the vagina) scan, in which case you will be asked to empty your bladder first.

MY TREATMENT OPTIONS

You may be given hormonal treatment to restart your periods; ask about potential side effects.

HOW CAN I HELP MYSELF?

Keep a check on your lifestyle. Avoid excessive exercise or dieting.

HAVE I GOT THE SYMPTOMS?

You should talk to a doctor if:
- You haven't started having periods by the age of 16
- You have missed 3 periods.

Heavy periods (menorrhagia)

Some women have heavier menstrual flows than others; it isn't necessarily a problem. However, leakage may be annoying and loss of iron through excessive bleeding can cause anaemia (see pp248–9).

WHAT IS IT?

Heavy periods may be due to disorders of the uterus (see pp98–9) or hormonal imbalances, but the cause is not always obvious.

WHAT NEXT?

Consult your doctor. He or she will examine you and may do blood tests to measure your iron and hormone levels. Your doctor may also take a sample of tissue from your uterus, using a speculum placed in your vagina. Other tests may include an abdominal or a transvaginal (through the vagina) ultrasound scan.

MY TREATMENT OPTIONS

Treatments could include the following. Ask your doctor to explain any possible side effects.
- Progesterone-coated IUD (see p132)
- Oral contraceptive pill (see p134)
- Iron medication (for anaemia)
- Tranexamic acid or anti-inflammatory tablets
- Laser surgery (for endometriosis, see p101)
- Surgery (for fibroids, see p99).

HAVE I GOT THE SYMPTOMS?

Heavy flow (with or without pain) is usually defined by one or more of the following:
- Bleeding that lasts for seven days or more
- Bleeding that cannot be controlled by sanitary towels or tampons
- Large blood clots being passed.

See your doctor if your flow fits these descriptions.

HOW CAN I HELP MYSELF?

If you are anaemic, try to eat plenty of iron-rich foods. These include lean meat, liver, green leafy vegetables, whole grains, and nuts.

Painful periods (dysmenorrhoea)

There are two types of painful periods: primary dysmenorrhoea, which occurs once ovulation is established; and secondary dysmenorrhoea, which affects women who have not had period pain before.

WHAT IS IT?

Primary dysmenorrhoea is linked to a rise of natural chemicals in the body at ovulation. Secondary dysmenorrhoea is usually a sign of an underlying disorder.

WHAT NEXT?

If you develop painful periods, see your doctor to make sure you have no reproductive disorder. You may have an internal examination, cervical swabs taken, and possibly an ultrasound scan. In addition, you may have an examination by laparoscopy (see p98).

MY TREATMENT OPTIONS

Drug treatment often relieves the pain. Ask your doctor about any possible side effects. He or she may suggest the following:
- Anti-inflammatory drugs such as ibuprofen (which block the action of the pain-causing chemical prostaglandin)
- Antispasmodic drugs
- Combined oral contraceptive.

HAVE I GOT THE SYMPTOMS?

Pain begins just before or just after bleeding starts and may be:
- Wave-like cramps in the lower abdomen
- Aches in the lower back and in the legs
- A dragging sensation in the pelvic area.

See your doctor if period pains become too uncomfortable.

HOW CAN I HELP MYSELF?

Taking over-the-counter painkillers may be enough. If not, try placing a covered hot-water bottle on your tummy for extra relief.

Premenstrual syndrome

In the week or so before their period starts, many women experience a collection of uncomfortable symptoms known as premenstrual syndrome. Bloating, migraine, and moodiness are just a few of the things that can make life miserable. But there are various ways in which you can ease the symptoms.

WHAT IS IT?

The symptoms of premenstrual syndrome (PMS) – once known as premenstrual tension (PMT) – are thought to be caused by hormonal changes just before menstruation. Approximately 90 percent of women experience some symptoms of PMS every month. These symptoms start to disappear with the onset of a period.

A more severe version of PMS, called premenstrual dysphoric disorder (PMDD, see opposite), can seriously impair a woman's ability to function normally. Some types of depression are also affected by PMS. If you suffer from depression (see pp210-11) most days of the month, you may find that you feel worse in the run-up to your period.

WHAT NEXT?

If PMS is affecting your lifestyle, talk to your doctor. You may be asked to make a symptom chart over several menstrual cycles in order for your doctor to confirm the diagnosis.

MY TREATMENT OPTIONS

The past 15 years have seen some developments in treating PMS but success isn't always consistent.

HAVE I GOT THE SYMPTOMS?

Over 150 symptoms of PMS have been identified. They may vary from month to month, but for a diagnosis, you must have at least one week every month without symptoms. These include:

- Breast tenderness or lumpiness
- Feeling bloated
- Feeling moody or irritable
- Depression and/or anxiety
- Tiredness
- Trouble concentrating
- Headaches or migraine, if you're a sufferer
- Back and muscle stiffness
- Disrupted sleep
- Food cravings
- Reduced libido.

Some women may also suffer from nausea, vomiting, cold sweats, hot flushes, and dizziness. **See your doctor** if you have any of these symptoms and they are causing you distress.

Your best option is to try different things over several months. Probably a combination of medications will work best. Ask your doctor to explain any side effects when discussing your treatment options.

Antidepressants SSRI antidepressants (see p227), such as fluoxetine and paroxetine, may be prescribed if your symptoms include fatigue, food cravings, mood swings, and sleeping problems. If your symptoms are approaching PMDD levels (see box opposite), you may be on a daily dose, but if you have more manageable symptoms you need only take the drugs for the two weeks before menstruation.

Diuretics If you can't control your weight gain, bloating, and fluid retention by diet and exercise alone, diuretics, such as spironolactone, can help your kidneys secrete excess water and make you feel less bloated.

Combined oral contraceptives The older oral contraceptives, which regulate hormone production, are surprisingly ineffective for dealing with PMS – in fact, some women actually have worse symptoms on the "pill". However, a newly developed progestin – drospirenone – has helped some women. As this drug is present in some of the newer oral contraceptives, it can be used for contraception at the same time as treating your PMS.

Synthetic steroid hormone
Danazol is occasionally prescribed for PMS. It decreases production of the hormones oestrogen and progesterone, which relieves the symptoms of PMS. However, doctors do not often choose danazol as this drug can have serious side effects.

HOW CAN I HELP MYSELF?
There are many self-help remedies for PMS. They may not all work for you, but it's worth experimenting because they're good for your health in general.

Aerobic exercise This has been the mainstay of PMS therapy for years. Aerobic exercise for at least 30–45 minutes three to four times a week, will help increase endorphins (the "feel good" hormones) in your brain, which are powerful natural pain-relievers. (See pp56–7 for advice on exercise.)

PMDD – SEVERE PMS, OR SOMETHING ELSE?

Doctors are divided in their opinions about PMDD. Is it a variant of PMS or is it a type of depression? The symptoms are severe manifestations of PMS. There are interesting differences in how SSRI antidepressants affect sufferers. Women with PMDD note improvement within a day of starting an SSRI, whereas a depressed woman may not notice any improvement for 3 to 4 weeks.

Women with PMDD need only take SSRIs for the 10 days when they have symptoms, whereas if you're depressed you'll need medication every day. Women with PMDD only seem to benefit from SSRIs whereas depressed women respond to other antidepressants. Women with PMDD are at higher risk of postnatal depression (see p215), so if you've recently given birth and are feeling depressed, talk to your doctor.

Change your eating Many experts recommend a low-salt, low-concentrated-carbohydrate, and high-complex-carbohydrate diet before your period. (See pp52–5 for advice on a healthy diet).

Calcium A few studies have shown that 1200mg calcium per day, in three doses, can be helpful.

Vitamins E and B6 Vitamin E, in doses of 200–400 units per day and vitamin B6, in doses of 100–200mg per day may reduce your symptoms of breast discomfort.

Herbal remedies Some women swear by herbal remedies (see below), but there are not sufficient scientific data to substantiate their effectiveness. One of the most popular is evening primrose oil, which is reported to improve breast pain; the usual dosage is 1000 units (2 standard capsules) per day. Herbal remedies aren't regulated in the same way as drugs, so make sure you buy them from a reputable supplier and always follow the manufacturer's advice on dosage.

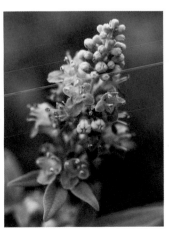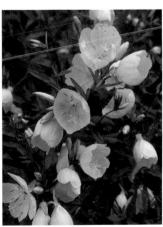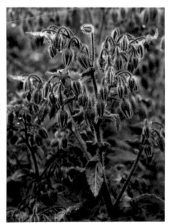

Herbal remedies to keep PMS at bay
Vitex agnus-castus (far left), usually taken as a tincture, is thought to help balance hormones; the seed oil from evening primrose (centre) and borage (left) contain omega-6 fatty acids that have anti-inflammatory properties, which may ease breast pain.

Ovarian disorders

The ovaries store all the eggs you will ever have, and are undoubtedly the key to reproduction. They also secrete female sex hormones that regulate your menstrual cycle and affect your physical and emotional wellbeing. Because the ovaries lie deep in your pelvis, problems are not always immediately obvious.

Ovarian cyst

This disorder is very common and nearly always harmless. Unless you have a very large cyst that presses on nearby organs, such as the bladder, you may not even know that you have one. It is comparatively rare for an ovarian cyst to become cancerous; this is something that is more likely to occur in women over 40.

WHAT IS IT?
Ovarian cysts are swellings that are usually filled with fluid and are found inside or on the ovaries. The most common type of cyst occurs in one of the follicles, or sacs, where the eggs develop. Another type, known as dermoid cysts, are

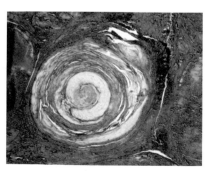

Dermoid cyst
This ovarian cyst arose from various body cells. It contains tissues usually found in parts such as bone and teeth.

formed from body cells and can contain teeth, hair, and bone.

Cysts range in size from tiny to so large that they can make your tummy look swollen. Most cysts occur singly; multiple cysts are caused by a hormonal disorder called polycystic ovary syndrome (see opposite).

WHAT NEXT?
If your doctor suspects you have an ovarian cyst, you'll probably have an ultrasound scan, either taken through your abdomen, or transvaginally (through your vagina). These scans can confirm the presence of a cyst, reveal its size, and, importantly, look at the blood flow to the cyst. Massive blood flow could indicate that a cyst is cancerous (new blood vessels often develop around cancer cells). However, in the vast majority of cases, ovarian cysts are not malignant.

MY TREATMENT OPTIONS
Quite often ovarian cysts disappear of their own accord, and no treatment is needed. However, you are likely to need regular check-ups to make sure that a cyst isn't growing larger.

HAVE I GOT THE SYMPTOMS?
Often there are no symptoms and a cyst is discovered by chance during a pelvic examination. If there are symptoms, you may have any of the following:
- Pelvic pain, or a sense of pressure in your pelvis
- Pressure on your bladder, which causes a frequent need to urinate
- Pressure on your rectum
- Pain during sexual intercourse
- Severe abdominal pain, if the cyst becomes twisted (torted).

See your doctor if you have any of these symptoms.

Drainage If a fluid-filled cyst continues to grow, your gynaecologist may drain it.
Surgery Sometimes it is necessary to remove a cyst surgically, especially if it is large. Occasionally, it is not possible to take out just the cyst and the ovary must be removed as well.

HOW CAN I HELP MYSELF?
Don't ignore any pelvic symptoms (see above). Talk to your doctor.

Polycystic ovary syndrome

This complicated disorder affects about 1 in 20 women in the UK. Polycystic ovary syndrome (PCOS) produces a variety of symptoms that may be difficult to diagnose.

WHAT IS IT?

In PCOS, a hormone imbalance results in lack of ovulation and overproduction of the male hormone testosterone, which is normally produced in minute amounts by the ovaries. Often, many small, fluid-filled cysts develop in the ovaries and the menstrual cycle is seriously disrupted or stops altogether. PCOS is a major cause of infertility and may also increase the risk of other diseases, including diabetes (see pp320–5) and cancer of the uterus (see p104). Because of the testosterone, male characteristics, such as excess facial hair, are common symptoms of PCOS.

WHAT NEXT?

If PCOS is suspected, your doctor will take some blood samples to test your hormone levels. You will probably also have an ultrasound scan to look for ovarian cysts.

MY TREATMENT OPTIONS

Treatment of PCOS will depend on how severe your symptoms are and whether you are planning to have a baby. Ask your doctor to explain any potential side effects.
Hormone therapy If you're not trying to get pregnant, you'll probably be prescribed an oral contraceptive to regulate your periods and suppress the growth of ovarian cysts. The "pill" will also help to control excess hair growth.
Infertility treatment If you are not ovulating and you want to have a baby, you'll need to be treated with fertility drugs, such as clomiphene. Many women with PCOS have successful pregnancies following infertility treatment.
Drugs to reduce the risk of diabetes Because PCOS can cause raised blood glucose levels, and possibly diabetes, your doctor may prescribe metformin, a drug used to lower glucose levels.

HOW CAN I HELP MYSELF?

Trying to keep your life on an even keel can help PCOS symptoms.
Watch your weight You are likely to have higher than normal levels of glucose in your blood as a side effect of PCOS, so you should be extra vigilant about weight gain.

HAVE I GOT THE SYMPTOMS?

You may not have any symptoms and the disease may only be diagnosed if you are being assessed for infertility. Possible symptoms include:

- Irregular periods, or even absence of periods
- Noticeable facial hair
- Very oily skin and acne
- Being overweight.

PCOS also puts you at a greater than average risk of developing diabetes.
See your doctor if you notice any of the above symptoms.

Eating healthily and taking plenty of exercise will help adjust your blood glucose levels and lessen your risk of developing diabetes.
Take control of stress Your hormone levels can be upset by stress. Try relaxation techniques to keep the stress in your life at a manageable level.

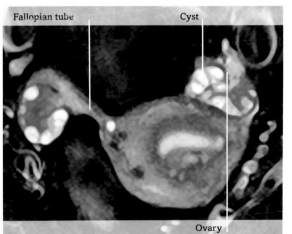

Multiple cysts
This MRI scan shows a large number of cysts (white spheres) affecting both ovaries (green) in a woman with PCOS. The condition is a major cause of infertility. The cysts are not cancerous.

Ovarian cancer

Around 7000 women are diagnosed with ovarian cancer every year, most of whom are past the menopause. Doctors don't know the causes, but various factors may marginally increase your risk.

WHAT IS IT?

Occasionally, a cancerous tumour develops from an ovarian cyst (see p94), but more often the disease occurs without any early warning signs. There are several types of ovarian cancer. The majority of these cancers form from the cells that cover the surface of the ovary. Less commonly, cancers develop from the cells that make eggs in the ovary. There are also other, rarer, cancers of the ovary that cannot be linked with any certainty to particular cell types.

A woman with ovarian cancer may not realize that anything is wrong in the initial stages. Often, symptoms arise only after the cancer has spread from the original site in the ovary (a process known as metastasis), when there may be pain and swelling in other organs.

WHAT NEXT?

If your doctor suspects you have ovarian cancer, you will probably be referred to a specialist for tests. These will include an abdominal or transvaginal (through your vagina) ultrasound scan. You may also have blood tests. There is one blood test that detects what is known as a "tumour marker" – in this case a protein, CA-125, which is produced by certain cancerous tumours. However, the test is by no means foolproof and can give a high reading, for example if you are menstruating or if you have endometriosis. Research is being carried out on other blood tests, but so far none is currently available for widespread screening.

If the results from the first round of tests are inconclusive, you will have more detailed investigations such as a CT or MRI scan, or laparoscopy (see p98). At the same time, your doctor may remove a small sample of tissue from one or more areas to test for cancerous cells.

If you have relatives with ovarian or breast cancer (see Am I at risk?, opposite), your doctor will discuss genetic testing with you. The breast cancer gene test can detect if you are carrying the BRCA gene, which is associated with a very high risk of ovarian cancer. If you do carry a genetic condition which predisposes you to ovarian cancer, you should discuss with a gynaecologist the benefits of removal of your ovaries once you have completed your family.

MY TREATMENT OPTIONS

As with most types of cancer, treatment is likely to involve several stages and will depend on how far the tumour has progressed and whether the cancer has spread to other organs. The mainstays of treatment are surgery and chemotherapy. You should discuss the risks and benefits of all treatment options with your doctor. Following treatment, you will be given regular check-ups to ensure that the cancer has not recurred.

Surgery The surgical option is a total hysterectomy (see p103) that includes a bilateral salpingo-oophorectomy, an operation in which your uterus, ovaries, and

---

HAVE I GOT THE SYMPTOMS?

This condition was once known as the silent killer, but many women do get symptoms at an early stage. These may include:

- Bloating/increase in abdominal size
- Pelvic/abdominal pain
- Difficulty eating/feeling full quickly
- Frequent or urgent urination
- Abnormal vaginal bleeding (this is rare).

See your doctor if any of these symptoms have come on recently and have occurred on more than 12 days last month.

"In women who have been taking oral contraceptives in the long term, the risk of ovarian cancer is reduced by 50 per cent."

> "A number of clinical trials are currently under way to try and improve the success rate of treatment."

fallopian tubes are all removed Although this is a major operation, it is relatively common – one in five women needs a hysterectomy and most recover without any complications. However, as with any surgery, there are slight risks involved with having an anaesthetic. In addition, bleeding, postoperative infection, developing a thrombosis (blood clot; see p252), or accidental damage to the bladder or bowel are other rare complications. If you are still menstruating, having your ovaries removed will cause instant menopause, and you could experience severe menopausal symptoms. If this happens, you should discuss your treatment options with your doctor.

Chemotherapy You are also likely to be given chemotherapy, either before the operation to reduce the size of the tumour, or afterwards to kill off any remaining cancer cells.

Other options Radiotherapy may be used to treat certain ovarian cancers or in specific situations. If the cancer recurs after you have had surgery and chemotherapy, you may be advised to have further chemotherapy or surgery.

Several clinical trials are in progress to try and find different therapies and combinations of chemotherapies to improve the success rate of treatments.

HOW CAN I HELP MYSELF?

As doctors have very little understanding of what causes ovarian cancer, it is difficult for them to recommend any lifestyle changes that might have a protective effect against the disease. However, it is estimated

AM I AT RISK?
You are possibly at higher risk of developing ovarian cancer if:
- You haven't had any children
- You've had infertility treatment
- You had a late menopause
- You have a family history of ovarian or breast cancer, such as one or two first-degree family members (mother, sister, or daughter) with the disease, or two second-degree family members (grandmother, aunt, or cousin), or one first-degree and two second-degree family members. Specialists vary in their analysis of what constitutes the greatest risk.

that in women who have been taking oral contraceptives in the long term, the risk of ovarian cancer is reduced by 50 per cent. You may want to discuss this with your doctor, if you are currently using other contraceptive methods.

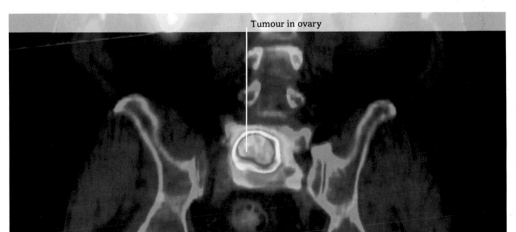

Tumour in ovary

Sites of cancer
This scan combines CT and PET (positron emission tomography) to get an accurate picture of ovarian cancer in this woman. The tumour (green) can be seen clearly on the surface of the ovary (red).

Uterine disorders

Problems with the uterus – which include infections, inflammation, and tumours – are common. Not all of these disorders are serious, but getting prompt treatment is important, particularly if you plan to become pregnant. Anything that affects your uterus may also affect your fertility.

Pelvic inflammatory disease

This is a common cause of pain in the pelvic and abdominal areas. However, pelvic inflammatory disease (PID) can often be present for some time without causing obvious symptoms.

WHAT IS IT?

PID is an inflammation of the uterus, fallopian tubes, and ovaries that is usually caused by a sexually transmitted infection (see pp114–19). If left untreated, PID can cause permanent scarring of the fallopian tubes, leading to infertility.

WHAT NEXT?

Your doctor will examine you and take a vaginal swab to diagnose the infection. A laparoscopy (see below) may also be recommended.

MY TREATMENT OPTIONS

PID is treated with drugs to fight the infection. Your doctor may also suggest that you take painkillers. Ask about any possible side effects.

Oral antibiotics You'll probably be prescribed oral antibiotics, unless your condition is severe.

Intravenous antibiotics If PID is making you seriously ill, perhaps because your immune system is

compromised, you'll receive intravenous medication in hospital.

HOW CAN I HELP MYSELF?

Practise safe sex and use condoms to protect against STIs. If you have an IUD and develop an infection, removal of the IUD may be needed, and other contraception used.

AM I AT RISK?

The risk factors include those for contracting STIs (see pp114–19). Other possible risk factors are having recently had an IUD inserted and the termination of a pregnancy.

HAVE I GOT THE SYMPTOMS?

Symptoms vary depending on the severity of the infection, but may include:

- Severe pain in the pelvic region
- Pain during intercourse
- Heavy, painful periods
- bleeding between periods
- Fever and feeling unwell.

See your doctor without delay if the symptoms come on suddenly or you feel very unwell.

LAPAROSCOPY

This procedure, performed under general anaesthetic, allows a gynaecologist to look at – and sometimes operate on – a woman's reproductive organs. Small cuts are made in the abdomen, through which a viewing instrument (called a laparoscope) and a probe to manipulate the internal organs are inserted.

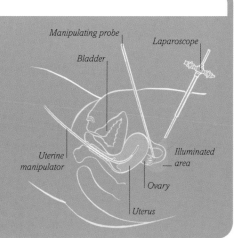

Manipulating probe

Laparoscope

Bladder

Uterine manipulator

Illuminated area

Ovary

Uterus

Fibroids

By the end of your reproductive life it is common to find non-cancerous growths called fibroids in the uterus. These won't give you any problems unless they grow very large or if they bleed heavily.

WHAT ARE THEY?

Fibroids are abnormal tissue growths that can form on the inner or outer wall of the uterus, or within the muscle layers of the wall. They vary in size from a pea to a grapefruit, and some are attached by stalks. Very large fibroids may distort the uterus.

WHAT NEXT?

If your doctor feels fibroids during a pelvic or abdominal examination and wants confirmation, you may have an abdominal or transvaginal ultrasound (through the vagina) scan. Other examinations could include hysteroscopy (see p100), laparoscopy (see opposite), or a CT or MRI scan.

MY TREATMENT OPTIONS

Unless your fibroids cause problems or you're being investigated for infertility, you probably won't need treatment. Fibroids depend on oestrogen for their growth, so after the menopause they start to shrink and no further action is necessary.

Gonadotropin-releasing hormone (Gn-RH) agonists These drugs, such as leuprolide, stimulate the pituitary gland (see p330) so that your ovaries produce less oestrogen and progesterone, and you experience a temporary menopause. This effect disappears once the drugs are discontinued, but your fibroids may return.

Synthetic androgens A male hormone, such as danazol, can help shrink fibroids, but it also reduces the size of your uterus and stops your periods. Such drugs have other unpleasant side effects, such as weight gain, headaches, unwanted hair growth, and a deeper voice. Discuss the implications with your doctor.

Surgery Fibroids can be removed in various ways: via the cervix with a hysteroscope, by laparoscopy (see opposite) or through a cut in the abdomen – myomectomy. Occasionally a hysterectomy (see p103) will be required. In a newer, highly effective procedure called uterine artery embolization, blood-clotting agents are released into a blood vessel in the uterus to starve the fibroids of their blood supply and make them shrink.

HOW CAN I HELP MYSELF?

You can't do anything to prevent fibroids, but you should report any unusual symptoms to your doctor.

HAVE I GOT THE SYMPTOMS?

Many fibroids are found incidentally during a routine pelvic examination or antenatal check-up, but they may cause you:

- Pelvic pressure
- Pelvic pain
- Heavy periods
- Frequent urination
- Constipation
- Backache.

See your doctor if your symptoms are worrying you.

TYPES OF FIBROIDS

Fibroids are classified by where they grow in the uterus. They can develop on the inner surface of the uterus (submucosal fibroids), in the middle of the uterine wall (intramural fibroids), on the outer surface (subserous fibroids), or in the neck of the uterus (cervical fibroid). Sometimes fibroids grow on a stalk (pedunculated fibroids).

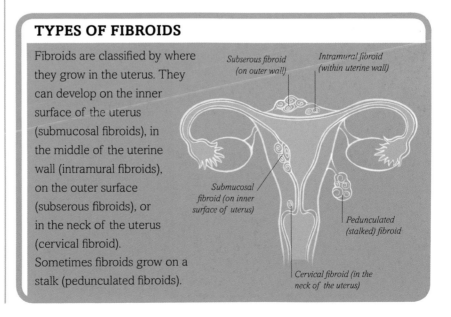

Subserous fibroid (on outer wall)

Intramural fibroid (within uterine wall)

Submucosal fibroid (on inner surface of uterus)

Pedunculated (stalked) fibroid

Cervical fibroid (in the neck of the uterus)

Endometrial polyps

These small growths in the uterus are usually harmless. They do sometimes cause bleeding, though – which needs investigating as it can be a symptom of more serious diseases. You're more likely to have endometrial polyps if you're between 40 and 60 years old.

WHAT IS IT?

An endometrial polyp is a tiny overgrowth of cells that is attached to the lining of the womb (the endometrium). Polyps may be as small as a sesame seed or as large as a golf ball, and you may have one or more. The most common type sits on top of a thin stalk.

WHAT NEXT?

To investigate polyps, your doctor may send you for a transvaginal (through the vagina) scan.

This may be combined with hysterosonography, in which saline is injected into your uterus to expand it for a better view. Alternatively, a hysteroscopy may be used. (see box below)

MY TREATMENT OPTIONS

If your polyps are very small and are not causing symptoms, you may not need treatment. The polyps may even disappear spontaneously. Otherwise, the only way to get rid of polyps is by removing them surgically. (Unfortunately, polyps can sometimes grow back, when they may require further surgery.)

If a polyp is protruding into your cervix, it may be possible for your doctor to remove it using a pair of forceps. If this is not an option, you may need one or both of the following procedures.

Curettage In this procedure, polyps are removed by scraping them off with a long loop-shaped instrument. If a polyp is found during a hysteroscopy investigation (see below) it will probably be removed there and then by curettage.

Hysterectomy Polyps that are removed by curettage are always sent for laboratory analysis. Very occasionally this reveals precancerous cell changes that cause concern. In such cases, and depending on your age, you may need a hysterectomy (see p103).

HOW CAN I HELP MYSELF?

To eliminate other disorders, report any unusual bleeding to your doctor as soon as possible.

AM I AT RISK?

Women taking HRT (see p137) or tamoxifen have a higher than normal risk. Other risk factors include high blood pressure, obesity, and a history of cervical polyps.

HAVE I GOT THE SYMPTOMS?

It's possible that you have no symptoms, but usually at least one of the following is present:

● Irregular periods
● Bleeding between periods
● Heavy periods
● Infertility
● Bleeding after the menopause.

See your doctor if any of these symptoms persist. They can be the symptoms of other problems, too. Bleeding after the menopause needs prompt investigation.

HYSTEROSCOPY

Gynaecologists use a device known as a hysteroscope, which is inserted through the vagina and cervix, to closely examine the inner lining of the uterus. The cavity of the uterus is filled with a gas or fluid to make viewing easier. During a hysteroscopy, tissue samples can be collected for further tests, and polyps and fibroids (see p99) can be removed.

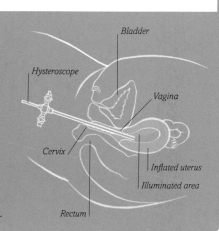

Bladder

Hysteroscope

Vagina

Cervix

Inflated uterus

Illuminated area

Rectum

Endometriosis

Although this condition is common, it is a bit of a mystery, as doctors do not know exactly why it occurs. The symptoms vary widely, which sometimes makes endometriosis difficult to diagnose.

WHAT IS IT?

In endometriosis, tiny fragments of the lining of the uterus (the endometrium) go astray and turn up in other parts of the body. The endometrial tissue may attach itself to any nearby organs, such as the ovaries, bowel, or bladder. This tissue is affected by the menstrual cycle in the same way as the uterine lining. When a period occurs, the stray tissue bleeds, too – but because it is trapped in the body it swells up and causes pain.

Eventually, scar tissue may build up. You are more likely to develop endometriosis if you delay pregnancy until your 30s, or if you never become pregnant. The condition usually eases up when you become pregnant and then disappears altogether when you reach the menopause.

Endometriosis can often be confused with other conditions that cause pelvic pain, such as pelvic inflammatory disease (PID; see p99), or inflammatory bowel disease (IBD; see pp310–11).

WHAT NEXT?

Your gynaecologist will give you a pelvic examination and you may have an ultrasound or MRI scan. Sometimes a laparoscopy is also needed (see p98).

MY TREATMENT OPTIONS

Your doctor will consider your age and the severity of your symptoms when deciding on treatment. If you are prescribed drugs, ask your doctor about possible side effects.

Oral contraceptives The standard treatment for many years has been birth control pills, which can be quite effective. You may be asked to take them continuously so that you avoid having a period.

Gonadotropin-releasing hormone (Gn-RH) agonists act on your hormones. When injected, they lower oestrogen levels, stop menstruation, and shrink the stray tissue. You may need repeat injections if your symptoms return, though this may not be for years.

HAVE I GOT THE SYMPTOMS?

Most women have a range of symptoms, with pain being the most common. You may have:
- Painful periods (dysmenorrhoea; see p91)
- Pain during intercourse
- Lower abdominal or low back pain during ovulation, bowel movements, or urination
- Irregular periods (oligomenorrhoea; see p90) or heavy periods (menorrhagia; see p91)
- Constipation and/or diarrhoea
- Infertility.

See your doctor if your symptoms are severely disrupting your life.

Surgery One surgical option is to destroy stray tissue with a laser during a laparoscopy. If you want to become pregnant, your gynaecologist will take as much care as possible to remove the tissue without damaging your reproductive organs. If you do not want a pregnancy, a hysterectomy, including removal of your ovaries (see p103), may be considered.

HOW CAN I HELP MYSELF?

You can take over-the-counter painkillers for the pain. Having a warm bath or putting a heating pad or hot-water bottle over your pelvis can help to reduce cramping pains. Some women find joining a support group enormously beneficial.

LOCATION OF ENDOMETRIOSIS

Stray endometrial tissue most commonly attaches itself to the areas shown below.

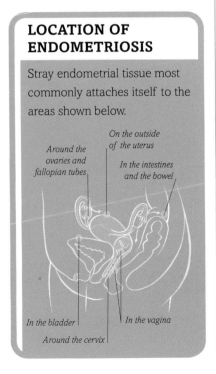

On the outside of the uterus

Around the ovaries and fallopian tubes

In the intestines and the bowel

In the bladder

In the vagina

Around the cervix

Adenomyosis

This is a less common version of endometriosis (see p101). Adenomyosis isn't dangerous, but it causes a lot of discomfort.

WHAT IS IT?

Adenomyosis occurs when stray pieces of the lining of the uterus (the endometrium) become embedded within the muscle fibres of the uterine wall. This tissue bleeds during menstruation, causing very heavy periods and abdominal pains.

WHAT NEXT?

Your doctor will take your medical history, carry out a pelvic examination, and possibly send you for an MRI or ultrasound scan of your uterus. Adenomyosis is very difficult to diagnose. Some of the symptoms are similar to those of other disorders of the uterus, for example polyps (see p100) or fibroids (see p99). These other conditions may have to be ruled out first. The only certain way of confirming the diagnosis is to examine the tissues of the uterus after hysterectomy (see opposite)

MY TREATMENT OPTIONS

Your treatment will depend on how close you are to the menopause, because adenomyosis disappears when you stop having periods. Ask your doctor about any side effects when discussing your options.
Anti-inflammatory drugs, such as ibuprofen, help to control the pain and may be the best treatment if you're nearing the menopause.
Hormone treatments such as oral contraceptives may ease pain and bleeding. The progesterone-coated Mirena IUS (see pp132, 135) can provide relief by stopping your periods completely.
Surgery If you have very severe pain and are a long way off the menopause, your gynaecologist may recommend surgery to remove your uterus (see hysterectomy, opposite).

HOW CAN I HELP MYSELF?

A hot-water bottle on your tummy may help to lessen severe pain.

HAVE I GOT THE SYMPTOMS?

You may have adenomyosis but no symptoms. However, one or more of the following symptoms is more usual:
- Heavy or prolonged menstrual bleeding, possibly containing blood clots
- Severe, piercing pelvic pain
- Bad cramps during your period
- Pain during intercourse
- Bleeding between periods.

See your doctor if any of these symptoms interfere with your everyday life.

HAVE I GOT THE SYMPTOMS?

The main symptoms of both acute and chronic endometritis are:
- Lower abdominal pain
- Vaginal bleeding
- Vaginal discharge
- Fever.

See your doctor if you have any of these symptoms and if you also feel unwell.

Endometritis

This condition (not to be confused with endometriosis, see p101) can affect women of any age, both before and after the menopause. Endometritis may develop over time or appear quite suddenly.

WHAT IS IT?

Endometritis is an inflammation of the lining of the uterus (the endometrium), usually following an infection of the genital tract.

Chronic endometritis This form of the infection develops gradually. Chronic endometritis can be a major part of pelvic inflammatory disease (see p98), which is itself usually the result of a sexually transmitted infection (see pp114–19). Sometimes, tuberculosis can also lead to chronic endometritis.
Acute endometritis The type of infections that cause acute endometritis, when symptoms develop very rapidly, are most likely to be complications from

gynaecological procedures, such as termination of a pregnancy, and delivery of a baby, especially by caesarean section. Having an IUD (see p132) inserted can also trigger an infection, but after 20 days, there is no longer any special risk

WHAT NEXT?
Your doctor will ask about your symptoms and how long you've had them. It is very important to find out whether you have acute or chronic endometritis so that the appropriate treatment can be

given. Your doctor will also give you a physical examination to establish if there is any abdominal tenderness. He or she and will probably do some blood tests and take a vaginal swab, which will reveal which infective organisms are causing the condition.

MY TREATMENT OPTIONS
Endometritis is treated with antibiotics. Your doctor will decide which drugs are best for you after taking into consideration whether you've just had a baby and how ill

the condition is making you. Most cases of mild endometritis are successfully treated with a course of oral antibiotics. If you're very ill, you may need to go to hospital for intravenous antibiotics. These are usually combined with – or followed by – a course of oral antibiotics. Ask your doctor about any likely side effects.

HOW CAN I HELP MYSELF?
To reduce the risk of infections, you should use condoms if you are sexually active.

Endometrial hyperplasia

This condition is most common in women who are perimenopausal. Sometimes, endometrial hyperplasia can lead to cancer of the uterus (see p104).

WHAT IS IT?
Endometrial hyperplasia is an overgrowth of the tissue lining the uterus. This can be due to hormone imbalances at the menopause or because of drug treatment.

WHAT NEXT?
Your doctor will examine you and may recommend a transvaginal scan (through your vagina). A tissue sample may be taken to look for precancerous cell changes.

MY TREATMENT OPTIONS
Treatment depends on what the biopsy reveals and may involve drugs or surgery. Ask your doctor about any potential side effects.

Hormonal therapy If there are no signs of cell changes, you'll probably receive hormonal therapy to remove the excess growth.
Hysterectomy If there are abnormal cell changes, or if you've reached the menopause, your doctor may recommend a total hysterectomy (see below) to prevent cancer developing in the future.

HOW CAN I HELP MYSELF?
Get symptoms checked at an early stage to reduce the risk of cancer.

HAVE I GOT THE SYMPTOMS?

Symptoms are similar to other uterine disorders and may include:
- Bleeding between periods
- Heavy menstrual bleeding
- Bleeding after the menopause.

See your doctor if you have a noticeable change in your periods.

WHAT IS A HYSTERECTOMY?

A hysterectomy is an operation to remove the uterus and cervix. It is used to treat conditions such as cancer and endometriosis. Sometimes the fallopian tubes and ovaries are also removed. Removal of both ovaries causes immediate menopause.

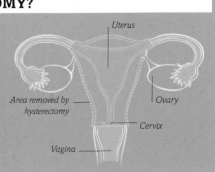

Uterus

Area removed by hysterectomy

Ovary

Cervix

Vagina

Cancer of the uterus

HAVE I GOT THE SYMPTOMS?

The symptoms depend on whether or not you've reached the menopause:

- Premenopause: increasingly heavy periods, bleeding between periods, or bleeding after sexual intercourse
- Postmenopause: renewed bleeding, which may vary from spotting to heavier bleeding.

See your doctor if you have any abnormal bleeding. Bear in mind that irregular bleeding is a common symptom of many noncancerous conditions.

Uterine cancer is the fifth most common cancer in women in the UK. If detected at an early stage, it can often be treated successfully.

WHAT IS IT?

This cancer usually develops as an abnormal growth in the lining of the uterus (the endometrium). Far more rarely, cancer occurs in the muscle wall of the uterus.

WHAT NEXT?

If your doctor suspects cancer, he or she will give you a pelvic examination, and may take a small tissue sample from your uterus for testing. You may need further tests such as a transvaginal scan (through your vagina) to look closely at your uterus, ovaries, and fallopian tubes.

Larger tissue samples may need to be taken at a hysteroscopy (see p100) and curettage (D & C). If cancer is diagnosed, you will have more tests to determine what stage it has reached (see box right).

MY TREATMENT OPTIONS

Treatment depends on the stage the cancer has reached. Talk to your doctor about potential side effects, which may be severe.

Surgery Removal of the uterus, ovaries and fallopian tubes (see hysterectomy p103), is the usual treatment. You may also have lymph nodes in your pelvic area removed at the same time.

Radiotherapy You may have radiotherapy after surgery to ensure that any remaining cancerous cells are destroyed.

Chemotherapy Treatment with anticancer drugs may be recommended if the cancer has spread to your lymph nodes.

HOW CAN I HELP MYSELF?

Be aware of the danger signs and do not delay in reporting unusual symptoms to your doctor.

THE FOUR STAGES OF UTERINE CANCER

Tests that analyse tissue samples of the uterus and lymph nodes reveal that there are four stages of uterine cancer as it grows and spreads. It is important for doctors to identify which stage the cancer has reached in order to decide the best treatment.

Stage I

The cancer is only found in the wall of the uterus

Stage 2

The cancer has spread to the cervix

Stage 3

The cancer has spread to the pelvic region, perhaps including lymph nodes

Stage 4

The cancer has spread to the bladder or rectum, and possibly also to distant tissues beyond the pelvic region, such as the lungs and liver

AM I AT RISK?

Your risk of developing uterine cancer increases if you have:

- Become overweight
- Reached your late 50s
- Never had children
- High blood pressure
- Taken oestrogen-only HRT
- Had breast cancer and have been treated with tamoxifen for more than two years.
- Endometrial hyperplasia (see p103), which can turn cancerous.

Uterine prolapse

Pregnancy and childbirth take their toll on your body. In many women the muscles and ligaments that hold the uterus in place become too overstretched to provide support.

WHAT IS IT?
In uterine prolapse the uterus drops down into the vagina. This displacement may be very slight but in severe prolapse the uterus may appear outside your vulva.

WHAT NEXT?
Your doctor can diagnose a prolapse by physical examination.

HAVE I GOT THE SYMPTOMS?

With a mild prolapse you may have no symptoms, but if the condition is more severe, you'll have some or all of the following:
- A feeling of heaviness or pulling in your pelvis
- Urinary incontinence: urge (needing to get to a toilet in a hurry) or stress (leaking when you cough or jump) or both
- Low back pain
- Difficulty with bowel movements
- A sensation of sitting on a small ball
- Pain during intercourse.

See your doctor if you have any of these symptoms, particularly if they are disrupting your life.

AM I AT RISK?

The risk factors for uterine prolapse include one or more vaginal births, being menopausal, doing a lot of heavy lifting, a chronic cough (for example, in COPD; see pp240-1), obesity, and constipation.

MY TREATMENT OPTIONS
If the symptoms aren't too annoying, your doctor may suggest self-help measures (see right). You may need treatment if you are in great discomfort.

Vaginal pessary You will be fitted with a ring pessary, which is inserted through your vagina to hold your uterus in the right place. The pessary will need to be replaced at intervals.

Surgery If your family is complete the most usual procedure is a vaginal hysterectomy. If you have not completed your family and you cannot manage with a ring pessary, advanced surgical techniques using mesh to reinforce weakened tissues may be considered. These techniques are also sometimes used when prolapse recurs after a hysterectomy (see p103).

HOW CAN I HELP MYSELF?
The following self-help measures can help you prevent or reverse mild uterine prolapse.

Lose weight if you're overweight.
Give up smoking if you smoke.
Get treatment for any chronic condition that causes coughing.
Avoid lifting heavy objects.
Avoid constipation – eat fibre, fruit, and vegetables, drink water, and take exercise (see also p303).
Strengthen your pelvic floor muscles with a regular daily routine of exercises (see p341).

PROLAPSE OF THE UTERUS

Compare a normal uterus (below left) with a prolapsed uterus (below right). With a prolapse, the uterus drops into the upper half of the vagina. This causes the bladder to bulge into the front vaginal wall and the rectum to bulge into the back vaginal wall.

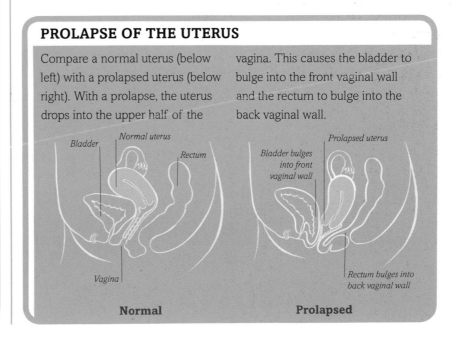

Bladder · *Normal uterus* · *Rectum* · *Vagina*

Normal

Bladder bulges into front vaginal wall · *Prolapsed uterus* · *Rectum bulges into back vaginal wall*

Prolapsed

Cervical disorders

The cervix is the lower part, or "neck", of the uterus. Muscles in the cervix keep it closed during pregnancy and allow it to expand in childbirth. Sometimes, the surface cells of the cervix show abnormal changes, which may develop into cancer. If detected early, cervical cancer is usually curable.

Cervical dysplasia

This condition is also referred to as cervical intra-epithelial neoplasia (CIN). Although cervical dysplasia can be an early warning of cancer, in most women the condition doesn't go on to become cancerous.

WHAT IS IT?

In cervical dysplasia, the cells of the cervix show abnormal changes. Most cases are caused by the human papilloma virus (HPV, see p366), which is transmitted by sexual intercourse. In mild dysplasia cells often return to normal. Severe dysplasia may develop into cancer if left untreated.

WHAT NEXT?

The condition is usually only picked up by a smear test. If your smear reveals precancerous changes, you'll probably be referred to a gynaecologist. He or she will examine your cervix through a viewing instrument called a colposcope, and may take a sample of tissue from the most abnormal-looking area. The tissue will be sent to a laboratory for testing and assessment.

MY TREATMENT OPTIONS

Treatment depends upon the severity of the condition. You may not need any treatment at all if you have only mild dysplasia – though you'll be monitored every six months to check for further cell changes. In more severe cases, you'll need treatment to remove or destroy all affected cells:

Cryosurgery This procedure uses extreme cold to freeze the affected cells, which will slough off. New, healthy cells are regenerated.

Laser therapy The affected cells are destroyed by laser treatment.

Surgery In loop electrical excision procedure (LEEP), a thin wire emitting low-voltage, high-frequency radio waves cuts away the affected area under local anaesthetic. In a cone biopsy, a cone-shaped section of cervical tissue is removed, usually under general anaesthetic.

HOW CAN I HELP MYSELF?

Always go for your routine smear test, stop smoking (see p64) and avoid unprotected intercourse.

HAVE I GOT THE SYMPTOMS?

You may have no symptoms, but some women have unusual vaginal bleeding as in cervical cancer (see opposite).

AM I AT RISK?

The following are possible risk factors for cervical dysplasia:
- Having unprotected sex before the age of 18
- Having unprotected sex with multiple partners.
- Smoking.

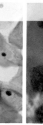
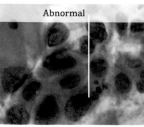

Dysplasia
These two smear test samples, seen under a microscope, show a comparison between normal and abnormal cervical cells.

Cervical cancer

This is the third most common cancer of the female reproductive system after ovarian and endometrial cancer. The UK's cervical screening programme, which has been running since 1967, has reduced the number of cases dramatically.

WHAT IS IT?

In cervical cancer, the cells of the cervix become severely abnormal. The disease is caused by the human papilloma virus (HPV) (see p366), which is transmitted by sexual intercourse. However, of the many types of HPV, only a few cause cancer. If left untreated, cervical cancer can spread to other organs in the pelvis, such as the bladder.

HAVE I GOT THE SYMPTOMS?

If you have cervical cancer you may have one or a combination of the following

- Unusual vaginal bleeding, such as after intercourse, between periods, or after your menopause.
- A heavy, watery vaginal discharge, which may be blood-stained and foul-smelling
- Pain during intercourse.

See your doctor if you experience any of the above symptoms.

WHAT NEXT?

If, having examined you, your doctor thinks that you may have cervical cancer, you will be referred to a gynaecologist. Your gynaecologist will examine your cervix through a viewing instrument called a colposcope and take a sample of tissue. This may be done by a punch biopsy (a small, circular section of cervix is removed) or a cone biopsy (a cone-shaped area of the cervix is removed). You may have additional tests, including blood tests, X-rays, and CT and MRI scans.

MY TREATMENT OPTIONS

Your doctor will advise you on the best treatment, taking into account your age, your general health, your own preferences and the stage the cancer has reached. If you are not suitable for surgery, chemotherapy and radiotherapy will be discussed. Talk to your doctor about the side effects of all your treatments.

Surgery Early disease may be amenable to a cone biopsy or hysterectomy (see p103). If you have a cancer confined to your cervix, your doctor will discuss either a radical hysterectomy with you or chemotherapy and radiotherapy. A radical hysterectomy means removal of the cervix, uterus, and tissues adjacent to these structures as well as the lymph glands that drain from these areas. The ovaries can be conserved. Some centres offer fertility-sparing procedures and you may wish to discuss this option.

Chemotherapy This may be used in combination with radiotherapy or before or after a surgical procedure. There are varying regimes used and this is dependent on whether the chemotherapy is being used in isolation or alongside other treatment.

Radiotherapy This may be given through your pelvis or internally.

HOW CAN I HELP MYSELF?

Always go for your routine smear test, stop smoking (see p64) and avoid unprotected intercourse. Women up to the age of 26 can benefit from a vaccination against cervical cancer.

AM I AT RISK?

The following can increase your risk of cervical cancer:

- Smoking
- Having a weakened immune system
- Taking the oral contraceptive pill; there may be a small increased risk associated with the pill
- Having unprotected sex with multiple partners.

"It's estimated that over a 10-year period, cervical screening by means of smear tests has saved the lives of 8,000 women in the UK."

Vaginal disorders

Your vagina connects the outside of your body to your cervix and uterus. The soft, moist folds of skin that line the vagina's thick, muscular walls produce secretions that help to keep it clean and protected against infection. Problems with the vagina are common but rarely serious.

Vaginitis

This condition, which causes itching and irritation, can affect any woman at any age. Vaginitis can be embarrassing and uncomfortable, but it's harmless and will go away with treatment.

WHAT IS IT?

Vaginitis is the inflammation of the lining of the vagina. It may be due to an infection, allergic reaction, or dryness resulting from low levels of oestrogen after the menopause (atrophic vaginitis). It often occurs with vulvitis (itching of the vulva).

HAVE I GOT THE SYMPTOMS?

You may have all the following symptoms, or just one or two:
- Burning
- Itching
- Soreness
- Vaginal discharge
- Unpleasant vaginal odour, often fishy
- Pain during intercourse.

See your doctor or sexual health clinic if your self-help measures don't bring relief.

Common infections that bring on vaginitis include the yeast *Candida albicans*, which causes thrush (see opposite), and a micro-organism called *Trichomonas vaginalis*, which causes trichomoniasis (see p119).

WHAT NEXT?

Your doctor will take a vaginal swab to check for infection. You may also need your urine tested for glucose to exclude diabetes mellitus (see pp320–5), which can sometimes lead to yeast infections of the vagina.

MY TREATMENT OPTIONS

Your doctor will recommend a treatment depending on what is causing your vaginitis. Ask about any side effects of medications.
For bacterial infections, you'll be prescribed antibiotics.
For fungal infections, you may be prescribed anti-fungal drugs to be taken either by mouth or as a vaginal cream or pessary.
To relieve itching, rub a cream onto your vulva. Your pharmacist can advise you on what to buy.
For atrophic vaginitis, you may be prescribed moisturizing cream, or a cream, tablets, or vaginal ring containing oestrogen.

AM I AT RISK?

You may be at risk of developing vaginitis if you:
- Use perfumed or scented bath products, sanitary protection, or detergents
- Use intimate deodorants
- Have recently taken a course of antibiotics
- Are diabetic or pregnant
- Eat a diet that is high in carbohydrates
- Sit around in a wet bathing suit or workout clothes, or wear jeans that are too tight.

HOW CAN I HELP MYSELF?

There are various self-help steps you can take to deal with vaginitis.
Avoid scented products, such as bath products, detergents, scented sanitary protection, and intimate deodorants.
Look after your genital region by keeping yourself clean, dry, and cool, and wearing cotton underwear and loose clothes.
Eating live yoghurt or taking acidophilus or probiotics can also help. Some women swear that inserting a tampon coated with plain, live yoghurt really works.

Vaginal thrush

Many women develop an uncomfortable vaginal itching accompanied by a thick, white discharge, especially during their childbearing years. This is vaginal thrush – a non-serious but sometimes recurrent disorder.

WHAT IS IT?

Thrush is caused by infection with a yeast known as *Candida albicans*, which lives naturally in the vagina and is normally kept in check by "good" bacteria. If the bacteria are killed by antibiotics or spermicides *Candida* can flourish unchecked. The bacteria can also be disrupted when the levels of female sex hormones change – for instance, before a period, during pregnancy, or as a result of taking the contraceptive pill. Intercourse with a partner who is infected with *Candida* can also lead to thrush.

WHAT NEXT?

If you're unsure about the discharge and itching, consult your doctor. He or she may give you a pelvic examination and take a swab of the discharge.

MY TREATMENT OPTIONS

Your doctor may suggest antifungal pessaries, creams, or pills. Some of these products are available over the counter. Ask your doctor or pharmacist about any side effects.

HAVE I GOT THE SYMPTOMS?

You may have developed vaginal thrush if you have:
- A vaginal discharge that has a "cottage-cheese" appearance
- Vaginal and vulval irritation.

See your doctor if you are worried about the symptoms or if self-help measures don't work.

HOW CAN I HELP MYSELF?

Wash your vagina with water only, and avoid spermicides and scented sanitary towels and tampons. Keep the outer vaginal area clean, and stay cool and dry by wearing cotton pants and loose clothing.

Dyspareunia (painful intercourse)

Thousands of women suffer from pain when they have sex, either all the time (when it is primary) or some of the time (secondary). It may be embarrassing to ask for help, but treatment can work well.

WHAT IS IT?

The causes of dyspareunia can be medical, resulting from:
- Pelvic surgery
- Radiotherapy or chemotherapy
- Pelvic inflammatory disease
- Endometriosis, ovarian cysts, fibroids.

They can also be psychological, resulting from:
- A bad experience, such as sexual abuse or rape.

WHAT NEXT?

Your doctor will take a full history and will ask about your sex life and medical history. You may have an examination and pelvic ultrasound.

MY TREATMENT OPTIONS

If an underlying medical cause is found, this will be treated. Ask about any possible side effects.

Hormone therapy If you're postmenopausal, you may be prescribed oestrogen in a cream, pill, or vaginal ring.

Desensitization Exercises to relax your vagina and pelvic floor may help to reduce the pain.

Counselling Talking to a sex counsellor may help.

HAVE I GOT THE SYMPTOMS?

Your sexual pain might occur:
- With any type of penetration, including tampons
- Under certain conditions, such as with particular partners
- After pain-free intercourse
- During thrusting movements
- As a burning or aching pain.

See your doctor if you have any of the above symptoms.

HOW CAN I HELP MYSELF?

Avoid scented bath products and douching, as they can cause irritation.

Try changing sexual positions and use a lubricant.

Vaginismus

If your vagina tightens painfully when you have sex or try to insert a tampon, you are suffering from vaginismus, a condition that affects many women. This disorder can cause untold distress, but the good news is that it's treatable.

WHAT IS IT?

Vaginismus occurs when your vaginal muscles contract against your will. This is usually caused by a subconscious fear of penetration, following such events as difficult childbirth or sexual assault.

A woman who is suffering from vaginismus finds sexual intercourse either impossible or very painful. The impact on her emotional health and relationships can be profound. What should be a pleasurable and loving act feels like violation. Feelings of dread, guilt, shame, and failure make the problem worse, especially if she is unable to talk about her problem.

HAVE I GOT THE SYMPTOMS?

The involuntary symptoms of vaginismus may include:

- Spasm of the muscles around the vagina
- Fear of pain
- Real pain
- Intense fear of penetration
- Loss of sexual desire.

See your doctor if you have any of these symptoms.

WHAT NEXT?

Despite the embarrassment, it's very important to see your doctor and be totally frank about your symptoms. Your sex life will be discussed in complete confidence. Your medical history and a physical examination, which could also be painful, will determine whether you require further tests. Your doctor will check for physical reasons, such as an infection or thinning of the vagina, that cause pain and therefore spasm.

MY TREATMENT OPTIONS

These may include one or all of the following:

Vaginal dilators You can try to gradually retrain the muscles around your vagina with a set of vaginal dilators. You can ask your partner to help you with this. Insert the smallest cone when you're relaxed; when you can do this without pain, move up a size. When you're confident with the largest cone, you may find you are ready to try sexual intercourse.

Medication You may need antibiotics to clear up an infection, or hormone drugs for vaginal thinning. Discuss any potential side effects with your doctor.

AM I AT RISK?

Several predisposing factors increase your risk of vaginismus:

- A vaginal or pelvic injury
- Dyspareunia (painful sex) (see p109)
- Bad early sexual experiences
- Sexual assault, abuse, or rape
- After-effects of childbirth
- Religious or cultural taboos about sex
- Strict upbringing where sex was never discussed.

Counselling Talking to a sexual health therapist or counsellor can often be helpful (see p225).

HOW CAN I HELP MYSELF?

You'll need plenty of patience, self-belief, and a supportive partner. **Know your body** Have a warm bath and relax on your bed. Touch yourself around your vaginal opening. If you tense up, stop, relax, and slow your breathing. Then try again. After a few days of doing this exercise, try inserting a finger – or ask your partner to insert his or her finger. Next, try a tampon. Finally, proceed to attempting intercourse.

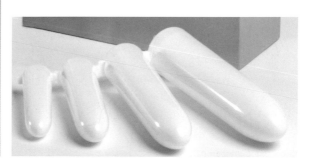

Vaginal dilators
Dilation therapy for vaginismus involves using four smooth cones of increasing width and length to retrain the vaginal muscles.

VAIN

Vaginal intra-epithelial neoplasia (VAIN) is a symptomless condition in which there are changes in the lining of the vagina. It is more common in women who are over 50. Rarely, VAIN may lead to vaginal cancer (see below).

WHAT IS IT?

In VAIN, abnormal cells are found in the skin lining the vagina. The condition is not fully understood, but infection with the human papilloma virus (see p117) may be a factor. In a very small number of women, the abnormal cells become cancerous. The severity of VAIN depends on the depth to which the cells are affected.

WHAT NEXT?

If VAIN is suspected, your doctor will use a viewing instrument called a colposcope for a magnified view of your vagina. A tissue sample may be taken at the same time.

MY TREATMENT OPTIONS

Mild cases of VAIN sometimes revert to normal without treatment. For more severe VAIN, you may need one of the following.

Ablation destroys the abnormal vaginal cells, either by laser or by loop electric excision procedure (LEEP) under a local anaesthetic.

Surgery may be used to remove the area of abnormal tissue. Sometimes, in severe cases, a larger area of surrounding vaginal tissue also has to be removed.

HAVE I GOT THE SYMPTOMS?

VAIN does not cause symptoms, and is detected by chance during other investigations, such as a smear test (see p106).

Radiotherapy is reserved for treating recurrences, or if the condition is widespread. It is carried out internally, using an applicator similar to a tampon.

Chemotherapy Anticancer drugs may be used in the form of a cream to be applied internally.

HOW CAN I HELP MYSELF?

Early detection is important, so keep up your routine smear tests.

Cancer of the vagina

Vaginal cancer is a rare disease that is most likely to affect women between 50 and 70.

WHAT IS IT?

The cause of this cancer is unclear. In the most common type, called squamous cell cancer (see p359), tumours tend to appear in the upper part of the vagina.

WHAT NEXT?

If cancer is suspected you'll have an internal examination, a smear, and investigations with a viewing instrument called a colposcope. Your doctor will also take a tissue sample for analysis.

MY TREATMENT OPTIONS

Your doctor will discuss the most suitable treatment depending on your age, tumour size, and whether it has spread.

Radiotherapy This is the usual treatment for most women. It may be applied externally through the pelvis, or internally via a tampon-like applicator inside the vagina.

Surgery removes the tumour and surrounding tissue, keeping as much of the vagina as possible. Occasionally, a larger part or all the vagina is removed and a new vagina made from other tissues.

Chemotherapy Intravenous anticancer drugs may be the only

HAVE I GOT THE SYMPTOMS?

You may have one of these:
- A blood-stained vaginal discharge
- Bleeding after sex
- Pain
- Problems passing urine
- Rectal pain.

See your doctor at once if you have any of these symptoms.

option for very advanced, or recurrent, vaginal cancer.

HOW CAN I HELP MYSELF?

Early detection is important, so keep up your routine smear tests.

Vulvar disorders

A woman's external sex organs, together known as the vulva, aren't susceptible to many disorders, but things do occasionally go wrong. This area is highly sensitive, and problems such as pain and itching can be uncomfortable. Don't ignore any symptoms because you feel embarrassed to see your doctor.

Vulvodynia

At some time in their lives, about 1 in 10 women may suffer from vulvodynia. The name of this disorder means "pain in the vulva", which can be so severe that having sex or even sitting down causes extreme discomfort.

WHAT IS IT?

Vulvodynia is a raw, burning pain that could be caused by a range of problems. Doctors don't know the cause for certain. Possible sources of the pain may include injury or irritation of nearby nerves, vaginal infection, local allergies, muscle spasm, and reduced oestrogen levels if you are post-menopausal.

WHAT NEXT?

This condition is often difficult to diagnose. Your doctor may want to refer you to a gynaecologist who will try to rule out any conditions that cause the same symptoms – for example, a sexually transmitted infection (STI) or skin condition.

You may also have a tissue sample taken from the affected area for investigation. This might reveal chronic inflammation.

MY TREATMENT OPTIONS

Even if all treatable medical conditions have been discounted, there are still a number of options. Your doctor will discuss the most suitable treatment for you.

Medications You may be prescribed a low dose of an antidepressant like amitriptyline, or an anticonvulsant drug such as gabapentin, both of which can be helpful in treating pain. You may also be offered a local anaesthetic ointment to use before intercourse to relieve any discomfort. Oestrogen cream may also help to alleviate the pain. Ask your doctor about potential side effects.

Biofeedback You will be taught to relax your pelvic muscles, which will help to reduce the pain.

Physical therapy A range of different therapies, including massage and transcutaneous electrical nerve stimulation (TENS), may also be recommended by your doctor.

HAVE I GOT THE SYMPTOMS?

It might be difficult for you to pinpoint the symptoms of vulvodynia, listed here, and the pain may be constant or intermittent (it can last for months or even years):

- Burning, soreness, and rawness in the genital area
- Sitting is uncomfortable
- Having sex is impossible
- The pain can't be alleviated.

See your doctor if the discomfort you feel fits one or more of these symptoms.

HOW CAN I HELP MYSELF?

These options may help to reduce the symptoms of vulvodynia:

- Cold compresses on the area
- Avoid tights and nylon pants
- Avoid hot baths
- Avoid washing the vulvar area too enthusiastically
- Take antihistamines
- Take regular exercise
- Use lubricants before intercourse.

"Over recent years, a number of specialist clinics have been set up to treat and investigate this particular condition."

Bartholin's gland cyst

At the base of your vagina is a pair of glands, called Bartholin's glands, which secrete a fluid that helps to keep your vagina moist and lubricated during sexual intercourse. Occasionally the ducts leading from the glands become blocked, which causes swelling.

WHAT IS IT?

Bartholin's glands are the size of a pea, and normally you cannot see them. If the duct opening out of one or both of the glands is blocked, a fluid-filled swelling called a Bartholin's cyst forms. The cyst can vary in size. It may remain small and painless, but it may swell up to the size of a lime and cause great discomfort if it gets infected. A painful abscess (an area of pus surrounded by inflamed tissue) may form as a result of the infection.

WHAT NEXT?

Your doctor will probably take your medical history and carry out a pelvic examination.

MY TREATMENT OPTIONS

Most cysts respond to self-help treatment or antibiotics; sometimes no treatment is needed at all.
Drainage of the cyst Your doctor may drain a large cyst under local anaesthetic.
Marsupialization In this procedure a permanent drainage hole is made in the cyst to prevent constant recurrence.
Removal of the gland In very rare cases the gland is removed.

HOW CAN I HELP MYSELF?

Most Bartholin's cysts occur for no apparent reason, and once a cyst develops you can try these options:

HAVE I GOT THE SYMPTOMS?

If the cyst is small and not infected, you may not experience any symptoms. Usually only one gland is affected, so if you have symptoms they'll be on one side of the vaginal opening:

- Tender or painful lump on one side of your vulva
- Discomfort, especially when you're walking or sitting
- Pain during intercourse
- Fever.

See your doctor if you think you have an infected Batholin's gland.

Warm baths Having a warm bath several times a day can sometimes help the cyst to burst and drain, easing the symptoms.
Painkillers You can buy over-the-counter remedies to relieve pain.

Vulvitis

Most women at some point in their lives are affected by vulvitis. This very common condition causes severe itching and soreness of the vulva. It has many of the same symptoms as vaginitis (see p108).

HAVE I GOT THE SYMPTOMS?

If you experience inflammation and itching of the outer genital area, consult your doctor.

WHAT IS IT?

Vulvitis is an inflammation of the vulva that produces itching, rawness, soreness, or a burning sensation. It can have variety of causes, including infections such as thrush (see p109), genital herpes (see p116), warts (see p117), pubic lice, or scabies. Vulvitis may also be an allergic reaction to soaps or detergents.

WHAT NEXT?

Your doctor will probably take your medical history and carry out a physical examination.

MY TREATMENT OPTIONS

Your doctor will recommend the treatment best suited to you:
Emollients help to ease itching.
Drugs applied to the vulva will help to treat the specific cause. Ask about any possible side effects.

HOW CAN I HELP MYSELF?

These simple procedures may help to prevent vulvitis:
Avoid contact of the vulva with bubble bath, soap, perfumes, personal deodorants, and so on.
Avoid tight garments that may chafe or overheat the area.

Sexually transmitted infections

The infections described here are usually passed from one person to another through sexual contact. Not all of them have obvious symptoms, especially in women. If you suspect that you have been at risk, see your doctor. Early treatment of sexually transmitted infections (STIs) saves later complications.

Gonorrhoea

While less common than it used to be, gonorrhoea is still a risk for anyone having unprotected sex. Men may have symptoms, such as pain on urinating, but many women have no symptoms.

WHAT IS IT?

Gonorrhoea is caused by a bacterium that is passed on through sexual contact, whether vaginal, anal, or oral. The infection can spread throughout the pelvic area and may even affect the joints.

HAVE I GOT THE SYMPTOMS?

You may feel well, but symptoms can appear suddenly.
They include:
- A vaginal discharge; burning feeling in the vagina and urethra
- A frequent need to urinate
- Anal irritation or discharge
- Bleeding between periods or heavier periods.

See your doctor or go to a sexual health clinic if you have any of the above symptoms.

WHAT NEXT?

If you or your partner suspect you have an infection, visit your doctor or sexual health clinic. The doctor or nurse will take a swab sample from the cervix, or any other area likely to have been infected, and send it for tests. You should have the results back within a couple of days. If you do have gonorrhoea, you may be tested for other STIs.

MY TREATMENT OPTIONS

You should get treatment as soon as possible. Gonorrhoea can have serious complications (see right).
Antibiotics The infection is usually cleared up with a single dose of antibiotics. This can be given orally or as an injection.
Surgery If you have a pelvic abscess associated with pelvic inflammatory disease (see right), it may need to be drained.
Your partner Any partner you have had in the last three months should be treated, too.

HOW CAN I HELP MYSELF?

Practise safer sex by using condoms, especially if you have many partners. If you are infected, avoid sex until your doctor gives you the all-clear.

AM I AT RISK?

You are at risk of contracting gonorrhoea if you have unprotected sex or genital contact with an infected partner. If gonorrhoea is left untreated, it can lead to the following complications:
- Gonorrhoea can cause pelvic inflammatory disease (PID, see p98); vaginal bleeding and infertility (see pp122–3)
- It can spread to the abdominal cavity and the liver, and cause perihepatitis (inflammation of the tissues surrounding the liver)
- It can spread via the bloodstream and lead to arthritis.

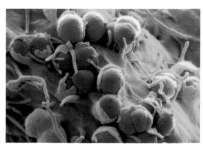

Gonorrhoea
This magnified image shows gonorrhoea bacteria (coloured red) infecting a human cell.

Chlamydia

A woman can have chlamydia without knowing it, as infection often causes no symptoms.

WHAT IS IT?

This bacterial infection can frequently go undetected for years, unless it leads to complications, such as pelvic inflammatory disease (see p98) and infertility. Once diagnosed, it's easily treated.

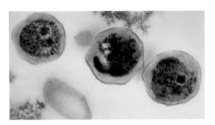

Chlamydia bacterium
Chlamydia trachiomatis (black areas) can cause serious damage if untreated.

WHAT NEXT?

If you suspect you have chlamydia, visit your doctor or sexual health clinic, where a sample swab will be taken from your cervix. The results are usually ready in 24 hours.

HAVE I GOT THE SYMPTOMS?

Although there often no symptoms, the following can be signs of the infection:
- Discharge from the vagina
- A frequent need to urinate
- A burning pain while urinating
- Lower abdomen pain.

See your doctor, family planning doctor, or visit a sexual health clinic, where you can be screened for chlamydia if you experience any of the above.

MY TREATMENT OPTIONS

Make sure both you and your partner are treated.
Antibiotics Chlamydia is treated with antibiotics. You will have a follow-up test in 3 to 4 months.

HOW CAN I HELP MYSELF?

Practise safer sex by using condoms, especially if you have many partners. You can buy home testing kits to check for chlamydia, if you need reassurance.

AM I AT RISK?

Chlamydia is a risk at any age, but it's most common in young women aged 15–25. You're at risk if you have unprotected sex or genital contact with an infected partner.

Syphilis

If left untreated, syphilis gradually progresses through three distinct phases. After the early stages, an infected person may show no further symptoms for many years.

WHAT IS IT?

Syphilis is a bacterial infection caught through sexual contact. A sore, called a chancre, is usually the first symptom. Other symptoms (see right) develop a few weeks later, and then often disappear. Third-stage syphilis, which causes widespread damage, may develop up to 20 years later.

WHAT NEXT?

Your doctor will examine you and take a blood sample and a swab of any sore to be sent for testing, or will arrange for this to be done at a sexual health clinic.

MY TREATMENT OPTIONS

Make sure both you and your partner are treated.
Antibiotics Syphilis is treated with antibiotics, given by injection. Ask your doctor about side effects.

HOW CAN I HELP MYSELF?

Use condoms, especially if you have many sexual partners.

HAVE I GOT THE SYMPTOMS?

The initial symptoms include:
- A painless sore on the vulva, anus, tongue, or lips.

Secondary symptoms include:
- Fever and aches and pains
- Rash
- Swollen lymph nodes in the groin
- Hair loss
- Flat warts on the vulva.

Third-stage symptoms include:
- Blindness
- Stroke and heart disease
- Paralysis.

Genital herpes

This disease is caused by the same virus that produces cold sores. Genital herpes, which is one of the most common STIs, tends to recur and needs to be controlled by careful management.

WHAT IS IT?

Herpes is caused by a strain of the herpes simplex virus, which is known as HSV2. A few days after infection, painful blisters may appear on the genitals, together with itching and burning sensations, and a feeling of general ill-health (see below). These symptoms usually disappear in two to three weeks, but the virus remains permanently in the body. This means that further attacks of may occur, and that the infected person can pass on the virus to a partner when suffering an attack. Some people only ever have one attack, while others may have several recurrences. Usually, the symptoms are milder in recurrent attacks and last for a shorter time.

WHAT NEXT?

If you suspect you have herpes, go and see your doctor as soon as possible. He or she will examine your genitals, take a sample of the fluid from the blisters, and send it away for testing. If your symptoms have disappeared, the doctor may take a blood test.

MY TREATMENT OPTIONS

Over-the-counter cold sore medication won't treat genital herpes, so always go to your doctor., who will prescribe the best treatment and will explain any side effects. Make sure your partner is evaluated, too. There are many ways to relieve herpes.
Ointment Anaesthetic ointment on blisters helps pain and itching.
Medication Antiviral medication is used during the initial attack. If you are prone to severe recurrent attacks, you can also take antivirals daily as a preventive measure to reduce the number and severity of the attacks.

HOW CAN I HELP MYSELF?

Bathing the affected area, having cool showers, and wearing loose clothing, as well as taking over-the-counter analgesics, can help relieve the pain and discomfort of blisters. If you have an attack, avoid even protected sex until all the symptoms have gone.

HAVE I GOT THE SYMPTOMS?

The following may occur:
- Painful blisters usually on the vulva but can occur anywhere
- Headache
- Fever and feeling unwell
- Aches and pains
- Swollen lymph nodes in your groin
- A burning sensation while urinating.

See your doctor if you have one or more of these symptoms.

AM I AT RISK?

You're at risk if you have oral or genital contact with an infected partner or partners.

DISPELLING THE HERPES MYTHS

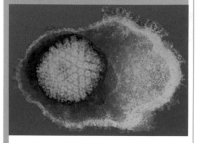

Herpes virus
This common virus infects a cell, then makes a copy of itself so it can go on to infect other cells.

Myth: herpes is forever While it's true that the herpes virus stays in your system, it's not true that outbreaks can't be treated or even prevented altogether. Antiviral drugs can reduce the likelihood of flare-ups from occurring.
Myth: herpes is a condition of promiscuity No it isn't – in fact, many women who catch herpes in the genital area actually have type 1 herpes (exactly the same kind that causes cold sores), which they may have caught through oral sex from their regular partner if he had a cold sore.
Myth: herpes gives you cancer There's no association at all between herpes infections and any type of cancer.

Genital warts

Genital warts are the most common STI in the world. They tend mostly to affect women aged 16 to 25. Treatment for them is simple, but they are stubborn and tend to recur. The infection cannot be cured but it can be controlled.

WHAT ARE THEY?

Genital warts are caused by infection with the human papilloma virus (HPV) (see p366). They grow as soft, painless lumps in and around the entrance to the vagina and anus. You may not realize that you have been infected, as the warts can take up to 18 months to appear. Some people have no symptoms at all. However, even if you have no visible warts, you can still pass on the infection to a sexual partner.

Fortunately, the types of HPV that cause genital warts (types 6 and 11) do not lead to cancer. However, it is essential to get regular cervical smear test to pick up precancerous changes (see p107).

WHAT NEXT?

If you think you may have genital warts, visit your doctor or sexual health clinic for an examination. A diagnosis will be made after a physical examination and you may be tested for other STIs as well.

MY TREATMENT OPTIONS

Don't try to treat genital warts with over-the-counter wart medication, as this will not work. Instead, talk to your doctor about the best treatment option for you with the fewest side effects. You should also make sure your partner is treated. Regardless of the type of treatment you have, genital warts often reappear.

Cream or liquid This kills the skin cells infected with the virus.

Laser treatment If medication does not work, your doctor may suggest that you have the warts removed by laser.

Vaccine It is possible to be vaccinated against contracting the HPV virus. Two vaccines are available, with the UK government recommendation being to use the vaccine Cervarix. Women aged 11 to 26 are advised to have the series of three injections prior to becoming sexually active. It is estimated that women who have the vaccine reduce their chances of developing cervical cancer by about 70 per cent.

HOW CAN I HELP MYSELF?

The main thing you can do to reduce your risk of contracting the HPV virus that causes genital warts, and of preventing the recurrence of warts, is to always practise safer sex with your partner.

HAVE I GOT THE SYMPTOMS?

Warts vary in size and shape from tiny lumps to cauliflower-like growths. They usually:
- Occur singly or in groups on the vulva, inside the vagina, on the cervix, and around the area of the anus (in men, they appear on the anus, the foreskin, and the penis shaft or head)
- Feel itchy.

See your doctor if you are worried that you or your partner may have genital warts.

Abstain If your partner or potential partner has visible genital warts then you should avoid sexual contact. However, as the virus has a long incubation period, it's possible to become infected by a new partner who does not show any signs of the infection, but who is a carrier of the virus.

Use a condom For up to three months after an infection, using a condom every time you have sex can help to prevent reinfection, and also give you protection against other STIs. However, as a condom may not cover all affected areas, it isn't a guarantee of complete protection against genital warts.

AM I AT RISK?

You're at risk if you have sexual or skin-to-skin contact with an infected partner.

"This highly prevalent STI is best avoided by practising safe sex with a new partner, even if he shows no obvious symptoms."

Hepatitis B

Hepatitis, or inflammation of the liver, can occur for a number of reasons. The most common causes are viral infections, of which there are several different types. The hepatitis B virus is spread through sexual contact and exchange of body fluids, including saliva, semen and blood.

WHAT IS IT?

The hepatitis B virus is a blood-borne infection that affects the liver. In most cases, hepatitis B causes a short-term, or acute, infection that may or may not produce symptoms (see right). Hepatitis often clears up within about three months. However, if the liver inflammation lasts for more than six months, it is regarded as a chronic, or long-term, form of the illness, and there may be permanent liver damage.

If you have hepatitis B and are pregnant, you can pass it on to your child while giving birth, so all pregnant mothers are now tested for the infection. Babies are vaccinated immediately after birth against hepatitis B.

WHAT NEXT?

If you think you may be suffering from hepatitis B, then visit your doctor who will carry out a blood test. You may also be given a test to check your liver function.

MY TREATMENT OPTIONS

Talk to your doctor about the best treatment option for you with the fewest side effects.

Lifestyle There's no specific treatment for acute hepatitis but rest and a healthy diet with no alcohol can help.

Medication For chronic hepatitis, antiviral medication may help to prevent more liver damage.

HAVE I GOT THE SYMPTOMS?

There may be no symptoms; if they do develop they can include:
- Mild fever
- Aches and pains
- Tiredness
- Loss of appetite
- Nausea and/or vomiting and diarrhoea.

See your doctor if you have symptoms that concern you.

Vaccination You should be vaccinated if you are at risk.

HOW CAN I HELP MYSELF?

Practise safer-sex methods and avoid anything, such as tattooing and injecting drugs, that may involve dirty needles.

AM I AT RISK?

You're at risk of contracting hepatitis B if you take part in unprotected sex or share needles with an infected partner, or if you have an open wound and come into contact with infected blood. If you are planning to travel to a country where hepatitis B is common, or to stay in a high-risk area for more than three months, then you may be at an increased risk through taking part in contact sports, and having medical or dental treatment where the equipment may not be sterile.

WHAT HAPPENS IN HEPATITIS

Hepatitis caused by a viral infection can be acute or chronic. Acute infection comes on suddenly and causes short-term inflammation of the liver. In chronic hepatitis, the inflammation of the liver lasts for six months or more and may continue for several years. For more information on hepatitis, including those forms of the disease that are not spread by sexual contact, see p296.

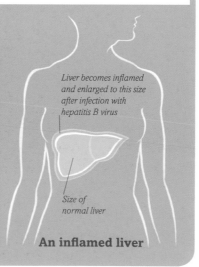

Liver becomes inflamed and enlarged to this size after infection with hepatitis B virus

Size of normal liver

An inflamed liver

Trichomoniasis

Trichomoniasis is a relatively common genital tract infection, which is usually, though not always, transmitted sexually. It's not normally serious and can affect both men and women of any age, but it is often easier to diagnose the condition in women.

WHAT IS IT?

Trichomoniasis is caused by a small organism called *Trichomonas vaginalis* and affects your vagina and urethra (the tube that carries urine from the bladder to the outside). Women's symptoms can start either a few days after infection or can take up to a few weeks to develop. The most easily recognized symptom is a frothy, smelly, yellow vaginal discharge. However, about half of women with the infection don't experience any symptoms at all, so you can be infected and not realize it. The organism may be found when you have your routine smear.

If you're pregnant and are infected, you run a slightly higher risk of having a preterm baby.

WHAT NEXT?

If you suspect that you have trichomoniasis, then you should visit your doctor or sexual health clinic, where a swab will be taken from your vagina for testing. Tests for other STIs may be carried out at the same time.

MY TREATMENT OPTIONS

Trichomoniasis is usually treated very quickly and easily. You should also make sure that your partner is tested and treated if necessary.

Antibiotics This is the usual form of treatment. Most cases are treated with the antibiotic metronidazole (Flagyl), which is very effective. You will need to take it twice a day for five to seven days, or as a single, concentrated dose. However, it may make you feel nauseous and you may vomit. If you vomit, tell your doctor, as it could be that the treatment is not working properly. If you're on the contraceptive pill or patch, and are prescribed metronidazole, check with your doctor to see if your contraception will be affected. If so, you'll need to take extra precautions. If you are pregnant, you will be unable to take the single concentrated dose of metronidazole.

Follow-up You may need a follow-up test if you still have symptoms after finishing the full course of antibiotics.

Avoid alcohol You must not drink alcohol while you are taking metronidazole or for at least 48 hours after finishing the course. Drinking alcohol while you are taking this medicine can cause severe side effects.

HOW CAN I HELP MYSELF?

Abstain from sex while taking medication, or at the very least use a condom, to avoid reinfection.

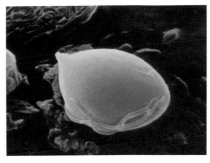

Trichomoniasis
The micro-organism that causes trichomoniasis infects cells in the vagina and urethra.

AM I AT RISK?

You are at risk if you have unprotected sex with an infected partner.

HAVE I GOT THE SYMPTOMS?

There may be no symptoms, but you could have:
- Inflammation and itching around the vagina
- Profuse, greenish-yellow, and smelly vaginal discharge
- A burning sensation when urinating
- Discomfort during intercourse
- Pain in the lower abdomen.

See your doctor, or alternatively visit your sexual health clinic if you experience any of the above symptoms.

"Always practise safe sex and use a condom."

HIV infection and AIDS

Worldwide, human immunodeficiency virus (HIV), which can lead to acquired immunodeficiency syndrome (AIDS), is one of the most feared diseases of modern times. However, early diagnosis and access to the right treatment can greatly improve the outlook of people who are infected with HIV.

HAVE I GOT THE SYMPTOMS?

The first symptoms of HIV infection usually appear within six weeks and may include:

- Fever
- Tiredness
- Aches and pains
- Rash across the chest.

The infection goes into a dormant phase and you may feel well. But if left untreated, HIV lowers the immune system and the following may develop:

- Weight loss
- Night sweats
- Persistent diarrhoea
- Persistent swollen glands
- Herpes infection, such as cold sores, for example
- Yeast infections of the mouth and vagina, such as thrush.

Once the immune system has been severely damaged, which can take up to 10 years, infections and cancers occur:

- Tuberculosis
- Pneumonia
- Kaposi's sarcoma (a form of skin cancer)
- Lymphoma (cancer of the lymph nodes).

WHAT IS IT?

HIV attacks the immune system, weakening the body's resistance to illnesses such as infections or cancers. HIV infection can be transmitted via blood, semen, vaginal fluids, and, to a certain degree, through breast milk. The virus enters the body more easily by anal sex than by vaginal intercourse. Once the virus is in the bloodstream, it enters special white blood cells called CD4 cells, which are responsible for fighting infections. HIV destroys these cells rapidly. Although the body can replace the CD4 cells, eventually the virus reduces the numbers of cells to such an extent that the immune system starts to fail seriously, which leads to the development of AIDS. Particular illnesses are associated with AIDS, and a person is said to have AIDS if she or he has developed one of them (see box, left.)

WHAT NEXT?

If you think you've been exposed to HIV infection, you should visit your doctor who will carry out a blood test to check for antibodies against the virus. If the test is negative, you may be advised to take another test three months later, as the antibodies can take a long time to develop. If the test is positive:

- You'll be referred to an HIV clinic, where you'll receive counselling and treatment from healthcare professionals
- You must tell your sexual partner, who should also be tested for the virus
- You'll need a smear at least once or twice a year, as HIV positive women are at high risk of developing cervical cancer.

MY TREATMENT OPTIONS

The HIV virus can change its form (mutate) fairly easily. This means

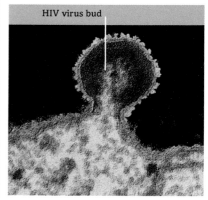

HIV virus
This HIV virus particle is "budding" out from the human body cell in which it has developed. Now it will infect other cells.

AM I AT RISK?

Anyone who has unprotected sex, especially with many different partners, may be at risk of contracting HIV. People at particularly high risk are those who have unprotected anal sex, or use intravenous drugs and share or reuse needles. Infection through contaminated blood transfusions is now rare as blood is always carefully screened.

that no vaccine to prevent HIV has been successfully developed because every time the virus mutates a different drug has to be used against it.

Medication Fortunately, over the last 15 years, antiviral drugs have been developed to keep HIV-infected people from progressing on to AIDS. In many people, these

drugs have reduced the virus to almost invisible levels in the body. Some of the drugs do have side effects, such as nausea.

However, antivirals are not a miracle cure for HIV, and can only help keep the disease under control. In many countries, people have no access to such medication.

HOW CAN I HELP MYSELF?

Most importantly, anyone diagnosed with HIV should always use a condom during sex (see box, right). Eating well, getting plenty of exercise, and stopping smoking, drinking, or taking drugs can help to improve general health.

PREGNANCY AND HIV-INFECTED WOMEN

In a pregnant woman, HIV is readily transmitted through the bloodstream to the unborn child. However, over the years, HIV

medications have progressed and are now extremely effective in preventing HIV from reaching the baby. In all parts of the world, it has been suggested that pregnant women should be tested routinely for HIV infection; and in many countries, HIV testing for pregnant women is already compulsory.

AVOIDING HIV INFECTIONS

Prevention is difficult, but blood testing for HIV is reliable and readily available. If you have a new partner, it is usually recommended that you do not have sex until he or she has had a negative HIV test.

- Even if a new partner has a negative HIV test, you should use a condom, because it can take up to three months after infection for a test to reveal a positive result
- Avoid having sex with many different partners
- Never share a needle with anyone to inject drugs
- Avoid practices such as tattooing unless you are sure that only sterile, disposable needles will be used
- If you're a healthcare provider and infect yourself with an HIV positive needle, or if you're sexually assaulted by an HIV positive person, you should take HIV medications immediately to reduce your chances of becoming infected.

HIV VIRUS PARTICLE

An HIV particle has an outer membrane with 72 tiny protein spikes and two strands of genetic material – RNA – in the core.

A spike attaches to a body cell and the virus enters the cell. Here the virus reproduces. The new viruses break out to infect other cells.

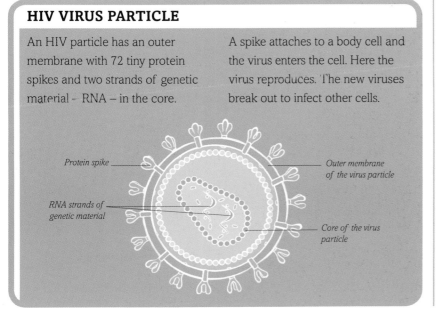

Protein spike

RNA strands of genetic material

Outer membrane of the virus particle

Core of the virus particle

Infertility

Once you've decided the time is right to have a child, it's easy to start worrying if you don't become pregnant straight away. But many couples take a few months to conceive, especially if they are over age 30, when fertility declines. If you have problems conceiving, either you or your partner may need help.

HAVE I GOT THE SYMPTOMS?

If you have not conceived after trying for a year, see your doctor to discuss possible problems.

WHAT IS IT?

If a couple fails to conceive after a year of having regular intercourse without contraception, they may be said to have a problem with fertility. The cause may be found in either the man or the woman – the chances are roughly equal. Some couples have no difficulty conceiving their first child, but encounter problems when they try for another child. This is known as "secondary infertility".

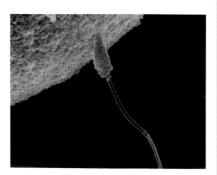

A sperm fertilizing an egg
Out of an ejaculation of semen containing up to 300 million sperm, just one sperm fertilizes a ripe egg in the fallopian tube.

There are many reasons why it may be difficult to conceive. The causes can include the following:

- Failure to ovulate, when no eggs are released by the ovaries
- Tubal infertility, where the fallopian tubes are blocked or damaged and the egg can't travel to meet a sperm
- Cervical mucus that destroys the sperm or is too thick for the sperm to pass through
- Sperm factors, such as too few sperm, abnormally shaped sperm, or sperm that fail to swim well. Blocked sperm ducts are another cause of infertility but this condition is rare.

WHAT NEXT?

It's advisable to see your doctor if you haven't conceived after a year of trying. However, if you are over 35 you should seek advice after six months. This is because the older you get, the less fertile both you and your partner become. You may have the following investigations:

- A blood test to check your levels of the hormone progesterone. If levels are high this means you are ovulating
- A check on your luteinizing (LH) and follicle-stimulating (FSH)

REASONS FOR INFERTILITY

Both male and female factors account for fertility problems, with the causes split fairly equally between the sexes.

Other causes

Ovulation problems

Problems with the sperm

Problems with the fallopian tubes

Cervical mucus problems

hormones, usually at the beginning of each menstrual cycle. These blood tests exclude the possibility that your ovaries have failed prematurely. The relationship between the LH and the FSH can suggest that you may have PCOS (see p95).

- A laparoscopy (see p98) may be carried out to examine your fallopian tubes, ovaries, and uterus. This can reveal such problems as endometriosis (see p101), scar tissue, or pelvic inflammatory disease (see p98)

During a laparoscopy, dye can be injected through the cervix to see if it spills through the fallopian tubes. This will show if the tubes are blocked or not.

- A hysterosalpingogram (HSG) test. This simple X-ray test also checks that your fallopian tubes aren't blocked. As in a laparoscopy (see left), dye is used to confirm the tubes are not blocked

- An analysis of your partner's semen to check the number and appearance of his sperm, and to see how fast they are moving. The test also checks the seminal fluid to see if it's thin enough and has the right acid balance for the sperm.

If the test results are all negative, your problems will be described as "unexplained infertility". The good news is that about half of couples with unexplained infertility will eventually conceive on their own. But if the tests reveal any possible problems, then your doctor will refer you to a fertility specialist.

MY TREATMENT OPTIONS

A number of treatments are available for infertility.

Clomiphene These pills can help improve ovulation.

Hormone injections If clomiphene doesn't work, you may be given injections of follicle-stimulating and luteinizing hormone to "kick start" the ovaries.

Surgery If your fallopian tubes are blocked, your doctors may suggest surgery to unblock them.

IN VITRO FERTILIZATION (IVF)

IVF is one of the most widely used fertility treatments. In this procedure, eggs are removed from the woman and mixed with her partner's sperm in a laboratory so that fertilization takes place outside the body. One or more fertilized eggs are then returned to the uterus. If all goes well and an egg implants in the lining of the uterus, a normal pregnancy should follow. Success rates depend on both the woman and the centre she is attending. Your doctor should be able to give you a success rate figure for three cycles of IVF at his or her centre.

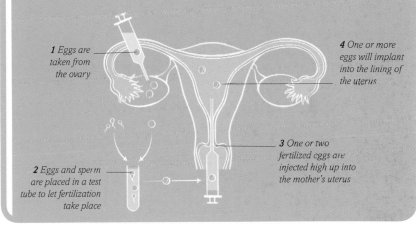

1 Eggs are taken from the ovary

2 Eggs and sperm are placed in a test tube to let fertilization take place

3 One or two fertilized eggs are injected high up into the mother's uterus

4 One or more eggs will implant into the lining of the uterus

In vitro fertilization (IVF) Some doctors recommend this treatment (see box above).

Improving your partner's sperm If your partner's sperm is the problem, he may be advised to make lifestyle changes such as stopping smoking, taking regular exercise, wearing loose-fitting underwear, and eating food that is rich in vitamins A, D and E.

- If the sperm can't be improved, a sperm may be injected directly into an egg. This is done outside the uterus and the embryo is put back into the woman's body using IVF (see box above).

Egg and sperm donation If other options fail, egg and sperm donation might be your next step.

HOW CAN I HELP MYSELF?

You can buy a kit that detects changes in your hormone levels, which indicate if you are ovulating. This information will also tell you the best time to have sex.

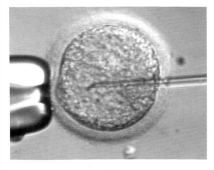

IVF
A human egg being fertilized by IVF. A micro-needle on the right injects the sperm while the egg is being held steady by a pipette on the left.

Complications of pregnancy

During the nine months of pregnancy, every woman worries about the things that could go wrong. However, for the majority of women – and their developing babies, too – all goes according to plan and without problems from conception to birth. But occasionally, complications do arise.

Miscarriage

Miscarriage occurs in about 15 per cent of all pregnancies, most commonly during the first 12 weeks. Having a miscarriage doesn't mean that you can't have a successful pregnancy next time.

WHAT IS IT?

A miscarriage is the spontaneous loss of a baby before 24 weeks. There are a number of factors that may cause miscarriage, including genetic abnormalities in the fetus or a disorder of the uterus such as fibroids, but often the reason is unknown. You may be at increased risk if you are:
- Aged over 35
- A heavy smoker
- Pregnant with twins or more.

If you've had a miscarriage, the emotional impact can be devastating and it is natural to feel grief. You may be advised to see a counsellor to help you come to terms with your loss. Although you can start having sex again once symptoms such as bleeding (see right) have cleared up, your doctor will probably advise you to wait for a couple of menstrual cycles before trying to conceive again.

WHAT NEXT?

If you experience bleeding during early pregnancy it may not mean you are having a miscarriage, but you should still see your doctor, who can arrange for an ultrasound scan to see if the pregnancy is continuing normally. From six weeks gestation, if all is well, it is usually possible to see a heart beat. The ultrasound scan can also exclude ectopic pregnancy (see opposite).

MY TREATMENT OPTIONS

In a complete miscarriage, the fetus is expelled naturally from the uterus. Provided the bleeding has stopped within 7 to 10 days, you'll need no further treatment.

Surgery If you have persistent or heavy bleeding you may need a hysteroscopy (see p100), usually performed under a general anaesthetic, to clear the uterus of any remaining pregnancy tissue.

Tests If you have three or more miscarriages in a row, your doctor will carry out some tests to find out if there's a specific cause.

HOW CAN I HELP MYSELF?

You should keep an eye on your weight as the miscarriage rate is higher in women who are seriously underweight or overweight. You can also take folic acid. This is recommended for any woman who is trying to conceive.

> **HAVE I GOT THE SYMPTOMS?**
>
> The most common symptoms of a miscarriage are:
> - Vaginal bleeding
> - Cramping pains in the lower abdominal area
> - Sudden cessation of pregnancy symptoms such as sore breasts and nausea.
>
> **Call your doctor** if you experience bleeding and/or cramping. If the bleeding is very heavy you should go to hospital straight away.

"As soon as you are ready, both emotionally and physically, you can start to try for another baby, usually after a couple of cycles."

Ectopic pregnancy

About 1 per cent of all pregnancies end in the first few weeks because of a complication known as ectopic pregnancy. The condition needs urgent diagnosis and medical attention.

WHAT IS IT?

An ectopic pregnancy occurs when the egg implants outside the uterus, usually in the fallopian tube, but sometimes in the ovary, abdominal space, or cervix. In many cases the pregnancy results in a spontaneous miscarriage. However, if an ectopic pregnancy continues undiagnosed it can rupture the fallopian tube and lead to a life-threatening situation.

An ectopic pregnancy is quite difficult to detect at first, as the symptoms are usually the same as for a normal early pregnancy, such as nausea and vomiting, tender breasts, frequently going to the toilet, and missed periods. But if you experience any bleeding and a sharp and stabbing pain in your abdomen, especially on one side, then it may suggest an ectopic pregnancy and you should see your doctor immediately.

Any woman can be at risk of having an ectopic pregnancy, but you may be at an increased risk if you've had:

- Pelvic inflammatory disease (PID, see p98)
- Endometriosis (see p101)
- Chlamydia (see p115)
- Pelvic surgery
- A previous ectopic pregnancy.

WHAT NEXT?

Your doctor may do a urine test to confirm that you're pregnant. If he or she thinks you may have an ectopic pregnancy you will have a ultrasound scan to investigate your uterus and fallopian tubes.

HAVE I GOT THE SYMPTOMS?

- Lower abdominal pain on one side
- Vaginal bleeding
- Shoulder tip pain.

See your doctor immediately if you suspect an ectopic pregnancy. If it is left untreated it can be life-threatening.

MY TREATMENT OPTIONS

As soon as an ectopic pregnancy is diagnosed, action is usually taken. Your doctor will explain what needs to be done and discuss the side effects:

Medication If the ectopic pregnancy is diagnosed before the fallopian tube ruptures, you may be given the drug methotrexate to stop the pregnancy from proceeding. The embryonic tissues will be absorbed by your body.

Surgery If the fallopian tube ruptures, you must have surgery immediately to remove the ectopic pregnancy. If the tube is damaged it will need to be repaired or, if repair is not possible, completely removed. You'll still have a good chance of having a normal pregnancy with one fallopian tube.

HOW CAN I HELP MYSELF?

If you get pregnant with an IUD in place, it is much likelier to be an ectopic pregnancy than under normal circumstances, so call your doctor immediately to rule out an ectopic pregnancy.

ECTOPIC PREGNANCY

Once an egg is fertilized it usually passes down the fallopian tube into the uterus, where it implants into tissue and begins to develop. In an ectopic pregnancy, however, the fertilized egg implants itself in tissue outside the uterus, most often in the fallopian tube. This may happen because the egg can't reach the uterus, perhaps due to a blockage in the fallopian tube.

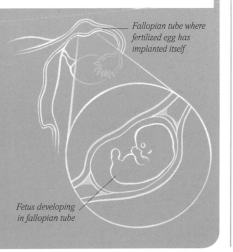

Fallopian tube where fertilized egg has implanted itself

Fetus developing in fallopian tube

Chromosomal abnormalities

In each cell of our body there are thread-like structures called chromosomes. These are made up of genes that control how cells work. Abnormalities in chromosomes or a faulty gene may result in a disorder in the fetus.

WHAT IS IT?

We each have 23 pairs of chromosomes. Sometimes eggs and sperm carry the incorrect number of chromosomes, or a defective gene, which causes abnormalities in a developing baby. The most common genetic disorder is Down's syndrome.

HAVE I GOT THE SYMPTOMS?

Only special tests, either on the fetus or on a baby after birth, can reveal chromosomal disorders.

Babies born with chromosomal abnormalities may have only mild problems and many lead normal lives. Others need life-long care.

WHAT NEXT?

When you meet your midwife she will discuss with you what tests are available to you to look for chromosomal abnormalities.

These range from simple blood tests to amniocentesis (see below).

MY TREATMENT OPTIONS

If the tests are abnormal you will be offered counselling in order to help you decide how best to proceed with your pregnancy.

HOW CAN I HELP MYSELF?

Joining a family support group can provide help and advice.

AMNIOCENTESIS TEST

Amniocentesis is a procedure used to obtain a small sample of the amniotic fluid that surrounds the baby in the uterus. This is carried out around weeks 16 to 18 of your pregnancy. Cells shed from the fetus into this fluid are tested for chromosomal or genetic disorders. The test carries a small risk of miscarriage.

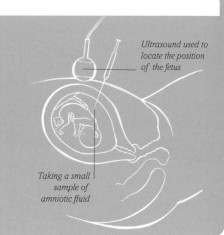

Ultrasound used to locate the position of the fetus

Taking a small sample of amniotic fluid

Incompetent cervix

This complication, which is unlikely to occur before about the 14th week of pregnancy, can be a cause of miscarriage.

WHAT IS IT?

The cervix – the neck of the uterus – normally stays tightly closed during pregnancy to keep the fetus in the uterus, and opens during childbirth. An incompetent cervix is one that starts to open too early.

Often there are no warning symptoms, so the fetus can just fall out. You may be at an increased risk of this disorder if you've had:
- Multiple dilatations and curettage procedures (D & Cs)
- Cervical or uterine surgery.

WHAT NEXT?

If you do experience such a miscarriage, you'll be monitored closely during your next pregnancy

HAVE I GOT THE SYMPTOMS?

Usually there are few symptoms. Some women have a blood-stained, watery vaginal discharge.

with pelvic examinations and ultrasound scans.

MY TREATMENT OPTIONS

If your cervix is seen to be opening, your doctor can place a stitch like a purse string around it, to sew it shut (a procedure called cerclage). It is carried out between 12 and 14 weeks gestation. The stitches are cut out late in pregnancy to allow delivery.

HOW CAN I HELP MYSELF?
If you have a cerclage you should avoid strenuous activity and rest as much as possible for the remainder of your pregnancy.

INCOMPETENT CERVIX

An incompetent cervix can be successfully held shut with stitches to keep the baby in the uterus. The stitches are left in place until just before the end of pregnancy. They are removed, without the need for an anaesthetic, to allow for a normal vaginal birth.

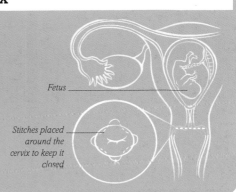

Fetus

Stitches placed around the cervix to keep it closed

Gestational diabetes

Diabetes can develop temporarily when you're pregnant. This is called gestational diabetes and usually occurs in late pregnancy. If you are already diabetic (see p320) and are contemplating pregnancy, then it's important to ensure that your condition is as well managed as possible beforehand.

WHAT IS IT?
Gestational diabetes occurs when there is too much glucose in your blood and your body cannot produce enough insulin to control it. This can happen in pregnancy because hormones produced by the placenta counteract the effect of insulin. You may be at an increased risk of developing gestational diabetes if you have a family history of diabetes, you are an older mother, or if you are very overweight. Some women who have gestational diabetes later go on to develop permanent diabetes.

WHAT NEXT?
All pregnant women have regular urine tests at their antenatal appointments to check their glucose levels. If you have risk factors (see above), you will be given a glucose screen test between 24 and 28 weeks – you have a sweet glucose drink and your blood glucose level is measured an hour later. If that shows elevated blood glucose, you will be given further tests.

MY TREATMENT OPTIONS
If you have gestational diabetes, reducing the sugar in your diet and eating more carbohydrates and fibre is usually recommended.

"Gestational diabetes usually disappears after childbirth."

HAVE I GOT THE SYMPTOMS?

Often, there are no specific symptoms but you may notice:
- Constant thirst
- A need to urinate more frequently
- Extreme tiredness.
See your doctor as soon as possible to have your glucose levels checked.

Tests Your doctor will regularly test your blood glucose levels. You may also be asked to carry out blood and urine tests yourself at home.
Insulin injections If your blood glucose levels remain high, you may need daily insulin injections. Your doctor or nurse will teach you how to do this correctly.

HOW CAN I HELP MYSELF?
Healthy eating, regular exercise, and keeping your weight down will help to stop you from developing permanent diabetes later in life.

Pre-eclampsia (toxaemia)

This potentially serious condition may affect 1 in 8 pregnancies by the end of the third trimester. The causes of pre-eclampsia are not completely understood, but the disorder can affect both the mother and her baby.

WHAT IS IT?

In pre-eclampsia, a pregnant woman develops high blood pressure, together with fluid retention and sometimes protein in the urine. The condition may be linked to problems with the placenta, but doctors are still uncertain. If pre-eclampsia is not treated, it may develop into eclampsia, a highly dangerous condition that can cause convulsions and coma, and at worst be a threat to life.

WHAT NEXT?

Pre-eclampsia is likely to be diagnosed during your routine check-ups, when your blood pressure is taken and your urine is tested as a matter of course. If you have severe symptoms (see box, right) you will probably be admitted to hospital for observation. If your symptoms are mild, your doctor may just recommend that you have more frequent check-ups than normal

MY TREATMENT OPTIONS

If you still have several weeks of pregnancy to go, your doctor may order bed rest, possibly in hospital. In severe cases your doctor will advise you to have your baby delivered. Pre-eclampsia usually disappears after delivery.

HAVE I GOT THE SYMPTOMS?

This condition is usually characterized by:
- High blood pressure
- Protein in your urine
- Oedema (swelling of tissues, often in the feet and ankles)
- Disturbed vision and headaches
- Pains in your stomach, sometimes with nausea or vomiting.

See your doctor or midwife immediately if you suddenly develop the last three symptoms.

HOW CAN I HELP MYSELF?

If you only have mild pre-eclampsia, you can try resting in bed as much as possible, while lying on your side.

Abruption

This disorder is a common cause of bleeding in late pregnancy. Abruption can be dangerous to both mother and baby and calls for swift medical treatment.

WHAT IS IT?

Normally, after your baby is born, the placenta, or afterbirth, peels off the wall of the uterus, and is delivered through the vagina in the final stage of labour. However, occasionally, the placenta partially separates from the uterus wall before delivery. This causes

bleeding, which may be vaginal but can also be concealed inside the uterus. If the bleeding is very heavy, this is an emergency situation that needs immediate attention in hospital. What causes abruption of the placenta is still unknown, but high blood pressure, smoking, excessive alcohol drinking, and cocaine usage may all increase a woman's risk.

WHAT NEXT?

Your doctor will usually make a diagnosis of your condition based on your history and by carrying out a physical examination.

HAVE I GOT THE SYMPTOMS?

The symptoms may include:
- Dark red vaginal bleeding
- Severe abdominal pain
- Uterine contractions.

See your doctor immediately if you think you have any of these symptoms.

MY TREATMENT OPTIONS

The treatment depends on the amount of bleeding and whether the fetus is showing signs of distress. If the placenta has separated only a small amount and bleeding is slight, bed rest may stop the bleeding and allow your pregnancy to continue as normal. If the condition is serious, the baby needs to be delivered either vaginally if the labour is advanced or by Caesarean section. You may need to have a blood transfusion to replace lost blood.

HOW CAN I HELP MYSELF?

Do a lifestyle check and cut out anything, such as smoking, that could put your pregnancy at risk.

WHAT HAPPENS IN ABRUPTION

The placenta contains many blood vessels and if it pulls away from the wall of the uterus before the end of pregnancy, vaginal bleeding may be very heavy. Sometimes there is no obvious bleeding, because the blood gets trapped between the placenta and the wall of the uterus. This is called a "concealed" abruption, which can cause severe pains in the abdomen as the blood continues to collect.

Placenta detached from wall of uterus

Bleeding from blood vessels of placenta

Blood flowing through cervix

Premature delivery

Babies born before the 37th week of pregnancy are considered to be premature. Provided these early babies are normally developed for their age, they often do very well with special care.

WHAT IS IT?

Sometimes, a woman goes into labour weeks before her baby is due. The cause of premature labour is often unknown, although in some cases there is a link to lifestyle factors such as smoking, drug abuse, and excess alcohol drinking. Occasionally, the membranes surrounding the baby rupture early, which can be caused by an infection in the pelvic area.

Women expecting more than one baby also have a high chance of going into premature labour.

WHAT NEXT?

If you start getting contractions or your waters break, you'll be admitted to hospital where they will carry out some tests and monitor you carefully.

MY TREATMENT OPTIONS

If your baby is still so immature that birth would be risky, you may be given intravenous drugs to stop the contractions, and you will have to rest in bed. If the birth is imminent, you'll be given steroid injections, which help to prepare

HAVE I GOT THE SYMPTOMS?

The symptoms may include:
- Regular contractions
- Breaking of the waters
- Vaginal bleeding.

See your doctor or midwife at once if you think you may be in premature labour.

the baby's immature lungs for the outside world. Often, premature babies are delivered normally through the vagina. However if the baby appears to be distressed or is in the breech position, your doctor may suggest a Caesarean section.

HOW CAN I HELP MYSELF?

You can reduce your risk of premature labour, by following a healthy diet, exercising regularly, stopping smoking if you are a smoker, and not taking drugs.

"If you don't have an infection in your uterus and the baby is doing well, then you will be given medication to stop the contractions."

Placenta previa

This is an abnormal positioning of the placenta that is potentially dangerous to mother and baby. However, careful monitoring usually keeps the situation under control and the baby is usually born with no ill effects.

WHAT IS IT?

In early pregnancy it is not unusual for the placenta to be placed low in the uterus. As the pregnancy progresses, and the uterus expands, the placenta usually repositions itself near the top of the uterus. It is then delivered after the baby in the final phase of labour. In placenta previa, the placenta remains low in the uterus throughout pregnancy and may cover part or all of the cervix (see box below). This condition can cause a lot of bleeding before or during delivery of the baby.

You may be at an increased risk of developing placenta previa if:

- You've had previous surgery on your uterus, including a Caesarean section
- You've had uterine fibroids or surgery to remove fibroids
- You are over age 35
- You have had several previous pregnancies
- You are expecting more than one baby.

WHAT NEXT?

Placenta previa is usually first diagnosed during a routine ultrasound scan. You will then be monitored to see if the placenta migrates upwards in your uterus as your pregnancy progresses. If you experience sudden, unexpected bleeding, you may have to go into hospital immediately for observation or treatment.

MY TREATMENT OPTIONS

Your treatment depends on the severity of the bleeding and how far your pregnancy has progressed.
Bed rest If you have had light bleeding then you will be advised to rest in bed and not to do any vigorous activities, including having sex. If the bleeding has been heavy, then you will need to be admitted into hospital.
Caesarean section If the bleeding is very heavy or won't stop, then you may need to have your baby delivered immediately. You may also need to have a blood transfusion to replace lost blood.

Caesarean section is sometimes the only delivery option if you have placenta previa, regardless of the severity of the condition. Even if your pregnancy has been proceeding without any other problems, you are likely to be delivered by Caesarean at 39 weeks or before. Giving birth vaginally, even if the placenta is not completely blocking the cervix, carries a high risk of causing uncontrollable bleeding.

HOW CAN I HELP MYSELF?

There is nothing you can do to prevent placenta previa. If it has been diagnosed, you need to stay alert for any signs of bleeding.

HAVE I GOT THE SYMPTOMS?

The most common symptom is:
- Vaginal bleeding, ranging from spotting to heavy blood loss, with no abdominal pain.

See your doctor or midwife immediately if you start to have bleeding at any time during pregnancy. If you have severe bleeding, your baby may need to be delivered straight away.

PLACENTA PREVIA

There are three types of placenta previa: where the placenta covers the whole of the cervix as shown below; where the placenta covers only part of the cervix; and where the placenta is located just near the edge of the cervix.

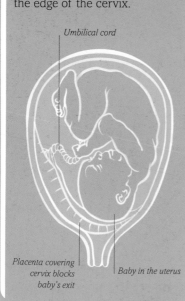

Umbilical cord

Placenta covering cervix blocks baby's exit

Baby in the uterus

Multiple births

If you are expecting more than one baby, you may be at a slightly higher risk of problems than women expecting just the one. However, your antenatal care team will make sure that you have any extra attention you need.

WHAT IS IT?

Multiple births can mean twins, triplets, and, rarely, even more. The babies may be either identical (produced from one fertilized egg that splits) or non-identical (produced when separate eggs are fertilized by different sperm). Some multiple pregnancies happen naturally, and may run in families. However, increasingly, the conception of twins or more is due to the use of treatments for infertility (see pp122–3). These procedures result in more than one egg at a time reaching maturity and being released from the ovary.

WHAT NEXT?

Multiple pregnancies are diagnosed by an ultrasound scan in early pregnancy. Usually the babies can be seen by the end of the second month. The chances are that your pregnancy will go well, but because of its complexity you may be at an increased risk of:
- High blood pressure
- Diabetes (see p127)
- Pre-eclampsia (see p128)
- Abruption (see p128)
- Premature labour (see p129)

Throughout your pregnancy you'll be monitored very closely and possibly put under the care of a specialist in multiple births. You will have more frequent check-ups and scans than usual, especially in

the later stages of pregnancy, to make sure that the growth and position of the babies are normal.

HAVE I GOT THE SYMPTOMS?

If you are carrying more than one baby you may:
- Get lots of morning sickness
- Look extra large for your dates
- Feel tired but unable to sleep
- Rapidly gain weight in the first trimester

See your doctor if you think that the symptoms of early pregnancy are worse than you would have expected.

MY TREATMENT OPTIONS

Most multiple babies are delivered early, often by Caesarean section. The vaginal birth of twins is possible in many cases, depending on their positions (see box left).

HOW CAN I HELP MYSELF?

If you are pregnant with more than one baby you need to make sure your body can cope with the strain:
Eat healthily (see pp52–5) Eat more, for your developing babies.
Increase your calcium intake Eat calcium-rich foods, such as dairy products (see p55 and p262).
Take iron supplements to prevent anaemia.
Exercise Avoid strenuous physical activity after 24 weeks. Walking or swimming may be fine, but check with your doctor.
Rest Get as much rest as you can.

DELIVERY OF TWINS

In a twin birth, if the baby nearest the birth canal is lying head downwards, you may be able to try for a natural (vaginal) delivery. A second baby lying head downwards is also likely to arrive without complications less than 30 minutes after the first. If the second baby is in the breech position (bottom first), a vaginal delivery is usually possible if the first baby has been delivered vaginally. You may be given an ultrasound scan during labour to check the babies' positions.

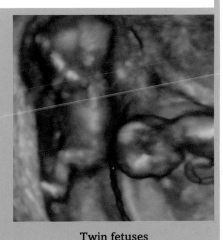

Twin fetuses
This coloured 3-D ultrasound scan shows non-identical twin fetuses at 16 weeks. Each baby has its own placenta.

Contraception

Many different contraceptives are now available and some are more reliable than others. Usually, the main responsibility for contraception falls on the woman. When deciding which method to use, you need to take various things into consideration, including your lifestyle, relationships, and any health issues.

NATURAL METHODS

Natural family planning This involves identifying your body's natural fertility signs, such as changes in your temperature and cervical mucus, on each day of your menstrual cycle, so you avoid sex when you are most fertile. When used correctly it may be effective, but is best used if you are in a long-term relationship and don't mind having an unintended pregnancy.

Advantages
- No hormones or devices involved
- No side effects
- Can be used to plan a pregnancy.

Disadvantages
- No protection against STIs (see pp114–21)
- Requires a regular menstrual cycle
- Must be taught by a professional
- Daily records must be kept
- Not very reliable.

Withdrawal Your partner withdraws his penis before ejaculating. As sperm can leak out beforehand, this method is not reliable.

BARRIER METHODS

Condoms have been available for many years and although they are not 100 per cent perfect, they are reasonably effective for preventing pregnancy and protecting against STIs. There are now two types of condoms, male and female. The male condom is usually made from latex, a form of rubber, and fits over an erect penis. Its effectiveness rates range from 88–95 per cent; of course, this assumes that a couple use the method correctly.

A male condom must be used early in sexual activity: the first drop of semen, which can appear during foreplay, contains millions of sperm that can result in a pregnancy.

The female condom, made from polyurethane, is placed in the vagina. If used correctly, it is as effective as a male condom.

Advantages
- Protection against pregnancy
- Protection against STIs
- No side effects
- Easily available and used only when having intercourse.

Disadvantages
- Can split or slip off during intercourse
- Some people are allergic to latex
- Can only be used once.

Intra-uterine devices (IUDs) or coils, and Intra-uterine system (IUS) IUDs are small T-shaped devices. The old type were made of copper and were called Copper Ts. Nova Ts and other brands are now used. They prevent sperm from travelling up into the fallopian tubes to reach the egg. Inserted into your uterus by your doctor, an IUD stays in place for several years.

An IUS – commonly called Mirena – is a newer, progesterone-coated plastic device. The progesterone is slowly released and deactivates the sperm as they enter the uterus so they cannot travel up the fallopian tubes. An IUS lasts for five years. Like an IUD, an IUS is inserted into your uterus by your doctor. Your doctor will review your medical history before prescribing any hormonal contraception. Do not have one inserted if there's any chance that you may be pregnant.

Advantages
- Your periods are lighter, or stop, although IUDs are associated with heavier periods

"Condoms are widely available, and protect against sexually transmitted infections (STIs)."

- Very effective at preventing pregnancy
- Last for several years.

Disadvantages
- Sometimes difficult to insert
- No protection against STIs
- Side effects may occur.

Diaphragms and cervical caps

The diaphragm is a dome-shaped device made from rubber that covers the cervix to prevent sperm from entering the uterus. It is inserted before having intercourse either immediately, or up to two hours beforehand. After intercourse the diaphragm must be left in place for at least six hours, or overnight. It can then be removed, washed, and used again.

Diaphragms are designed to be used with spermicidal creams or gels (see p134). If you have sex more than once with a diaphragm in place, you should add more spermicidal gel into the vagina. If used correctly, their effectiveness ranges from 85–95 per cent.

A cervical cap is somewhat smaller than a diaphragm, and fits right over the cervix. It should be filled with a spermicide prior to use, and may be left in place for several days. Caps are slightly less effective than diaphragms.

Advantages
- Only need to be used while having intercourse
- Easy to use, and no health risks
- May help prevent STIs and cervical cancer
- Reliable against pregnancy if used correctly.

YOUR CONTRACEPTIVE BARRIER METHODS

Some contraceptives are more effective than others. One of the major factors you have to consider is how reliable your preferred method needs to be. With any barrier contraceptives, always use a spermicide as well. If you use a diaphragm or cap, it will need to be checked regularly by your doctor or a nurse to maintain the correct fit

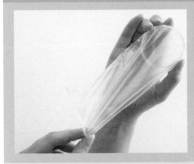

Female condom
Lightly lubricated for easier use, this sheath contains two rings that help to keep it in place inside the walls of the vagina. It must inserted before intercourse, and used only once. Female condoms are thought to be 95% effective if used correctly.

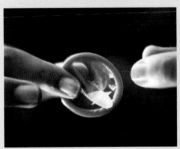

Male condom
This sheath should be unrolled carefully over an erect penis before intercourse (the roll of rubber should be on the outside, not the inside). Any air at the end should be squeezed out. Male condoms can provide reliable contraception if used carefully.

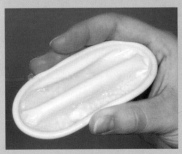

Diaphragm
This dome of thin rubber has a metal spring in the rim. It fits diagonally across the front wall of the vagina so that the cervix is covered during intercourse. The diaphragm is thought to be about 90% effective when used with a spermicide.

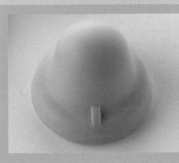

Cervical cap
The cap, smaller and more rigid than a diaphragm, is held in place by suction over the cervix. Caps are usually used by women who can't use diaphragms because of a prolapse or cystitis. Used properly with a spermicide, caps are thought to be 85% effective.

Disadvantages

- May increase risk of cystitis (see pp336–7)
- May increase risk of pelvic inflammatory disease (see p98)
- May cause an allergic reaction
- Diaphragms and caps are available in different sizes, so you'll need to be fitted for the correct size by your doctor or a nurse.

Spermicides There are several chemicals, known as spermicides, that are known to kill sperm, but are not toxic to vaginal tissue. They are available over the counter in a gel, cream, pessary, and foam form. Used in conjunction with barrier methods, they give added contraceptive protection; some experts believe that if a woman inserts a spermicide and a man uses a condom, they will achieve about 97–98 per cent protection from pregnancy. Some experts also believe that spermicides protect against HIV transmission; however, the evidence here is less clear.

Advantages

- Widely available over the counter
- Can increase the effectiveness of diaphragms and caps.

Disadvantages

- Can cause allergic reactions
- No protection against STIs
- Not reliable if used alone in protecting against pregnancy.

HORMONAL CONTRACEPTIVES

Oral contraceptive pills first appeared in the early 1960s, and are one of the most popular forms of contraception. Taken correctly, they

> ## "If taken correctly every day, the pill is thought to be 99 per cent effective."

are 99 per cent effective. There are many types available to women. The combined pills all contain the hormones oestrogen and progestogen, which stop the ovaries from producing eggs. They also thicken the mucus in the cervix, so it is difficult for sperm to reach the egg, and they thin the lining of the uterus so it doesn't accept a fertilized egg readily. Follow your doctors instructions regarding taking your pill. If you forget a pill you probably won't have a failure, but you should consider using a barrier method and following the instructions in your pill packet. If the combined pill is unsuitable, you may be given the progesterone-only pill (mini pill), which contains just progestogen.

Advantages

- Protection against pregnancy
- Your periods are usually regular, lighter, shorter, and less painful
- Some pills can help reduce PMS (see pp92–3)
- May help against acne
- May help with perimenopausal symptoms (see p136).

Disadvantages

- No protection against STIs
- You may have minor side effects when starting them
- Sometimes, serious side effects, such as heart attacks, deep vein thrombosis, or strokes, can occur as a result of taking the pill. Heart attacks and strokes mainly

happen to smokers, which is why older smokers should not take the oral contraceptive pill.

Injections You may prefer an injection of long-acting progestogen. Depo Provera is an injection of a synthetic progesterone, which prevents ovulation and is effective for three months. It is 99 per cent reliable, and only requires you to have an injection four times a year.

Advantages

- Protection against pregnancy for 12 weeks
- You don't have to remember to take daily pills.

Disadvantages

- Possible breakthrough bleeding
- Weight gain.

Implants If you prefer a very low-maintenance hormonal method, you could try an implant, called Implanon. This is a piece of plastic, about the size of a matchstick, that is coated with progestogen and works in a similar way to the injection. It's inserted beneath the skin of your upper arm under local anaesthetic by your doctor or nurse, and provides three years of contraception. Your doctor must take it out either at the end of three years, or if you decide you would like it out sooner.

Advantages

- You don't have to remember to take daily pills.

Disadvantages

- Your periods may be irregular

- You may have mood swings and tender breasts.

Patches Adhesive skin patches have recently become available, and work in much the same way as the combined pill. The patch is attached to a non-hairy part of your skin and lasts for seven days. After three weeks there's a break for a week, and during this time you will have a period.

Advantages
- You only need to remember to replace the patch once a week
- Your periods are usually regular, lighter, and less painful.

Disadvantages
- Visible on the skin and there may be some skin irritation
- Possible breakthrough bleeding.

PERMANENT METHODS

Sterilization If you don't want any more children, then you can be sterilized. During the procedure, which is carried out under general anaesthetic, your fallopian tubes are cut or blocked with rings or clips. There are no changes in your sex hormone levels, or in your femininity afterwards.

Advantages
- Very effective.

Disadvantages
- No protection against STIs
- Not usually reversible
- Not as easy an operation to perform as male sterilization.

Male sterilization This procedure, called vasectomy, is as reliable as female sterilization and carries fewer potential health risks than female sterilization.

YOUR OTHER CONTRACEPTIVE METHODS

If contraceptives are to work effectively, they must be used correctly. Oral contraceptive pills, condoms, and diaphragms, which rely on being taken daily or used immediately before intercourse, will not work if they stay in a drawer, while an IUD, for example, will be effective all the time for up to five years.

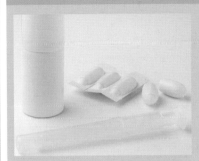

Spermicide
Some spermicides are recommended for use with barrier methods. Others are used alone; they are inserted into the vagina as near to cervix as possible with an applicator, and are about 70% effective if used correctly.

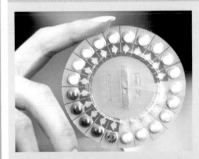

Oral contraceptive pills
If taken at approximately the same time every day, the pill will give maximum contraceptive effect – about 99%. The first course of pills is started on the first day of a period, or on the fifth day after bleeding starts.

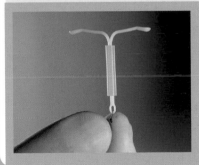

IUS
The progesterone-covered plastic IUS device is inserted into the uterus through the cervix by a doctor or nurse. As long as it is replaced every five years, an IUS is thought to be more than 99% effective.

FEMALE STERILIZATION

A usually permanent method of contraception in which the fallopian tubes are sealed with clips, cut, removed or blocked with plugs. The procedure can be performed laparoscopically (see p98), during another open abdominal procedure, for example Caesarean section, or hysteroscopically (see p100). This method has a very small failure rate.

The menopause

The menopause is when our fertility comes to an end and menstruation stops. It is a perfectly natural part of getting older. This time of life brings many hormonal, physical, mental, and emotional changes, some of which can be very trying. The good news is that plenty of help is available.

HAVE I GOT THE SYMPTOMS?

All women will experience the menopause differently. You may have several symptoms, or you may suffer relatively few. Of all the various symptoms that women experience the most common ones include:

- Hot flushes and night sweats
- Irregular periods and/or heavy bleeding
- An inability to sleep at night
- Vaginal dryness and discomfort during intercourse
- A loss of sex drive
- Bladder problems, such as incontinence and urinary tract infections (e.g. cystitis, see pp336–7)
- Mood swings, depression, and anxiety
- Poor concentration
- Short-term memory problems
- Feeling tired and lethargic
- Dry and itchy skin
- Thinning hair
- Weight gain
- Headaches
- Palpitations.

See your doctor if your symptoms are causing problems.

WHAT IS IT?

The menopause is the stage in your life when your ovaries stop working. Having released an egg each month since you reached puberty, they now cease to do so. At the same time, they also stop producing both oestrogen and progesterone. It is the drop in the level of these hormones in your bloodstream that gives rise to the symptoms of the menopause. As a result of these changes, you stop having periods and can no longer conceive.

The menopause usually happens gradually. A few years before, perhaps as early as your 40s, you may notice that your periods become irregular and bleeding is heavier. This stage is called the perimenopause and usually lasts about four years.

Some women can go through the menopause without experiencing any problems at all, while others suffer from one or more symptoms, such as hot flushes, night sweats, and insomnia (see box, left). Hot flushes are often worse during the perimenopausal stage, but then, within two years of their last menstrual period, many women notice a significant improvement and experience fewer hot flushes.

About 20 per cent of women never experience hot flushes, but if you have had a sudden menopause – for instance, after having your ovaries removed – your symptoms may be more severe. Few women get every menopausal symptom, but certain risk factors, such as smoking and being overweight, can make your symptoms worse. Once you have gone for a full year without having a period, you are said to be "menopausal", or "postmenopausal". Until this time you should continue to use your chosen method of contraception.

If you have gone for a year without a period, but then start bleeding again, you should see your doctor. It's important to make sure there is nothing abnormal happening in your uterus that is causing you to bleed.

Although some women have menopausal symptoms much

"Women experience the menopause differently and you may not suffer from any symptoms at all."

"POSTMENOPAUSAL ZEST"

The anthropologist Margaret Mead described this syndrome, whereby women feel much better once they have passed through the menopause. Particularly in societies that revere older women as wiser and more experienced, menopausal symptoms seem much less bothersome.

Many of the medical disorders and conditions in this book are likely to get better after you have passed through the menopause. These include fibroids (see p99), endometriosis (see p101), and heavy bleeding (see p91). If you have always been worried about getting pregnant, you can now stop worrying and enjoy a hassle-free sex life, which is good news as you can hopefully expect to live 30 or more years beyond the menopause!

earlier than others, the average age of the menopause is about 51. Most women have reached the menopause by the age of 59. There are some exceptions:

- If your ovaries are removed surgically you will have an instantaneous menopause
- If you have chemotherapy or radiotherapy treatment, your periods usually stop, but they normally start again after finishing treatment
- If you smoke you are more likely to go through the menopause about one to two years earlier than non-smokers
- About 1 per cent of women will go through the menopause before the age of 40. If you think that you may be experiencing an early menopause you should visit your doctor for advice.

After the menopause, lower levels of oestrogen and progesterone in your body may increase the likelihood of some long-term health problems. These include:

- Osteoporosis, or bone thinning (see pp260–2)
- Heart disease (see pp158–74)
- Stroke (see p196).

If you are suffering from any unexplained symptoms or feel concerned about these health problems, then talk to your doctor.

WHAT NEXT?

If you are having uncomfortable menopausal symptoms, or want to know if you are still fertile, talk to your doctor. He or she may be able diagnose the menopause by your symptoms, age, and patterns of your period. Sometimes doctors use hormone tests, but none of these is definitive. They include a follicle-stimulating hormone (FSH) test to measure the level of FSH – the hormone that stimulates ovulation – in your blood.

MY TREATMENT OPTIONS

There are many ways to deal with menopausal symptoms, from lifestyle changes to hormone replacement therapy (HRT) and complementary therapies. Your doctor can advise you on the best course of treatment. You may find one particular treatment that suits you, though many women get good results by using a combination of therapies together with self-help measures (see pp139–41).

Hormone replacement therapy (HRT) This is the most effective way to treat the symptoms of the menopause, including hot flushes, night sweats, vaginal dryness, and infections of the urinary tract.

Hormone therapy works by replacing some of the hormones that your body naturally stops producing during and after the menopause. It usually means that you regularly take a combination of oestrogen and progestogen (synthetic progesterone).

IS HRT RIGHT FOR ME?

HRT may be ideal for your particular symptoms and your doctor may suggest that you follow this treatment. However, there are circumstances when HRT isn't suitable, including if:

- You've had breast cancer or cancer of the uterus
- You've had a heart attack or angina
- You've had deep vein thrombosis (DVT)
- You have liver disease
- You have abnormal vaginal bleeding.

If you've had your uterus removed in a hysterectomy (see p103) you can take oestrogen-only HRT. This was commonly offered to any woman until the 1970s, but then it was found that women with a uterus were more likely to develop uterine cancer if they only took oestrogen. To make HRT more closely resemble the natural menstrual process, when the ovaries make both oestrogen and progesterone, progestogen was added, and the increased risk of uterine cancer disappeared.

HRT was extremely popular in the 1980s and 1990s, and was used not only to treat symptoms of the menopause, but also to reduce the risks of heart disease and osteoporosis. However, some studies done in the UK and the US, and released in 2002 and 2003, showed that women who take HRT with the combination of oestrogen and progesterone for more than five years have a slightly increased risk of breast cancer, heart disease, and stroke. Many experts feel that the increased breast cancer risk is greatest after taking HRT for more than five years and that in otherwise healthy women with moderate to severe menopausal symptoms, the benefits may exceed the risks. Women considering HRT should discuss their risks and benefits carefully with their doctors.

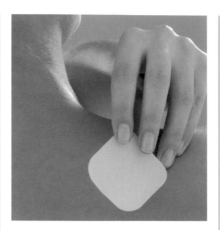

Oestrogen skin patch
The skin patch slowly releases oestrogen into the bloodstream, which helps to relieve menopausal symptoms.

Combined HRT comes in many forms – pills that are taken orally, adhesive skin patches that are placed on your stomach, chest (not breasts), back, upper arm or buttocks, implants, and skin gels. Vaginal creams, pessaries, and vaginal rings, which are applied or inserted into your vagina are very effective if you have problems such as vaginal dryness. All these different forms are also available in many different combinations of oestrogen and progesterone and in different strengths. So if one type of HRT doesn't seem to agree with you, you can try another. There is truly no "one size fits all" for this type of therapy.

There are many benefits, but also some side effects, when taking HRT, so you should discuss these with your doctor before you start the therapy. The benefits include the following:

- Relief from hot flushes and night sweats
- Relief from vaginal dryness
- Improved quality of sleep
- Potential delay in the onset of Alzheimer's disease
- Protection against osteoporosis
- Reduced risk of colon cancer.

You may also suffer from some of the side effects when taking HRT and these include:

- Tender breasts
- Heavier periods
- Water retention
- Weight gain
- Depression
- Irritability.

Taking HRT in the long term is also associated with certain medical conditions; these include the following:

- Breast cancer
- Cancer of the lining of the uterus and ovaries
- Deep vein thrombosis
- Heart disease
- Gallstones
- Stroke.

If you take HRT for a long time these risks increase and some may even continue after stopping treatment. If you do decide to take HRT then you will need to see your doctor for regular check-ups to make sure there are no problems and side effects.

Vaginal therapy If you only have problems with vaginal dryness, topical lubricants and moisturizers are readily available over the counter at pharmacies.

"Hormone therapy is one of the most effective ways to treat menopausal symptoms."

> "Herbal remedies may offer an alternative treatment for relieving the symptoms of the menopause."

However, for many women these really aren't sufficient to relieve dryness and pain with intercourse, so vaginal oestrogen creams, suppositories, and rings are available by prescription. The amount of oestrogen absorbed from vaginal tablets and rings is minuscule; most oncologists will allow their breast cancer patients to use vaginal oestrogens for moisture. If you use HRT patches or oral tablets, you may need to supplement them with some form of vaginal therapy.

Antidepressants These may be prescribed for women who prefer not to take hormonal therapy, but for whom natural self-help remedies don't work.

Commonly used antidepressants include drugs known as selective serotonin reuptake inhibitors (SSRIs) and serotonergic noradrenergic reuptake inhibitors, both of which can be helpful in relieving menopausal symptoms. Women who have had breast cancer, and for whom treatment with oestrogen is unsuitable, may find significant relief with these medications. However, the exact role of these drugs on the menopause has yet to be clarified.

Natural therapy Herbal remedies may offer an alternative to conventional treatments for menopausal symptoms, and can sometimes be used in addition to mainstream medicine.

There is some data that shows that preparations of black cohosh, which is a member of the buttercup family, may be helpful in alleviating mild hot flushes. Two other commonly suggested herbal remedies are *Vitex agnus-castus* and sage. However, you should be cautious about self-dosing with any herbal remedy. Very few such remedies have been subjected to rigorous clinical trials. If you are on other medication, always check with your doctor before taking any additional remedy. He or she will work with you to find the best treatment for your particular needs, taking into account your individual symptoms and the possible side effects of each treatment.

HOW CAN I HELP MYSELF?

If you're reluctant to use either hormonal or herbal therapies to relieve menopausal symptoms, there are plenty of non-medical options that you may be more comfortable with.

Lifestyle habits Often, simple lifestyle habits are helpful. For example, to help relieve hot flushes and night sweats:

- Wear light clothing made of natural fibres, such as cotton
- Dress in layers that are easy to remove if a flush comes on
- Take regular exercise
- Reduce stress with relaxation techniques
- Eat a balanced diet

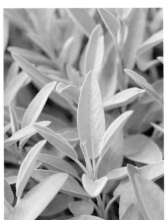
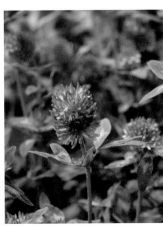
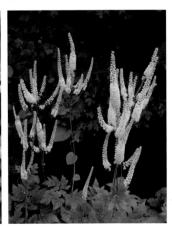

Herbs for hot flushes
Three herbs that may help to reduce hot flushes are sage (far left), red clover (middle), and black cohosh (left). Herbal remedies aren't regulated the same way as drugs, so make sure you buy them from a reputable supplier and always follow the manufacturer's advice on dosage.

- If you are suffering from night sweats, do all you can to keep your bedroom cool
- Avoid nightclothes and bed linen made from nylon or polyester
- Avoid known triggers, such as red wine and spicy foods.

Soya-based foods If none of the above lifestyle habits help, try adding soya-based foods to your diet (see opposite). However, some specialists do not regard soya as particularly helpful if you are already taking oestrogen replacement therapy.

Other lifestyle measures The following medication-free, self-help measures may relieve symptoms such as irritability, anxiety, depression, and mood swings:
- A diet high in vitamin B, zinc, and magnesium (see pp54–5)
- 30 minutes of strenuous exercise to release endorphins (the body's natural stress-relieving chemicals)
- Relaxation techniques, such as yoga (see below) or meditation.

"Regular weight-bearing exercise, such as walking and dancing, is great for reducing your risk of osteoporosis."

To improve your quality of sleep:
- Go to bed at a regular time every night
- Avoid exercising at night
- Have a warm milky drink before you go to sleep.

To help relieve skin dryness:
- Avoid using soap, which dries out your skin
- Avoid direct sunlight
- Wear a sunblock
- Make sure your diet includes vitamins A, B, C, and E as well as potassium, zinc, magnesium, iron, calcium, and essential fatty acids (see pp52–5).

HOW TO PREVENT OSTEOPOROSIS

Osteoporosis (see pp260–2) is a greater risk in menopausal women. To reduce your risk of fracture:
- Stop smoking

- Keep your alcohol consumption within reasonable limits
- Do regular weight-bearing exercise, such as walking, running, and dancing
- Eat a well-balanced diet
- Eat foods that are rich in calcium and vitamin D (see p262)
- Ask your doctor about taking supplements of calcium and vitamin D. It is recommended that menopausal women have 800mg of calcium daily and 5mcg–10mcg of vitamin D.

HOW TO PREVENT HEART DISEASE

Another health risk that increases after the menopause is heart disease (see pp158–174). To reduce this risk:
- Maintain a healthy body weight
- Eat a healthy diet that is low in saturated fats and rich in fruits and vegetables
- Take regular aerobic exercise, ideally every day, but at least three to four days a week for 30–40 minutes minimum
- Stop smoking
- Have the level of cholesterol in your blood checked. If your cholesterol level is very high, then you may need to take medication to lower it
- Get your blood pressure checked regularly. You may need drugs to lower it (see pp161, 170).

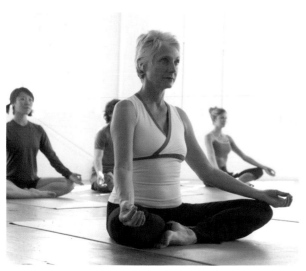

Relaxation techniques
Holistic practices such as yoga are ideal for helping to deal with the range of issues that the menopause can bring, whether they are emotional or physical and mental. Yoga aims to harmonize mind and body to help you achieve an equilibrium.

Phytoestrogens and the menopause

A number of foods contain chemical compounds that act like oestrogen. Called phytoestrogens, these compounds may help to reduce menopausal symptoms, although the medical evidence to support this is inconclusive, and phytoestrogens have not been proven to reduce the risk of diseases such as osteoporosis and heart disease. Two of the main groups of phytoestrogens are isoflavones and lignans. These should be eaten as part of a healthy, well-balanced diet (see pp52–5)

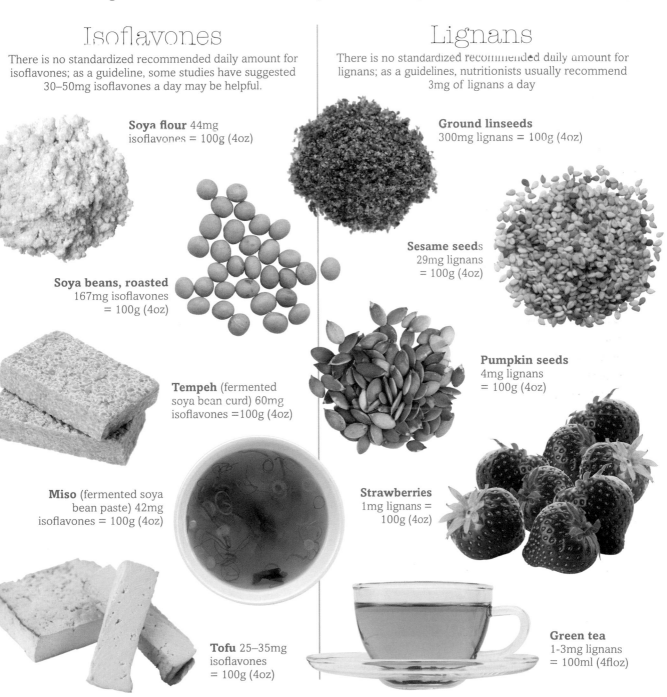

Isoflavones

There is no standardized recommended daily amount for isoflavones; as a guideline, some studies have suggested 30–50mg isoflavones a day may be helpful.

Soya flour 44mg isoflavones = 100g (4oz)

Soya beans, roasted 167mg isoflavones = 100g (4oz)

Tempeh (fermented soya bean curd) 60mg isoflavones =100g (4oz)

Miso (fermented soya bean paste) 42mg isoflavones = 100g (4oz)

Tofu 25–35mg isoflavones = 100g (4oz)

Lignans

There is no standardized recommended daily amount for lignans; as a guidelines, nutritionists usually recommend 3mg of lignans a day

Ground linseeds 300mg lignans = 100g (4oz)

Sesame seeds 29mg lignans = 100g (4oz)

Pumpkin seeds 4mg lignans = 100g (4oz)

Strawberries 1mg lignans = 100g (4oz)

Green tea 1-3mg lignans = 100ml (4floz)

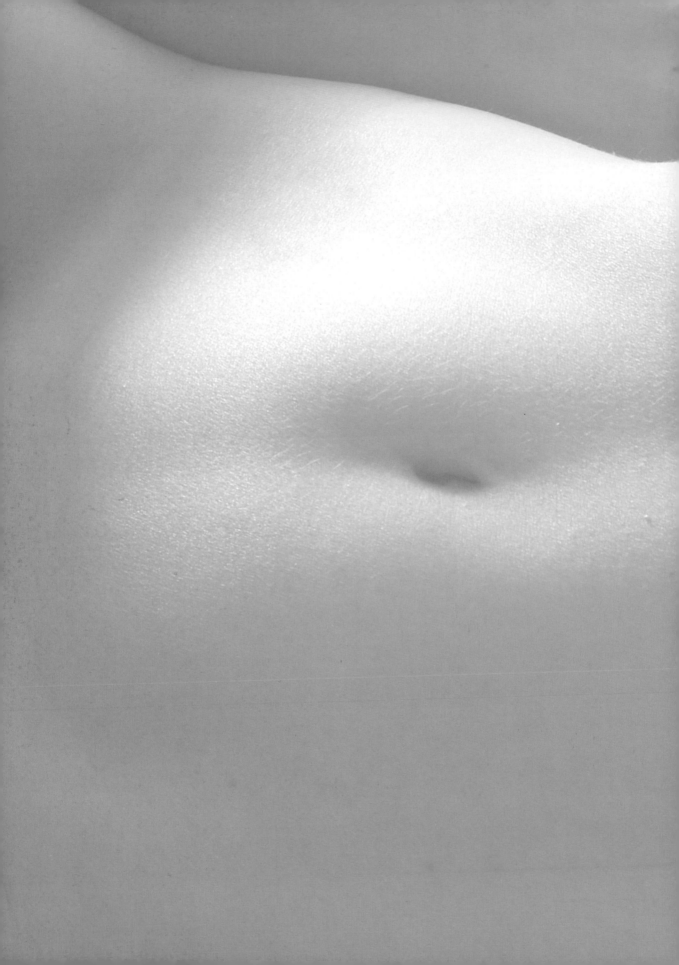

Breast health

Dr Fiona MacNeill MBBS FRCS MD

Breast health

Your breasts are a vital feature of your body and are an important part of your life as a sexual being. Although the appearance of breasts helps to distinguish women from men, their main purpose is to feed a baby from the time it is born until it is around a year old. If you are able to breast-feed and choose to do so, breast-feeding can bring you great satisfaction and will benefit your baby. However, especially as you age, your breasts can be a source of tremendous anxiety, both in terms of how you look and your health.

CROSS-SECTION OF THE BREAST

The breast is made up of lobules (glands) that produce milk, and ducts that carry milk to the nipple. These lobules and ducts are supported by thick fibrous connective tissue and fat.

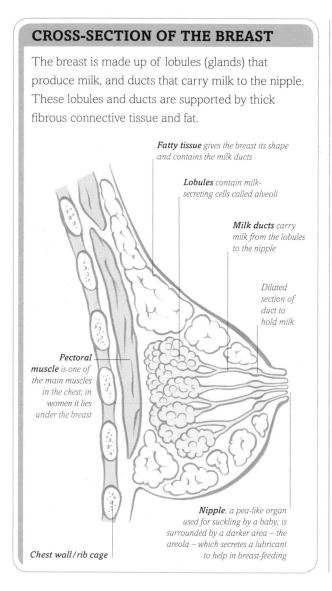

Fatty tissue gives the breast its shape and contains the milk ducts

Lobules contain milk-secreting cells called alveoli

Milk ducts carry milk from the lobules to the nipple

Dilated section of duct to hold milk

Pectoral muscle is one of the main muscles in the chest; in women it lies under the breast

Nipple, a pea-like organ used for suckling by a baby; is surrounded by a darker area – the areola – which secretes a lubricant to help in breast-feeding

Chest wall / rib cage

THE ANATOMY OF A BREAST

The breast is made up of lobules (glands) that produce milk, and ducts that carry the milk to the nipple. These lobules and ducts are surrounded and supported by thick fibrous connective tissue and fat. The amount of fat and fibrous tissue varies, which accounts for differences in breast shape and texture. The younger you are, the greater the proportion of dense, fibrous connective tissue. The amount of fatty tissue also varies depending on your age, body shape, and weight.

HOW YOUR BREASTS CHANGE DURING YOUR LIFETIME

The breast buds in girls start to grow at the menarche (a girl's first period) and the breasts then develop during puberty (when girls are between the ages of nine and 14). This growth continues until a girl is 17 or 18, but the breasts only fully mature after pregnancy.

Breasts change in shape and size depending on the levels of female sex hormones in the body. They usually get larger during puberty, just before a monthly period, and during pregnancy and breast-feeding. You may be aware of breast pain and general lumpiness at these times.

It is the dense fibrous tissue in breasts that makes them firm and gives them a youthful appearance. After pregnancies and breast-feeding, and as a woman gets older, this dense fibrous tissue is slowly replaced by fatty tissue and the breasts become softer and droop. This is why mammography works so well for the over-50 age group: the fat appears black on a mammogram,

"Our breasts bring us satisfaction when we are nurturing our children and are an important part of our sexual lives."

which makes it easier for your doctor to spot any abnormalities, while the dense fibrous tissue appears white, which can hide abnormalities.

Some women experience general concern, even anxiety, about the size and shape of their breasts, which can lead them to contemplate breast surgery (see p150).

THE INFLUENCE OF HORMONES

Your breasts, particularly the ducts and lobules, are constantly being affected by your body's hormonal changes. Every month, oestrogen and progesterone prepare your breasts for the possibility of pregnancy and milk production. If you don't get pregnant, the breast tissue returns to its normal state. These hormonal fluctuations can make your breasts feel swollen, tender, and lumpy, especially before the onset of your monthly period (see p146).

As the result of complex hormonal changes during pregnancy and breast-feeding, the breasts and nipples grow considerably, with the skin around the nipples becoming larger and darker. All of these symptoms and changes are normal and not a sign of disease.

The fluctuation of female hormones as well as increasing age cause many other normal changes in your breasts. For example, it can cause fluid-filled sacs, or lumps, called cysts to form. Nine out of 10 breast lumps are innocent, but any lump that remains after your monthly period needs to be checked out by a nurse or doctor. Any woman who has undergone the menopause and develops a lump must have it checked out immediately.

Your ovaries are the main source of oestrogen before the menopause, yet your breasts continue to change after the menopause. This is because excess body fat is converted to oestrogen compounds in the adrenal glands as well as in the adipose (fat) tissue itself. In fact, breast changes are closely related to your body fat content.

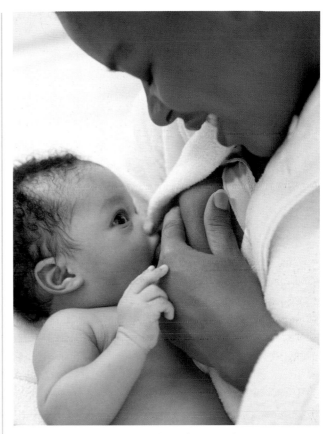

Enjoying the benefits of breast-feeding
If you can and wish to breast-feed, do so in the knowledge that breast-feeding is what our breasts were designed for. It can bring you deep satisfaction and offers many benefits to your baby.

THE IMPORTANCE OF BREAST-FEEDING

Our breasts are the most visible sign of our femaleness, but their main function is to provide nutrition in the first few years of a baby's life. In some cultures, however, breasts are more often seen as sexual objects, overshadowing our appreciation of their amazing life-sustaining function. Breast-feeding has a number of benefits for both babies and their mothers. The benefits for babies include: protection from gastrointestinal trouble, respiratory problems, ear infections, and allergies; improved sleep patterns and a lowered risk of SIDS (sudden infant death syndrome). The benefits for the mother include: helping to lose pregnancy weight and reducing post-partum bleeding; helping to bond with the baby; and possibly helping to reduce the risk of breast and ovarian cancer.

Breast pain

Many of us feel the odd twinge of breast pain from time to time, but it usually subsides quickly and we forget about it until the next time we feel it. For some women, though, breast pain causes considerable discomfort and has an impact on their daily lives. Breast pain can have a number of causes.

Breast pain, often called mastalgia, is very common and is usually linked to the menstrual cycle. The good news is that breast pain on its own is rarely a sign of a serious condition, such as breast cancer, but if you are worried about it, consult your doctor. Often lifestyle changes (see pp148–9) are enough to help you manage the pain.

WHAT IS IT?

If your breast pain is linked to your menstrual cycle, it's a response to changing levels of oestrogen in your body (see p89) and is known as "cyclical" breast pain. If you suffer from this type of pain you may be more aware of it in the days before your period. Another sign of cyclical breast pain is that it tends to be generalized, affecting both your breasts, and sometimes radiating out to your arms.

In nearly one-third of women with breast pain, the pain is unrelated to the hormonal changes of their menstrual cycle. This is referred to as "noncyclical" breast pain and is more likely to occur in just one area of your breast, and may be constant or may occur at random intervals. Noncyclical breast pain can have a variety of causes, either related to your breast or to another part of your body. One possible cause is muscle strain, which can mean you feel pain between your breasts and towards your arms.

Other causes of noncyclical breast pain include:
- Being overweight
- Producing too much oestrogen
- Having had breast surgery
- Having an inflamed vein in the breast
- Infection
- Having a breast duct that is abnormally wide.

Noncyclical breast pain has also been linked to some types of medication, including drugs used in fertility treatments, the oral contraceptive pill, and hormone replacement therapy (HRT) drugs.

Infection and inflammation of the breast (when the breast becomes red, hot, and painful), known as mastitis, are common during breast-feeding (see box, p148).

> **"Breast pain is rarely the sign of a more serious condition, such as breast cancer."**

HAVE I GOT THE SYMPTOMS?

The pain you feel in your breast depends on whether it is cyclic or noncyclical:

- If your pain is cyclical, you may feel a pain that affects both breasts, and radiates out towards your armpits. This type of pain becomes more intense before your period
- Cyclical breast pain may be accompanied by swelling and lumpiness
- If your pain is noncyclical, it usually occurs in one breast only and is often localized. The area may feel sore or achy.
- Noncyclical pain can be constant or intermittent.

See your doctor if your pain continues for some time, or if you also notice other changes in your breast.

In a non-breast-feeding woman, signs of infection can occasionally indicate an inflammatory cancer. This can develop quickly and without warning (see p153). Although infections in the breast are far more common than

> **"Most breast pain is connected with the menstrual cycle and is not a cause for concern."**

cancers, this form of cancer needs to be ruled out quickly as it requires urgent medical treatment, so if you develop these symptoms you must see a nurse or doctor.

Occasionally, noncyclical breast pain may be caused by some underlying condition that isn't related to your breast. It is possible that the pain is associated with coronary heart disease (see pp162–73), gastro-oesophageal reflux (see pp290–1), or gallbladder disease.

Noncyclical breast pain may also be the result of an injury or inflammation in your chest wall or rib joints. More commonly, it may be linked to a cyst, or more rarely to breast cancer (see pp152–7). And occasionally there are times when a doctor cannot find a cause for noncyclical breast pain.

WHAT NEXT?

Monitor the pain and if it doesn't improve, or it gets worse, over four to six weeks, make an appointment to see your doctor or nurse. If you can manage to do so, try to keep a diary of the times and occasions when you experience the pain. Your doctor will take your full medical history and will ask you about your experience of the pain. Try to describe the pain as accurately as you possibly can. Your doctor will want to know when and how your symptoms started, how the pain feels, and when and how often you feel it.

Your doctor will also examine your breasts and armpits and may also check your chest wall and listen to your heart and lungs with a stethoscope to determine whether you are suffering from a non-breast-related condition. If your doctor discovers that you are, you will be given the treatment that is appropriate for that condition.

However, if it appears that the pain is definitely coming from your breast, your doctor will try to determine the pattern of the pain, and decide whether it is either cyclical or noncyclical

If it turns out that you have noncyclical breast pain, your doctor must rule out the possibility of breast cancer. He or she will check for any lump or change in your breast tissue and if you are over 35 or have a family history (either mother's or father's side), your doctor will recommend that you have a mammogram and an ultrasound (see p155).

AM I AT RISK?

You are more likely to experience breast pain if:

- You are premenopausal; most breast pain is associated with the menstrual cycle
- You are over 40 (if the cause is noncyclical).

DECIDING THE CAUSE OF BREAST PAIN

True breast pain comes from the tissue of either breast. If the pain is around an armpit or from your breastbone it is probably musculoskeletal in origin – a muscle strain or an injury or inflammation in the wall of your chest.

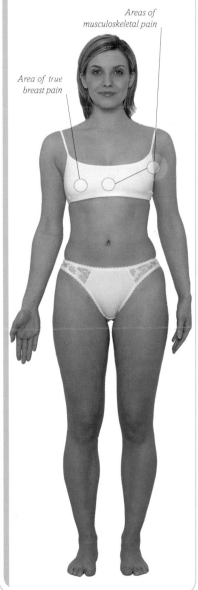

Areas of musculoskeletal pain

Area of true breast pain

MY TREATMENT OPTIONS

Usually, no specific treatment is recommended for breast pain, but if you do need treatment, your doctor will find the best option for you – the one with the greatest benefits and the fewest side effects.

Reassurance If investigations have ruled out the possibility of breast cancer (see pp152–7), then reassurance from your doctor is often enough to help you manage the pain and relieve the symptoms.

Medications If your breast pain is particularly severe, your doctor can prescribe one of several different medications. However, the range of drugs that are currently available has significant side effects so this form of treatment should be overseen by a breast specialist who is familiar with the risks as well as the benefits of each medication.

HOW CAN I HELP MYSELF?

For severe noncyclical breast pain, there are several lifestyle changes, together with supplements you can take, that can help you to alleviate your symptoms.

Decrease dietary fat Excess fat in the diet is thought to increase the amount of oestrogen that circulates in the body. Oestrogen can stimulate the breast tissue and cause pain. Reducing your fat intake – for example, by switching to low-fat or nonfat foods – may greatly reduce the severity of your breast pain.

Take a supplement Evening primrose oil (which contains gamma linoleic acid) may help to balance fatty acids in the breast tissue and decrease the sensitivity of the breast ducts to hormones such as oestrogen. It is thought that taking the recommended dose of 1.5 grams twice a day for up to three months at a time can alleviate discomfort. Some women swear by taking vitamins E, B1, and B6, but placebo trials have indicated that these do not effectively reduce breast pain.

Reduce your caffeine intake Although not proven, it has been suggested that restricting your caffeine intake or not having any caffeine-containing drinks may help to reduce breast pain.

Stop smoking If you do smoke, now is the time to reduce the amount you smoke or to stop completely, if you possibly can (see p64). Ask your doctor to tell you about local support groups that can help you stop smoking.

Support your breasts You may be able to ease the breast pain considerably by wearing a bra that supports your breasts properly. Getting your breasts measured professionally and wearing a well-fitted, firm-support bra can help to reduce pain and discomfort. If your breasts are particularly heavy, and your pain is severe, then you may find that wearing a bra at night makes a difference.

Lose weight If you are overweight for your height (see pp58–9), you will find that losing weight – using a

---

MASTITIS

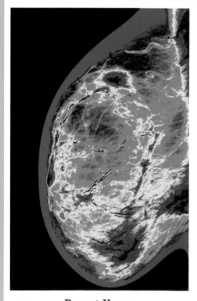

Breast X-ray
This specially coloured breast X-ray shows inflamed breast tissue caused by mastitis

Mastitis is a painful inflammation in one or both breasts and affects 1 in 10 breast-feeding mothers, often during the first six weeks. Redness spreads from the nipple and is accompanied by swelling, tenderness, and possibly fever and fatigue. Mastitis is caused by an infection in a blocked milk duct. It is usually managed with antibiotics, warm compresses, and standing under a hot shower. Mothers with mastitis shouldn't stop breast-feeding or expressing milk, otherwise the breast will become painfully engorged, encouraging an abscess to develop. Rarely, the abscess needs to be surgically drained.

Eating for breast health

A diet for healthy breasts means eating plenty of fresh vegetables, fruits, and fibre-rich foods, and choosing cold-water fish for the good fats they contain (see pp52–5). It's also important to reduce the amount of saturated fats and trans fatty acids you eat (see p172).

Vegetables

Allium vegetables such as onions, leeks, and particularly garlic, contain sulphur compounds, which may support healthy blood vessels.

Cruciferous vegetables include broccoli and cauliflower, which are packed with nutrients, including vitamin C.

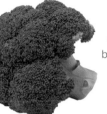

Green leafy vegetables such as spinach, Swiss chard, and kale, also contain many essential minerals and vitamins.

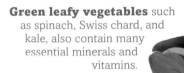

Yellow-orange vegetables such as peppers and carrots, are rich in carotenoids that may keep the body's cells healthy

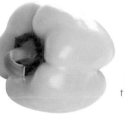

Beverages

Green tea contains polyphenols and flavonoids, powerful antioxidants that may neutralize damaging compounds in the body.

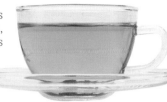

Fruit

Citrus fruits such as oranges and grapefruits, contain carotenoids and flavonoids, which may be immune boosters.

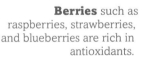

Berries such as raspberries, strawberries, and blueberries are rich in antioxidants.

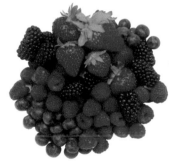

combination of sensible diet control and increasing the amount of regular exercise you take – will help to reduce the size of your breasts. When you start to lose weight, the weight loss often occurs first in the breasts.

Direct therapies Alternating hot and cold compresses on your breasts is thought to reduce the discomfort. Massaging your breasts may help unless you can't tolerate the pressure. Another effective treatment is to stand under a hot shower. Try to direct the shower head at full strength on to your breast for as long as you can stand it. You may need to do this several times before you start to feel better and the pain eases.

Reduce stress It is thought that stress and anxiety can contribute to breast pain, so trying relaxation techniques may bring you some relief. There is a wide range of relaxation therapies on offer – for example, yoga and meditation – and you may need to explore several to find one that works for you. Other excellent therapies include acupressure, massage, reflexology, reiki, and Pilates. If there is any part your life that you experience as stressful, think about reducing it or, better still, eliminating it altogether.

Breast reduction and augmentation

The pressure to look good means that many of us worry about the size of our breasts. Cosmetic surgery can make you happier with your body, but it can have major complications. Think very carefully about whether you really do want surgery, and discuss it with your doctor or surgeon before making a decision.

Breast reduction

Pain in the shoulder, neck, or back, as well as breasts that are too large, are the main reasons why women choose to have their breasts made smaller. This is one surgical procedure that has the highest patient satisfaction.

Macromastia is the term given for breasts that are too big. If you suffer from this problem, you might well be feeling pain caused by the weight of your breasts pulling on the muscles of your neck, back, and shoulders. You might also have some soreness caused by the skin rubbing under your breasts.

If you decide that surgery is what is needed to make you feel better, you should be aware that, unless your life is seriously affected by the size of your breasts, it is best to wait until you've had children. Although breast-feeding is possible after breast reduction, surgery can block the milk ducts. It is also recommended that women wait until after their breasts are fully developed (aged 18 minimum).

The surgery takes between two and four hours (see box, left). As far as possible, the surgeon will try to ensure that you still have sensation in your nipples after the operation. The incisions look like an inverted "T". It's difficult to predict how you are going to scar, but scarring can range from barely perceptible to more defined.

A number of complications might occur, including:

- Fat necrosis – fat cells die and clump together. This may appear as a lump that is found during a breast exam, or a calcium deposit (microcalcifications) on a mammogram
- Microcalcifications on a mammogram that may require biopsy
- Loss of nipple sensation.

SURGERY FOR BREAST REDUCTION

During this procedure, which takes place under general anaesthesia, the surgeon makes an incision around the areola and a keyhole incision. After removing excess tissue, the surgeon transplants the nipple and moves it upward.

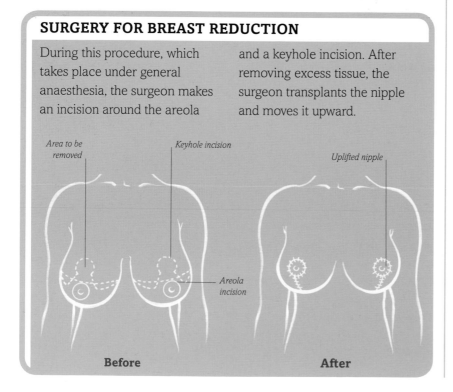

Area to be removed

Keyhole incision

Uplifted nipple

Areola incision

Before

After

Breast augmentation

If you are self-conscious that your breasts are too small or sagging, or if you have lost the volume and size of your breasts after breast-feeding and childbirth, then you may decide that you need breast augmentation (breast enlargement). Of course, you may want the operation for cosmetic reasons.

Medically, the main candidates for breast augmentation are women with genetically underdeveloped breasts (micromastia) and women who have no breast tissue because they have a congenital condition called Poland's Syndrome.

There are other medical reasons for breast augmentation. One is making a woman's breasts symmetrical after she has had a breast removed in a mastectomy. Another is breast reconstruction (see p157).

During surgery (see box, below) the breast is enlarged by adding an implant filled with saline (salt water), silicone gel, or silicone composite gel. You may need an overnight hospital stay – longer if you need a breast lift (mastopexy) as well.

A number of complications might occur, including:

- Deflation and/or rupture of the breast implant
- Pain and/or infection
- Changes in sensation in the nipple and breast
- Wrinkling of the implant after a period of time
- Blood or fluid in your breasts
- A feeling of dissatisfaction with the way your breasts look that continues after the operation
- Calcium deposits in the tissue surrounding the implant
- Delayed wound healing
- Extrusion of the implant, in which the implant emerges through your skin
- Further surgery may be needed as the result of complication.

ARE BREAST IMPLANTS SAFE?

Breast augmentation has come under tremendous scrutiny, and controversy as the safety of silicone implants has created a stir in both medical and legal communities. The implants were used for breast reconstruction and enhancement between 1962 and 1992, but fear of leakage, formation of calcium deposits, and systemic autoimmune diseases (see pp266–71) resulted in their removal from the market between 1992 and 2006.

Now though, silicone implants can be used in reconstruction after breast cancer and for enlargement or augmentation in a healthy breast. There are no studies linking breast implants with an increased risk of breast cancer or other breast diseases. The National Cancer Institute has published data to show that there is a lower risk of breast cancer among patients with breast augmentation.

SURGERY FOR BREAST AUGMENTATION

Breast implants may be positioned in front of (below left) or behind (below right) the pectoral muscle. Mammography is possible in either implant position, as implants do not hinder the detection of breast lumps. However, needle tests can be more difficult and risk damaging the implant if it is positioned in front of the pectoral muscle.

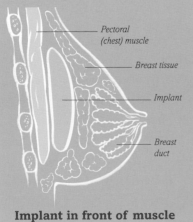

Pectoral (chest) muscle

Breast tissue

Implant

Breast duct

Implant in front of muscle

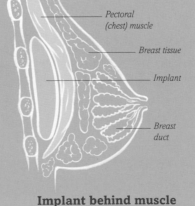

Pectoral (chest) muscle

Breast tissue

Implant

Breast duct

Implant behind muscle

Breast cancer

A diagnosis of breast cancer can be frightening, but with early detection and modern treatments many women do recover from the disease. Regardless of the outcome, breast cancer is a life-changing experience. Understanding what can be done to treat this disease is the first step in overcoming any fears.

HAVE I GOT THE SYMPTOMS?

The classic signs of breast cancer are described here, but it can present in many different ways. These signs usually only affect one breast:

- Lump in a post-menopausal woman
- Skin changes – indentation of the breast skin (dimpling) associated with a lumpy ("orange-peel") appearance of the skin, especially around the nipple area and lower breast
- Nipple changes – recent indrawing of the nipple and eczema type rash (crusting, bleeding, etc) on the nipple. Nipple discharge is rarely a sign of cancer, but it does require further investigation
- Signs of inflammation and infection when you are not breast-feeding. **See your doctor** if you notice any change in your breast that doesn't improve after you have had your monthly period.

Breast cancer is one of the most anxiety-producing conditions that women have to contend with and many of us have friends who have had the condition. Your likelihood of getting breast cancer increases with age, but there are also other risk factors at play.

There are various methods of assessing your risk, but the one most often used is the GAIL risk assessment model. You can access it online. It asks you a series of questions concerning, for example, your age, race, and the age you were when you gave birth to your first child. This method provides you with useful personal pointers.

The most important thing of all in the treatment of breast cancer is early detection. Women (and a very few men) die of the disease only when it has spread beyond the breast area, settled in distant organs, and failed to respond to chemotherapy or radiation. If your breast cancer is diagnosed before it has spread, treatment is far more likely to be successful and the cancer is less likely to return later on in your life.

The main tool for the early detection of breast cancer is mammography, which uses low-dose X-rays to produce two-dimensional images of your breast tissue. When you have a mammogram, each breast is compressed from top to bottom between two plates while a brief pulse of X-ray produces the image. This procedure is repeated on the area of tissue from your breastbone to your armpit.

Mammograms can often detect lesions years earlier than clinical examination, so although having them regularly won't stop you getting breast cancer, it may prevent you from dying from it. Studies show that mammograms decrease the chance of dying from breast cancer by 40 per cent (see graph opposite).

However, there are differences from country to country as to the age at which you will be offered your first screening mammogram. There are also differences between countries as to how long the

"Around 1 in 9 women develop breast cancer; if it is detected early and treated, the possibility of a complete recovery is much higher."

HOW HAVING A MAMMOGRAM COULD SAVE YOUR LIFE

Screening saves lives. A 40 per cent decrease in death from breast cancer was found in women who were diagnosed with breast cancer and who participated in mammographic screening in Sweden between 1979 and 1999 (B). The death rate remained the same for women who did not have screening mammograms (A).

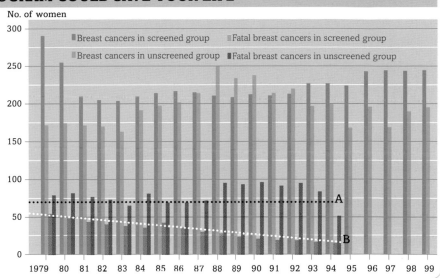

No. of women

Legend:
- Breast cancers in screened group
- Fatal breast cancers in screened group
- Breast cancers in unscreened group
- Fatal breast cancers in unscreened group

intervals between your screening mammograms will be. Although screening mammography is key, around 10 per cent of all breast cancers cannot be picked up by it, so it is vital to get to know your breasts and to check yourself at regular intervals (see p154). The more aware you are of how your breasts normally look and feel, the more easily you can pick up changes early.

If you discover a lump in your breast, either when you undertake your own breast exam or via any other method, a surgeon will need to do a breast biopsy (see p155) to determine whether your lump is benign or malignant, or if it needs further investigation.

AM I AT RISK?

Only 25 per cent of all breast cancers occur in women who have one or more family members with breast cancer. Of these women, only six per cent are carriers of a specific genetic mutation. Therefore, 75 per cent of all breast cancers occur in women who have no family history of it at all. For this reason it is extremely important for you to understand what the risk factors are in your own particular case.

Your chances of developing breast cancer are increased if:
- You are aged over 50
- Relatives have had breast cancer
- You had an early menarche or a late menopause
- You gave birth to your first child late in life
- You don't have children
- You have had biopsies already
- Atypical cells have been found on a biopsy.

INFLAMMATORY BREAST CANCER

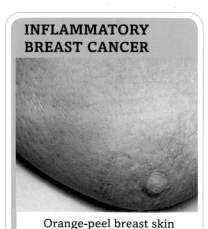

Orange-peel breast skin
The skin becomes swollen with fluid, producing an "orange-peel" effect.

Inflammatory breast cancer (IBC) is a rare cancer that can develop suddenly. The symptoms mimic infection (mastitis) and include: the breast turning red, purple, pink, or bruised; orange-peel skin (see above); a thickness in the breast; swelling; warmth; pain, tenderness, or itching; swelling in the armpit; inverted nipple.

HOW TO BE BREAST AWARE

Get to know how your breasts look, feel, and change during your cycle. Maintain this practice for life. The more you know about what is normal for you, the better placed you'll be to spot abnormalities.

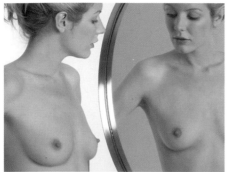

1 Look in the mirror Stand with your arms on your hips, then over your head. Each time look to see if your breasts are the usual shape and size, then check the skin of your breasts for any changes, such as dimpling, pulling in, puckering, or bulging. Is there any redness, soreness, thickening, or swelling? Is the nipple inverted rather than protruding? Has the nipple changed position? Is there a spontaneous discharge from just one breast? Is the discharge bloody or a clear, watery fluid (old blood can stain the bra or night clothes and look like tea stain)? Is the discharge associated with nipple retraction?

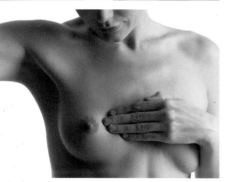

2 Feel your breasts for any changes Use body oil or gel on your hands. Begin with one arm over your head and use firm but gentle pressure with the other hand, gliding the pads of your fingers over your breast. Move your fingers from the top of the breast to the fold below it, moving from the breastbone toward the armpit. Use your right hand to examine your left breast and vice versa. Pay particular attention to the nipple region, feeling for any peculiar changes, such as a pea-like or marble-like lump, a thickening or a ridge, or "gravel" in the breast.

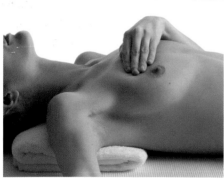

3 Repeat the hand examination lying on your back Place a folded towel beneath your shoulder blade. Use the flat of your hand rather than the tips of your fingers to check each breast from the armpit to the breastbone and from the collarbone to your abdomen. Most breasts are lumpy or grainy so get to know what is normal for you and then any changes or lumps will become obvious.

IMPROVING YOUR RISK FACTORS

Many risk factors for breast cancer cannot be changed (see p153), but be aware of those that can. The following are some suggestions. **Breast-feed** if you have a baby of the appropriate age. It is believed that breast-feeding clears the ductal cells. **Control your weight** (see pp58–9) since fat is converted to oestrogen compounds in the adrenal glands. **Take exercise.** If you do some cardiovascular exercise for at least three hours each week your risk of developing breast cancer decreases by 20 per cent. **Control your alcohol intake** (see p65). Your risk increases with the volume you consume.

WHAT IS IT?

Invasive breast cancer is the disorderly or chaotic growth of cells in the ducts or lobules of the breast. These cells have lost their ability to be regulated by the body and so divide uncontrollably. In the process they form tumours, which are also called carcinomas. Cancer can destroy the cells in an increasing proportion of normal breast tissue over time. If left untreated it can spread outside the breast to other organs.

Breast cancer does not come about overnight. There are gradual changes in the breast ducts, which can continue to invasive ductal carcinoma – the most common kind of breast cancer.

WHAT NEXT?

If you have found a lump in your breast, see your doctor or breast specialist. He or she will determine which test you need.

A mammogram is the preferred tool for detecting breast cancers early. The smaller and earlier stage the tumour is at diagnosis, the better the chance of curing the cancer. If your mammogram shows a change, you may be given additional diagnostic mammography, breast ultrasound, and, occasionally, breast MRI.

Ultrasound is a non-invasive tool that evaluates the density of your breast tissue and of any masses (lumps) in it.

Magnetic Resonance Imaging (MRI) uses the energy of very strong magnets, combined with a dye, to create an image that helps to determine the nature of a breast lesion.

After the dye has been injected into your blood, you are placed inside the MRI cylinder where the scan is taken. The scan should be performed between days seven and 14 of your menstrual cycle to eliminate any changes in your breasts that are due to normal hormonal variations.

A breast biopsy may be needed when a mammogram, ultrasound, or MRI reveals an abnormality, or if a lump is found. A small amount of tissue is removed for analysis.

There are four main types: fine needle aspiration (FNA), core, vacuum-assisted and open-surgical. In FNA, cells are withdrawn via a thin needle. In a core biopsy, a needle is inserted several times to obtain tissue. In a vacuum-assisted biopsy, the device is inserted once and several samples are removed. An open-surgical biopsy requires an operation for either an incisional biopsy (a piece of breast tissue is removed) or an excisional biopsy (the entire lesion is removed).

A biopsy might reveal one of the following results:

- A benign lesion. This can be safely left, as it won't increase your risk of developing breast cancer.
- A lesion that may pose a risk – e.g. atypical ductal hyperplasia (ADII), lobular neoplasia (LN), or lobular carcinoma in-situ (LCIS). This type of lesion usually requires removal, as it might put you at risk of invasive breast cancer later.
- Non-invasive breast cancer – ductal carcinoma in-situ (DCIS). This is the very earliest stage of breast cancer, where cancer cells are confined to the milk ducts. They cannot spread to vital organs, but require treatment as they may develop into invasive breast cancer.
- Invasive breast cancer. This is cancer that has broken through the milk ducts into the surrounding fibrous and fatty tissue of the breast. The cancer cells then move into blood and lymph channels and spread to vital organs.

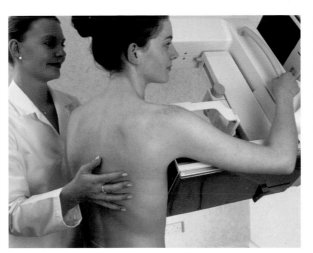

Mammography
Each breast is compressed between a plastic cover and the X-ray plate so that X-rays pass through the breast and onto the plate.

WHAT SHOULD I ASK MY DOCTOR?

After you have been diagnosed with breast cancer, it is a good idea to become as well-informed as you can about your condition by talking to your doctor. There are several questions that you can ask:

- What type of breast cancer do I have?
- What type of tumour do I have?
- What stage is my tumour?

- Has my tumour spread away from my breast?
- What are my treatment options?
- What is the risk of the cancer returning after treatment?
- Do I need chemotherapy?
- Do I need radiation therapy?
- How can I decrease the risk of my cancer returning?
- Do I have the breast cancer gene?

MY TREATMENT OPTIONS

Your tumour may be "staged" to see how developed it is, although this is not routinely done. Several staging tests can be performed: bone scan, liver function tests, chest X-ray, and possibly a PET (positron emission tomography).

Breast cancer treatment usually requires a combination of surgery, chemotherapy, radiotherapy, and tablets such as tamoxifen or an aromatase inhibitor, which block or suppress oestrogen. Your specific regimen will depend on the stage of your cancer. Your doctor will tell you about different treatment options and together you can decide the best course of action.

Wide local excision (see right) conserves the breast and only removes the tumour (lump), plus some surrounding normal tissue.

After a lumpectomy, you will have about six weeks of radiation therapy and then your doctor may prescribe oral medication to help prevent the cancer from returning. If you have large breasts, you may

not notice a difference in the shape. If you have small- or medium-sized breasts, the procedure may change their shape visibly.

Mastectomy involves the removal of 95 per cent of breast tissue (it is impossible to remove it all) and

breast skin, including the "tail" of tissue that extends into your armpit (the axillary tail). The remaining skin edges are closed together as a neat line across the chest, leaving the chest wall flat so that an external implant can be fitted.

A skin-sparing mastectomy is only done when reconstructing the breast (see opposite). It can preserve the breast skin in various ways – like an incision around the areola.

Axillary staging Your doctor also checks if the tumour has spread outside the breast. The standard way of doing this is to remove and examine (evaluate) the lymph nodes in your armpit. Lymph node evaluation is required in all cases of invasive cancer and some cases of DCIS (see p155). This can be done

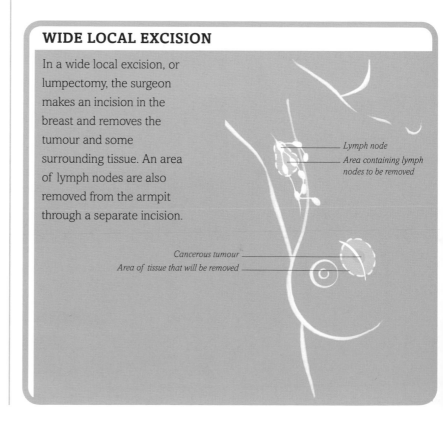

WIDE LOCAL EXCISION

In a wide local excision, or lumpectomy, the surgeon makes an incision in the breast and removes the tumour and some surrounding tissue. An area of lymph nodes are also removed from the armpit through a separate incision.

Lymph node

Area containing lymph nodes to be removed

Cancerous tumour

Area of tissue that will be removed

at the same time or before you have surgery to your breast. Nodes with the highest risk of cancer are evaluated. If they contain cancer, additional nodes are removed.

For many women, only a small number of lymph nodes will need to be removed, using a technique called sentinel lymph node biopsy. But women with cancer in their sentinel nodes, or those at high risk of lymph node spread, will be advised to have most of the lymph nodes removed (axillary clearance). Sentinel nodes are the first in line to be attacked by any cancer cells that have spread from the tumour. Removing the lymph nodes can cause lymphoedema, or swelling of your arm, which can occur months or years after treatment.

Chemotherapy is generally given after surgery. But occasionally it is given before surgery, as in the case of inflammatory breast cancer and with large tumours – the aim is to shrink them prior to surgical removal of the cancer.

During chemotherapy, drugs are given intravenously in hospital or taken by mouth. There are many different chemotherapy drugs and combinations of drugs, all with their own side effects. You usually have a few weeks between treatments to recover from the side effects. Chemotherapy lasts 4–6 months and you may need surgery and radiation therapy afterwards.

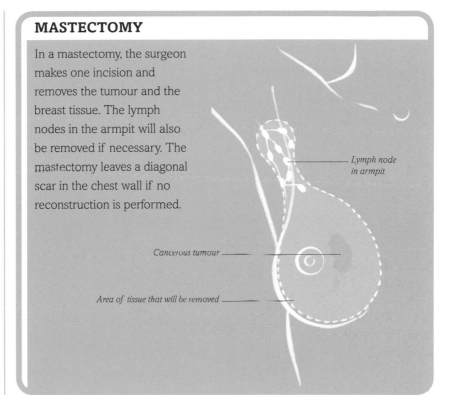

MASTECTOMY

In a mastectomy, the surgeon makes one incision and removes the tumour and the breast tissue. The lymph nodes in the armpit will also be removed if necessary. The mastectomy leaves a diagonal scar in the chest wall if no reconstruction is performed.

Lymph node in armpit

Cancerous tumour

Area of tissue that will be removed

Breast reconstruction can be done at the time of a mastectomy or delayed until you are ready. If you are likely to have radiotherapy, reconstruction is delayed for a year or more to let the tissue recover. There are many techniques, ranging from an implant under the pectoral muscle to the more complex free tissue transfer.

HOW CAN I HELP MYSELF?

Although surgery and medication are key to treating breast cancer, there are measures you can take yourself: being well-informed about your particular breast cancer can help allay any fears you may have and make you feel more positive.

Complementary therapies These therapies complement but do not replace conventional medicine, and can help to enhance healing. For example, Reiki, massage, yoga, acupuncture, reflexology, meditation, and other holistic therapies can help you to release fears you might be holding on to. They can help speed recovery and be supportive once treatment is over.

Alternative therapies When you have been diagnosed with breast cancer, you're very vulnerable and may be tempted by "treatments" offered as alternatives to standard medical practice. However, there are no effective "alternatives" to surgery, chemotherapy, and radiotherapy.

"Knowing as much as you can about your breast cancer will help you feel more positive."

Heart and circulation

Dr Ghada Mikhail BSc MBBS MD FRCP
Vascular disease Dr Sarah Jarvis MA BM BCH DRCOG FRCGP

Your heart

Although your heart is a small portion of your body weight, it is one of your most vital organs. This important pump – the size of a fist – beats continuously, on average, 60–100 times a minute, around 100,000 times per day. Each minute it pumps all of your blood – about 5 litres (9 pints) – around the body via a system of arteries, veins, and capillaries (see p246). This system, together with your lungs, serves to oxygenate your blood, and ensure that every cell in your body receives the oxygen it needs to function.

HOW YOUR HEART WORKS

Your heart weighs approximately 250–340g (9–12 oz). It is divided into four sections, or chambers, with two chambers on either side. The top two chambers are the right and left atrium (plural, atria), and the bottom two are the right and left ventricles.

For your heart to beat normally, electrical impulses make the atria contract. This electrical activity then travels to the ventricles, which then contract.

The right side of the heart receives deoxygenated blood (without oxygen) that has travelled, via the veins, from the rest of your body. With every heartbeat, the heart pumps this blood to the lungs, where carbon dioxide is removed and the blood is reoxygenated (see pp230–1). The oxygenated blood then travels from the lungs through your blood vessels to the left side of your heart. From here it travels to the rest of the body through the aorta (the main artery) and other arteries. Blood then returns to the heart via the veins, continuing the cycle.

Valves in the heart – the tricuspid and pulmonary valves on the right and the mitral and aortic valves on the left – control the flow of blood (see opposite). The blood vessels also have valves to ensure that blood flows in the right direction through them.

HOW WOMEN ARE DIFFERENT

When it comes to heart disease, women differ in their risk factors (see p163), and in the diagnosis (see pp168–9) and treatment (see pp170–1).

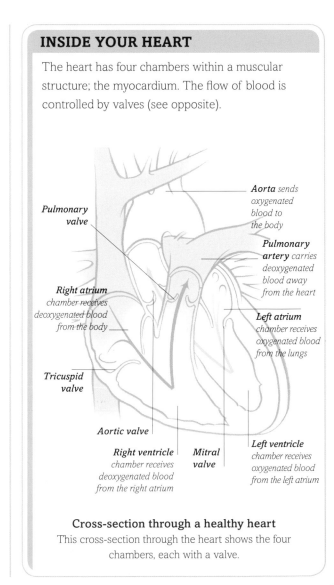

INSIDE YOUR HEART

The heart has four chambers within a muscular structure; the myocardium. The flow of blood is controlled by valves (see opposite).

Pulmonary valve

Aorta sends oxygenated blood to the body

Pulmonary artery carries deoxygenated blood away from the heart

Right atrium chamber receives deoxygenated blood from the body

Left atrium chamber receives oxygenated blood from the lungs

Tricuspid valve

Aortic valve

Right ventricle chamber receives deoxygenated blood from the right atrium

Mitral valve

Left ventricle chamber receives oxygenated blood from the left atrium

Cross-section through a healthy heart
This cross-section through the heart shows the four chambers, each with a valve.

VALVES IN THE HEART

Valves in the heart keep the blood flowing in the correct direction. Atrioventricular valves (mitral and tricuspid) lie between the atria and ventricles; semilunar valves are at the openings of the pulmonary artery and aorta. The valves have cusps or leaflets that open under pressure as the heart contracts to force the blood through. Then the cusps or leaflets shut, closing the valves and stopping the blood from flowing backwards.

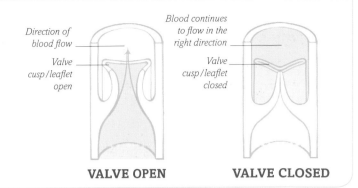

Direction of blood flow

Valve cusp/leaflet open

Blood continues to flow in the right direction

Valve cusp/leaflet closed

VALVE OPEN   **VALVE CLOSED**

BLOOD PRESSURE

Every time your heart beats, it pumps blood into your blood vessels. Blood pressure is the pressure of the blood as it flows through the blood vessels. Your blood pressure is at its highest – known as the systolic pressure – when the heart contracts and pumps blood to the rest of the body. When the heart is at rest, between beats, your blood pressure falls. This is the diastolic pressure.

Your blood pressure should not be higher than 140/90mmHg (140 is the systolic pressure and 90 is the diastolic pressure). In certain conditions, such as diabetes, you should be aiming to reduce your blood pressure below this.

Both your systolic and diastolic pressures are important, and if either one is raised this is known as high blood pressure, or hypertension. Low blood pressure is known as hypotension. There are several ways to measure blood pressure.

Shygmomanometer The doctor or nurse will wrap a cuff around your upper arm and will inflate the cuff. He or she then listens to your pulse with a stethoscope. When the pulse is first heard, the systolic pressure is measured. The pressure in the cuff is then gradually released and the sound of the pulse becomes faint until it disappears, at which point the diastolic pressure is measured.

Electronic blood pressure machines These devices measure blood pressure electronically. They are often used by patients to monitor their blood pressure at home.

24-hour ambulatory blood pressure monitoring

This involves wearing a blood pressure cuff for 24 hours. It measures blood pressure periodically day and night and calculates the average blood pressure for certain periods. This method is useful if your blood pressure is borderline, or to monitor the effect of a medication. It's sometimes used if your blood pressure is thought to be high because you get anxious when a doctor or a nurse measures it. This is known as "white coat hypertension".

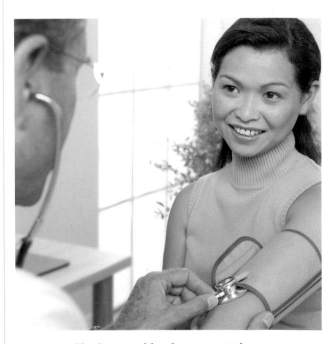

Having your blood pressure taken
This method of checking blood pressure involves using a shygmomanometer, or cuff that is inflated.

What is coronary heart disease?

Although in the UK coronary heart disease (CHD) leads to one in five deaths in men and one in six in women, there's still a common misconception that it's a disease of men. Women may fear breast cancer more than CHD, yet CHD kills almost four times more women than breast cancer does.

WHAT IS IT?

Coronary heart disease, or CHD, is a disease of the coronary arteries caused by a build up of fatty material that can lead to narrowing and blockages in the coronary vessels. The process is called atherosclerosis and the fatty deposits are known as atheroma.

Once the coronary arteries are narrowed by atheroma, the blood flow to the heart muscle is obstructed, which can cause angina (see p164). A sudden blockage of a coronary artery can lead to a heart attack, or myocardial infarction (see p166).

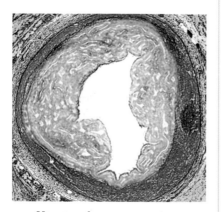

Narrowed coronary artery
Atheroma plaque (yellow area) has almost completely blocked this coronary artery, so blood flow will be obstructed.

DIFFERENCES IN WOMEN

Many women lack the basic awareness that heart disease is their biggest killer and that it can affect them as well as men. In addition, women's symptoms may be different from men's (see p164), so women do not always recognize that they may be having symptoms that could be related to heart disease. Women, therefore, tend to seek medical help later than men.

In addition, because basic cardiac investigations, such as electrocardiograms and exercise tests, tend to be less sensitive and less specific in women compared to men (see pp168–9), making a diagnosis in a woman more challenging than it is in a man.

Also, since women tend to be protected by their hormones, especially by oestrogen, until the menopause, CHD is a disease of the older woman. So by the time a woman goes to the doctor or hospital with anginal symptoms, not only is she older, but she is also likely to have more risk factors for CHD, such as diabetes, high cholesterol (hypercholesterolaemia; see opposite), and high blood pressure (hypertension).

Women also tend to have smaller coronary arteries than men, so when it comes to treating women with either coronary angioplasty or coronary artery bypass surgery (see pp170–1) the treatment can be more challenging.

DENTAL TREATMENT AND HEART CONDITIONS

Until recently, antibiotics were recommended prior to dental treatment for people with certain heart conditions, as it was thought that bacteria in the mouth could enter the bloodstream during invasive dental treatment, causing infection in the heart, known as subacute bacterial endocarditis. However, using preventive antibiotics is no longer recommended as it's felt there is insufficient evidence that dental treatment specifically can lead to infection in the heart.

AM I AT RISK?

There are a number of risk factors that increase your likelihood of developing coronary heart disease. These include:

Smoking This significantly increases your risk of coronary heart disease. Smoking reduces the amount of oxygen carried in the blood. It also increases the tendency of the blood to clot by raising the levels of fibrinogen and platelets, both of which are involved in the clotting process of the blood.

High cholesterol (hypercholesterolaemia) Cholesterol is a fatty material made in the liver, mainly from the fatty foods that we eat. It is present in the membrane of cells and is important for their healthy functioning. However, there are good and bad types of cholesterol – "bad cholesterol" is known as LDL and "good cholesterol" is referred to as HDL. Having high levels of LDL and low levels of HDL increases your risk of developing cardiovascular disease.

High blood pressure (hypertension) Having high blood pressure increases your risk of CHD as well as your risk of having a stroke (see p196).

Diabetes increases your risk of getting CHD. If you have diabetes it is important that you monitor and keep your blood sugar levels under control.

Being overweight Being overweight can lead to high blood pressure, raised cholesterol, and diabetes, all of which increase your risk of CHD. In particular, it's thought that weight accumulated around your waist increases your risk (see pp58–9).

Lack of exercise Inactivity increases your risk of CHD as well as a myriad of other conditions (see pp56–7). Regular exercise reduces your risk.

Stress Studies suggest that chronic stress can increase your risk of CHD. In particular, stress can result in high blood pressure, which is a risk factor for CHD.

Being postmenopausal Following the menopause (see opposite), women's risk for CHD increases, and by the time of the menopause, they may have also developed other risk factors for CHD.

A family history of cardiovascular disease Having a family history of heart disease in first-degree relatives can increase your risk of CHD, especially if you also have other risk factors. It's therefore important to try and modify all your other risk factors to reduce your risk of CHD.

Modify your risk factors

It is imperative that women start modifying their risk factors when they are younger in order to reduce the risk of developing heart disease once they are older. Better awareness and education, more aggressive control of risk factors as well as early diagnosis and treatment are all desperately needed.

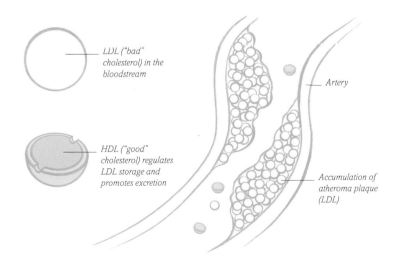

LDL ("bad" cholesterol) in the bloodstream

HDL ("good" cholesterol) regulates LDL storage and promotes excretion

Artery

Accumulation of atheroma plaque (LDL)

HDL ("good") and LDL ("bad") cholesterol

CHD: Have I got the symptoms?

Chest pain is a common symptom in people with CHD. Women, however, may experience other, atypical, symptoms that they may not associate with CHD. That is why it is important for women to be aware of the whole range of possible symptoms so they can seek help at the earliest opportunity.

There is no doubt that CHD is the biggest killer in women: it kills more women than breast cancer. Women need to be aware of the risk of this potentially fatal disease and realize that it is not just a man's disease. They can help protect themselves by modifying any risk factors they may have, and by learning to recognize the symptoms and seek medical help early. This is the key to successful treatment (see p170).

The main symptom of CHD is chest pain. This is usually described as a heavy, crushing, or squeezing discomfort in the centre of the chest. At times, pain or discomfort can also be felt in the arms, neck, or jaw. Chest pain can occur on exertion (angina) or at rest. The chest pain of a heart attack (myocardial infarction) is usually intense and prolonged, and can be associated with sweating, nausea, and vomiting.

Women with heart disease can have various symptoms that are not always typical and can differ from those of men – there are many other symptoms apart from chest pain (see box, opposite).

Angina

It's easy to dismiss chest pain and other less typical symptoms. However, if you have any symptoms that you think may be related to heart disease and you have risk factors, it's best to consult your doctor who can help to determine whether the pain is a cause for concern.

WHAT IS IT?
When the heart's blood flow is obstructed due to fatty deposits in coronary arteries, the heart muscle receives insufficient oxygen, which can lead to chest pain, known as angina. When you rest, the heart may be able to cope with a reduced oxygen supply. Angina arises once you increase the heart's oxygen demands, for example, after physical exertion or emotional stress.

WHAT NEXT?
Your doctor will take a medical history to assess your symptoms and any risk factors that you may have. After performing a medical examination, he or she will suggest tests, such as an electrocardiogram (ECG) or a stress test (see p168), to help towards diagnosing CHD. If your exercise test is positive, your doctor will advise that you have a coronary angiogram to assess whether you have any narrowings or blockages in your coronary arteries.

HAVE I GOT THE SYMPTOMS?

The pain is often described as a dull, heavy feeling in the centre of the chest that can also extend to the throat, jaw, neck, back, or arms. It usually occurs on exertion – when you walk or take exercise, for example – although it can also occur at rest. The pain usually improves when you rest or take medication such as a nitrate spray, or nitrate tablet under the tongue (see p170). If the pain persists, you need to seek medical help.
See your doctor if you have these symptoms.

MY TREATMENT OPTIONS

The treatment your doctor recommends will depend on the extent and severity of your CHD.
Medication Angina can be treated with medications such as nitrates.
Other treatments In some cases, coronary angioplasty and stenting or bypass surgery may be recommended (see pp170–1).

"A heart attack is a medical emergency – if you think you may be having a heart attack, don't delay, seek help immediately."

HOW CAN I HELP MYSELF?

It is important that you start modifying your risk factors from a young age to reduce the risk of developing heart disease when you are older. Modifiable risk factors include stopping smoking, eating healthily, exercising regularly, and having your cholesterol, blood sugar, and blood pressure checked.

ANGINA AND HEART ATTACK SYMPTOMS

Note these symptoms for angina and heart attack (see p166) and if you have risk factors for CHD, do not delay – you must get medical treatment fast.

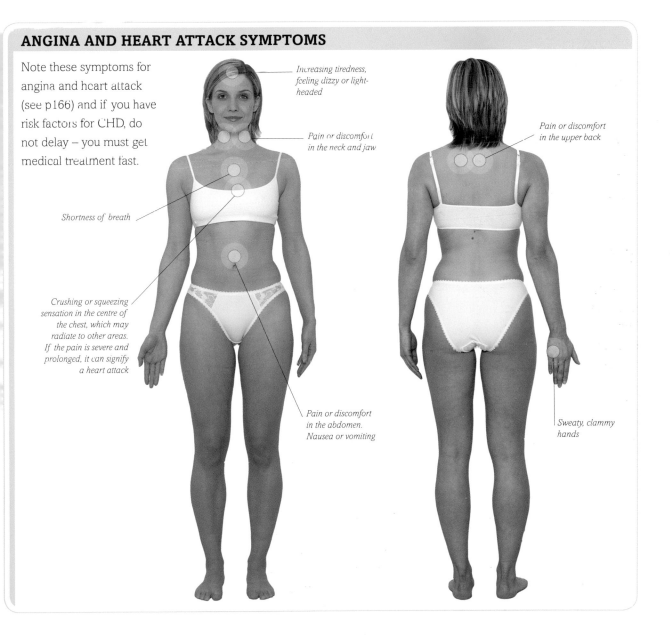

Increasing tiredness, feeling dizzy or light-headed

Pain or discomfort in the neck and jaw

Pain or discomfort in the upper back

Shortness of breath

Crushing or squeezing sensation in the centre of the chest, which may radiate to other areas. If the pain is severe and prolonged, it can signify a heart attack

Pain or discomfort in the abdomen. Nausea or vomiting

Sweaty, clammy hands

Heart attack

A heart attack occurs when there is a sudden blockage in an already narrowed coronary artery. Although heart attacks can be fatal, treatments have improved and the degree of damage caused by a heart attack often depends on how quickly a person receives the necessary treatment.

WHAT IS IT?

Narrowing of the arteries occurs over a period of years as fatty deposits gradually accumulate on the arterial walls. A heart attack occurs when a blood clot suddenly forms on the fatty deposits in a coronary artery, blocking the blood supply to the heart.

WHAT NEXT?

A heart attack is an emergency that requires urgent medical attention, so seek help immediately.

MY TREATMENT OPTIONS

Medications for a heart attack mainly include aspirin and clot-busting drugs. Some hospitals offer a primary coronary angioplasty service, in which the person having a heart attack is taken without delay to the cardiac catheter lab where a coronary angioplasty is performed to unblock the artery responsible for the heart attack (see p170).

HOW CAN I HELP MYSELF?

If you think you are having a heart attack, you should call an ambulance immediately.

HAVE I GOT THE SYMPTOMS?

Chest pain that is prolonged often indicates a heart attack. The pain is described as a heavy or squeezing sensation and can spread to the arms, jaw, neck, back, or stomach. It can also be associated with sweating and a feeling of nausea. In women, however, the symptoms may be different (see p165). Women may therefore be unaware that they might be having a heart attack, take longer to seek help, and may be more ill by the time they do. **Get medical help immediately** if you think you are having a heart attack.

Heart failure

Heart failure can be the result of coronary artery disease, valvular heart disease (see p174), high blood pressure (see p161), or cardiomyopathy (disease of the heart muscle). It can also be caused by alcohol excess, certain drugs or toxins, and some infections.

WHAT IS IT?

Heart failure occurs when the heart weakens and its pumping action becomes less efficient. It may be acute, when symptoms come on suddenly, or chronic, when symptoms are milder and build up over time.

WHAT NEXT?

Your doctor, after taking your medical history and examining you, is then likely to organize certain investigations, such as an ECG (see p168), an echocardiogram (ultrasound of the heart, see p169), and a chest X-ray, to help make a diagnosis of heart failure.

MY TREATMENT OPTIONS

There are different treatment options available to treat heart failure. Talk to your doctor about which is the most suitable for you.
Medication Patients with heart failure will require a combination of tablets to help the heart pump more efficiently and to reduce fluid overload, which leads to leg swelling and breathlessness. You are likely to need diuretics (water tablets), which will help reduce fluid retention.
Other treatments Depending on the underlying cause of your heart failure, you may be offered other

HAVE I GOT THE SYMPTOMS?

Common symptoms and signs of heart failure include:
- Breathlessness
- Fluid retention, including swollen legs
- General fatigue.

See your doctor if you have any of these symptoms.

"There are different treatment options available to treat heart failure, so talk to your doctor about which option is most suitable for you."

treatments. For example, you may have a pacemaker inserted (see below) to improve the pumping action of your heart. People with pacemakers require regular follow-up in pacing clinics to ensure that the pacemaker is functioning correctly. If you are a younger person with severe heart failure, a heart transplantation or a heart mechanical assist device may be an option.

HOW CAN I HELP MYSELF?

Always take the medication that has been prescribed by your doctor. Make an appointment to see your doctor if you feel that your weight is increasing, you are retaining fluid (when the lower legs or ankles swell), or you notice that you are becoming more breathless when you perform your normal everyday tasks.

Palpitations

A racing, or thumping, heart can cause the sensation known as palpitations. Although, often, these aren't a cause for concern and don't require treatment, they can be a sign of a problem with the heart or its blood vessels – known as arrhythmias – and should therefore be investigated.

WHAT IS IT?

Arrhythmias of the heart occur if the electrical impulses in the heart that co-ordinate the pumping action don't function correctly, so the heart beats too fast, too slow, or irregularly.

HAVE I GOT THE SYMPTOMS?

You are experiencing symptoms of palpitations if you feel that your heart is beating too fast, too slowly, or irregularly.
See your doctor if you have any of these symptoms.

WHAT NEXT?

If you have palpitations that your doctor thinks may be due to an arrhythmia, your doctor may recommend an electrocardiogram (ECG) and a 24-hour monitor (see p168). You will be asked to keep a diary of the times when you experience palpitations. When your doctor analyses the recording, he or she will check if there was an abnormal heart rhythm at the time you felt the palpitations.

MY TREATMENT OPTIONS

Palpitations may not always require treatment. Your doctor will advise on the most appropriate treatment:
Medication Some people's symptoms settle by taking tablets that suppress the arrhythmia.
Pacemakers These are generally used to correct a slow heartbeat. There are a number of different types of pacemaker that can be used depending on the rhythm abnormality. Pacemaker implantation is normally carried out under local anaesthetic and requires electrical leads to be passed through a vein in the chest to the heart. The electrical leads are then attached to a small pacemaker box, which sits underneath the skin.
Electrophysiological studies and ablation therapy People with troublesome palpitations may be offered an electrophysiological study and ablation therapy. Electrophysiological study involves passing tubes known as electrode catheters into the heart via a vein or artery in the groin. The electrode catheters are positioned in different areas of the heart to try to detect the abnormal heart rhythm. Once detected, ablation therapy can then be used to destroy or ablate the affected area that is producing the arrhythmia.

HOW CAN I HELP MYSELF?

If you are experiencing symptoms of palpitations (see box, left), it is important that you see your doctor.

CHD: How is it diagnosed?

A diagnosis of CHD will require a number of investigations. In women, the diagnosis can be more challenging because women can have more unusual symptoms than men (see pp164–5) and because certain investigations can be less sensitive and less specific in women compared to men.

HOW HEART DISEASE IS DIAGNOSED

Simpler tests, such as blood tests, can be done by a doctor or nurse. The more complex tests are usually carried out by a cardiac physiologist in the cardiology department of a hospital, while scans of the heart (CT, MRI, and myocardial perfusion scans) are performed by a doctor or radiographer in the radiology department. The tests are then reviewed by a cardiologist. Scans of the heart are usually reviewed by a radiologist specializing in cardiac imaging. The cardiologist will discuss the results with you.

Blood tests These are done to measure your blood sugar and cholesterol levels. If the results are high, you are at increased risk of heart disease. If you have had a suspected heart attack (see p166), a blood sample will be taken to look for the presence of and to measure specific enzymes, such as Troponin T and Troponin I, that are released into the bloodstream at the time of a heart attack.

Electrocardiogram (ECG) This test is used to record the electrical activity of your heart, including the heart rate and rhythm. During the

procedure, sticky pads known as electrodes are placed on your chest, wrists, and ankles. These are connected to a machine that records the readings. The test takes less than 10 minutes, but although the result is available immediately, a cardiologist will need to report on the test. If you have had palpitations, you may need a 24-hour recording to look for evidence of an abnormal heart rhythm, or arrhythmia (see p167).

Exercise test This test combines exercise with an ECG to see how your heart responds to exercise and exertion. During the test an ECG reading is taken while you exercise on a treadmill. Any symptoms of chest pain or undue breathlessness are noted, together with any changes in the ECG reading. Your blood pressure is also recorded. The length of the test depends on how long you are able to exercise for.

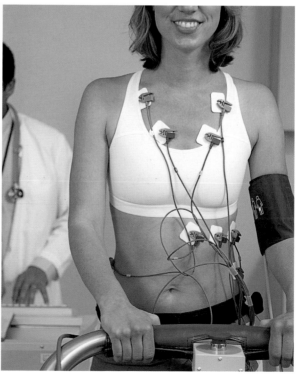

Exercise treadmill test
This woman is exercising on a treadmill with electrodes attached to her chest. The electrodes record the electrical activity of her heart and can detect any changes that occur with exercise. These can indicate that there may be disease of the coronary arteries.

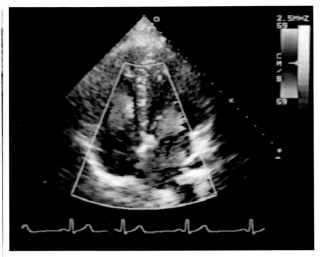

Echocardiogram with Doppler ultrasound
The echocardiogram gives an image of the heart, while the Doppler ultrasound (the coloured area within the triangle) shows the blood flow through the valves.

Echocardiogram This is an ultrasound of the heart used to assess the size of the heart, and how well its four chambers and its valves are working. The test takes around 30 minutes.

Stress echocardiogram This is similar to an echocardiogram (see above), but your heart is made to beat faster and stronger using medication injected into your arm. This test assesses how the muscle of the heart responds to stress and exercise.

A stress echocardiogram helps to identify certain areas of the heart that may not be receiving a good blood supply from the coronary arteries. It indicates, therefore, whether there may be narrowings or blockages in the coronary arteries.

Myocardial perfusion scan This two-phase test is used to investigate the function of your heart muscle, both when it is at rest and during exercise. A small amount of radioactive substance (radioisotope) is injected into the bloodstream then, during the first phase of the test, images of the heart at rest are taken using an ultrasound scanner.

During the second phase of the test you are given a further injection of radioisotope and the function of your heart is then reassessed, either after you have exercised on a treadmill (see opposite) or after you have been given an injection of a medication which increases your heart rate (as in a stress echocardiogram; see above). A second set of images are then taken and a direct comparison of the heart muscle at rest and after exercise can be made to help in the diagnosis.

CT (computerized tomography) scans (which include a coronary calcium scoring test and CT coronary angiogram; see right).

These tests involve taking images of the heart and coronary arteries using a CT scanner. The amount of calcium deposits (atheroma) in the coronary arteries can then be measured.

Cardiac MRI (magnetic resonance imaging) scan This test involves taking images of the heart to give a detailed picture of its structure, including its chambers, valves, the muscle of the heart and the coronary arteries as well as the great blood vessels.

Coronary angiogram This more invasive test is done by a cardiologist in the cardiac catheter lab. It is normally performed under local anaesthetic and takes approximately 30 minutes but can take longer.

It is used to image the coronary arteries to assess any narrowings or blockages within the coronary vessels. During the procedure, a needle is inserted in one of your blood vessels, either in the groin or in the arm, then hollow plastic tubes, or catheters, are passed along the blood vessel and into your heart. A dye is then injected into the coronary vessels and a series of X-ray images are taken (see p171). If you do have narrowings or blockages in the coronary arteries, these are seen as soon as the dye is injected. The cardiologist performing the procedure can then discuss the results with you.

"All investigations are reviewed by a cardiologist who will discuss the results with you."

CHD: How can I help myself?

Anyone at risk of CHD (see p163) should take preventive steps to avoid developing it. For women, who typically get CHD later in life when they may have other risk factors, prevention early on is key and they need to modify their risk factors when they are young. Fortunately, there is a lot you can do.

Preventive measures are geared towards preventing the build up of fatty deposits in your arteries.

WATCH YOUR LIFESTYLE

Follow these simple lifestyle rules for a healthy heart:

Stop smoking Smoking significantly increases your risk of developing CHD (see p163), so stopping is a major step to improving your heart health.

Eat healthily You should make sure you eat a healthy, low-fat diet (see opposite).

Reduce your salt intake Salt raises your blood pressure. You should not eat more than 6g a day (see p54).

Moderate your alcohol intake A small amount of alcohol is unlikely to cause harm, although you should keep within the recommended limits (see p65). Excessive drinking may increase your risk of CHD (see p163).

Keep fit Keeping active is important in preventing the development of heart disease. This is because exercise helps to control your blood pressure and cholesterol levels, helps you maintain a healthy body weight, and reduces stress. If you're diabetic (see pp320–5), a healthy weight helps towards managing your blood sugar levels.

Reduce your stress Learning relaxation techniques can help you to cope with and reduce the harmful effects of long-term stress.

GET CHECKED OUT

As well as taking steps to improve your lifestyle, it's also important to have your cholesterol levels and blood pressure checked regularly. You can often have high levels of cholesterol and high blood pressure – two major risk factors for developing CHD – yet be symptom-free. Asking your doctor for regular checks can highlight a problem, which can then be treated early.

Cholesterol Your cholesterol levels can be checked with a simple blood test. If your "bad" cholesterol, or LDL, level (see p163) is high, your doctor will recommend lifestyle changes to lower it (see opposite), and in some cases may suggest medication (see p170).

Blood pressure It's sensible to have your blood pressure checked regularly, at least every year (see pp28–47), and more frequently if you suffer from a condition such as diabetes, have other risk factors for CHD (see p163), or already have heart disease.

Diabetes If you suffer from diabetes (see pp320–5), you are already at an increased risk of developing CHD and so it's even more important to make sure that your diabetes is kept under control and that you take preventive lifestyle measures.

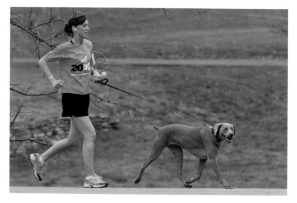

Keeping fit
Being active and building exercise into your weekly routine helps to keep your heart healthy. Aim to do a 30-minute exercise programme at least three times a week.

Foods to eat for a healthy heart

Eating a healthy, low-fat diet, with a minimum of saturated fats (see pp52–5) can help to prevent the build up of plaque deposits in your coronary arteries. Eating healthily also helps you to maintain a healthy weight, which in turn lowers your risk of heart disease as well as of other dangerous conditions such as diabetes.

Soluble fibre

Increases the feeling of fullness, which can help with weight control. RDA of dietary fibre = 30g

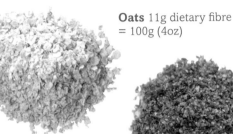

Oats 11g dietary fibre = 100g (4oz)

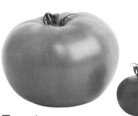

Ground linseeds 27g dietary fibre = 100g (4oz)

Oily fish

Provides the heart-healthy omega-3 fatty acids, which may help reduce LDL cholesterol and triglycerides
RDA of essential fatty acids = currently, no amount set

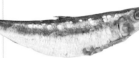

Sardines (canned in oil) 1480mg (total omega-3 fatty acids) = 100g (4oz)

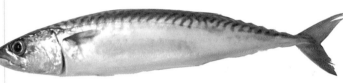

Mackerel (cooked) 1422mg (total omega-3 fatty acids) = 100g (4oz)

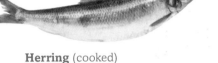

Herring (cooked) 1729mg (total omega-3 fatty acids) = 100g (4oz)

Antioxidants

Antioxidants (beta carotene, vitamin C, and vitamin E) may help protect the cardiovascular system from damage. RDA of beta carotene = none set, vitamin C = 60mg, vitamin E = 10mg

Tomatoes
beta carotene 0.5mg, Vit C 17mg, Vit E 1.2mg = 100g (4oz)

Carrots
beta carotene 9mg, Vit C 5.9mg, Vit E 1.6mg =100g (4oz)

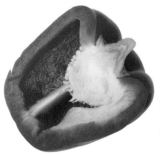

Red peppers beta carotene 1-2mg, Vit C 140mg, Vit E 0.8mg = 100g (4oz)

Magnesium

Important for the function of nerves and muscles. RDA of magnesium = 300mg

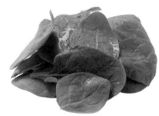

Green vegetables such as spinach (cooked) 34mg magnesium = 100g (4oz)

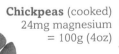

Chickpeas (cooked) 24mg magnesium = 100g (4oz)

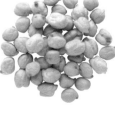

Almonds 270mg magnesium = 100g (4oz)

Valvular heart disease

Your heart valves help to control the flow of blood between the four chambers of the heart as well as the blood entering and leaving the heart (see p160). Sometimes a valve can be narrowed or doesn't close fully. Your doctor will be able to hear a heart murmur and you will need to undergo investigations.

WHAT IS IT?

Valvular heart disease occurs when there is an abnormality or dysfunction of one or more of the four heart valves. If a valve is narrowed, blood flow will be obstructed. This is known as valve stenosis. If a valve does not close fully, there will be leakage of blood, known as valve regurgitation.

Either problem can be caused by an anatomical abnormality of the valve from birth, as a result of having had rheumatic fever, or simply as part of the ageing process.

Valve stenosis or regurgitation can affect the pumping action of the heart. This means that the heart will work less efficiently or may become enlarged, which can result in heart failure.

Endocarditis is a condition which results from infection of heart valves. If the valve is abnormal the risk of endocarditis is greater than in a normal valve.

WHAT NEXT?

It your doctor suspects valvular heart disease, he or she will examine you to check for a heart murmur. You will also need other tests, including an ECG, (see p168) an echocardiogram (see p169), and a chest X-ray.

MY TREATMENT OPTIONS

Patients with mild forms of valvular heart disease may not require any treatment but will need regular follow-up. Some patients only require treatment with

medication, for example diuretics and ACE inhibitors.

Surgery Patients with severe disease and who have symptoms are likely to require surgery, which involves repairing or replacing the existing heart valve using either a metal or a tissue valve. Your cardiologist and surgeon will advise on which is the most suitable for you. Transcatheter valve procedures are new techniques that are used to treat some valves without the need for open heart surgery. However, they are only available in certain hospitals.

HOW CAN I HELP MYSELF?

If you think you may have the symptoms of valvular heart disease, you should make sure you seek medical help.

VALVULAR HEART DISEASE AND PREGNANCY

Valvular heart disease can get worse during pregnancy, so if you have been diagnosed with this condition you should consult your doctor if you are planning a pregnancy.

HAVE I GOT THE SYMPTOMS?

Symptoms may be minimal, but can include the following:

- Breathlessness
- Chest pain
- Dizzy spells
- Swollen ankles.

See your doctor if you have any of these symptoms.

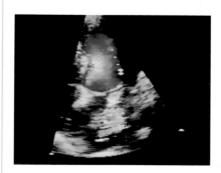

Valve regurgitation
This echocardiogram with Doppler ultrasound (coloured area within the triangle) shows a leaking valve (valve regurgitation).

Vascular disease

Varicose veins rarely cause serious complications, but they're at best unsightly, and at worst, uncomfortable. They don't significantly increase your risk of deep vein thrombosis (see pp252–3), but they can cause aching and swollen ankles and can make you more prone to eczema and possible leg ulcers.

Varicose veins

Achy legs are common after you have been standing for a long time, but varicose veins may be to blame.

WHAT ARE THEY?

Varicose veins are enlarged, twisted veins, usually in the leg. Blood runs through superficial veins, then through one-way valves into deeper veins. As the valves become less efficient, blood may flow backwards, then pool, enlarging and making the superficial veins visible.

WHAT NEXT?

Your doctor will examine the veins while you are standing. He or she may arrange for a scan to assess the blood flow in the vessels to confirm the diagnosis.

MY TREATMENT OPTIONS

If self-help measures (see right) fail to bring relief, talk to your doctor about the best treatment for you. However, you should be aware that varicose veins can recur after any of the treatments below.

Injections (sclerotherapy) Small veins may be treated with an injection of a chemical, which sticks the vein walls together to stop blood from entering.

Surgery This may be considered for larger varicose veins. Either the vein is tied and cut, or a long vein may be removed, a procedure known as "stripping".

Laser surgery This may be used to treat superficial "thread" veins, but works less well for varicose veins.

HOW CAN I HELP MYSELF?

Several self-help measures may relieve the symptoms.

Compression stockings These help the blood to flow through the veins more efficiently.

Regular exercise This improves your circulation so that blood flows more effectively.

Keeping your weight down This takes pressure off your veins.

Avoiding standing for long periods This can help swelling and aching, as can resting with your legs raised.

Red vine leaf extract This can relieve achy, swollen legs.

ANEURYSMS

Aneurysms are rare, occurring where there is a weak area in a blood vessel that balloons out. Most aneurysms are small and symptomless, often going undetected, but the danger is that a larger one may burst, causing a life-threatening haemorrhage. Aneurysms can occur throughout the body but are most common in the aorta, known as an aortic aneurysm. If an aortic aneurysm is found, it will be monitored and surgery may be planned. A burst aortic aneurysm is an emergency; its symptoms include pain or tenderness in the abdomen or chest, a pulse-like sensation in the abdomen, and backache.

HAVE I GOT THE SYMPTOMS?

Visible bulging veins are a clear indication of varicose veins. Other symptoms include:

- Aching or painful legs that continue to ache during rest
- In severe cases, itchy skin and ulceration.

See your doctor if you have symptoms that are painful or concern you.

Brain
and nerves

Professor Karen Morrison MA BMBCh DPhil FRCP

Dizzy spells and falls

Dizziness usually passes quickly, but if you aren't careful, it can make you fall over unexpectedly, which can be dangerous and cause injury. It's common to feel dizzy or off-balance if you change positions suddenly and this can happen, for example, if you stand up too quickly after bending over.

Dizziness

Dizziness is the feeling of being off-balance and light-headed, as if you're about to faint.

WHAT IS IT?

Dizziness has a great many causes, some of which are:

- Low blood sugar
- A disorder that causes low blood pressure, such as severe bleeding and overmedication with drugs for high blood pressure
- Episodes of very slow heart rate, known as "vasovagal attacks"
- Disease of the blood vessels in the neck
- Neurological diseases such as Parkinson's disease (see p197) and epilepsy (see pp194–5)
- Side effects of medications
- Panic attacks and hyperventilation (over-breathing).

HAVE I GOT THE SYMPTOMS?

You may be suffering from dizziness if you feel:
- Off-balance and light-headed
- Sweaty and pale.
See your doctor if you have the above symptoms.

WHAT NEXT?

Your doctor will diagnose the problem, recommend tests, and review your medications.

MY TREATMENT OPTIONS

Treatments depend on the cause. For example, low blood pressure may require elastic stockings and a drug such as fludrocortisone. Ask your doctor about side effects.

HOW CAN I HELP MYSELF?

Some simple self-help measures include the following:

Take regular, balanced meals to combat bouts of low blood sugar (see pp52–7, 325).

If you're elderly, hold on to something solid when you stand up from a chair. Use a sturdy walking stick when you're out and about.

Vertigo

Vertigo is the feeling that you or your surroundings are spinning.

WHAT IS IT?

Vertigo occurs when the brain fails to coordinate sensory information from your ear, eyes, and joints. It is often accompanied by nausea and vomiting. Vertigo can be caused by ear disease, Ménières disease (see box, below), migraine (see pp182–3), multiple sclerosis (see p198), head injury, viral infection, diabetes (see pp320–5), and stroke (see p196).

WHAT NEXT?

Your doctor will recommend tests to help with diagnosis.

MY TREATMENT OPTIONS

Your doctor may prescribe sedatives, such as diazepam; ask about side effects. Head and eye exercises with a physiotherapist can help, too.

HOW CAN I HELP MYSELF

If you have an attack of vertigo, lie still and avoid sudden movements.

HAVE I GOT THE SYMPTOMS?

Attacks of Ménières disease are sudden, and last minutes or days.
- Sudden dizziness and loss of balance
- Nausea and vomiting
- Jerky eye movements
- Buzzing or ringing in the ear
- Loss of hearing
- Pressure or pain in the ear.
See your doctor if you have any of the above symptoms.

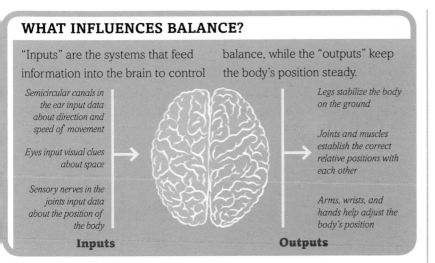

WHAT INFLUENCES BALANCE?

"Inputs" are the systems that feed information into the brain to control balance, while the "outputs" keep the body's position steady.

Semicircular canals in the ear input data about direction and speed of movement

Eyes input visual clues about space

Sensory nerves in the joints input data about the position of the body

Legs stabilize the body on the ground

Joints and muscles establish the correct relative positions with each other

Arms, wrists, and hands help adjust the body's position

Inputs

Outputs

HAVE I GOT THE SYMPTOMS?

These symptoms of vestibular neuritis may be mild or severe:

- Vertigo, which may range from a subtle dizziness to a violent spinning sensation
- Nausea and vomiting
- Unsteadiness and imbalance
- Vision impairment
- Impaired concentration
- Inability to sit, stand, or walk.

See your doctor if you have any of the above symptoms.

Falls

Giddiness sometimes makes us fall, though of course not all falls are preceded by giddiness. The elderly are particularly vulnerable.

WHAT IS IT?

You might develop a tendency to have falls because you have:

- Dizziness or vertigo (see opposite)
- Faintness
- A lack of coordination
- Weakness affecting a leg or ankle, or in the muscles, nerves, brain, or spinal cord
- Sensory nerve problems, such as numbness or tingling in the feet
- Poor vision
- Become intoxicated with drugs or alcohol.

WHAT NEXT?

Talk with your doctor if you are worried that you are prone to falls.

MY TREATMENT OPTIONS

Treatment is aimed at addressing the root cause of the problem.

HOW CAN I HELP MYSELF?

Improve the lighting in your home so that you can see better. Remove slippery mats and fix uneven floors that might make you lose your footing. If you wear glasses all the time, make sure that you have the correct prescription.

Vestibular neuritis and labyrinthitis

These are two disorders of the vestibulo-cochlear nerve, which connects the inner ear to the brain.

WHAT IS IT?

Vestibular neuritis and labyrinthitis result from infections that inflame the vestibulo-cochlear nerve. Symptoms of labyrinthitis are similar to vestibular neuritis (see above), but may include tinnitus and/or hearing loss (see p188).

WHAT NEXT?

Discuss your symptoms with your doctor. He or she may prescribe

medications to try to control the nausea and suppress the dizziness during the acute phase, after other illnesses have been ruled out.

MY TREATMENT OPTIONS

If a middle-ear infection is present, possible medications are steroids, an antiviral drug (e.g. aciclovir), or antibiotics (e.g. amoxicillin). Ask your doctor about the potential side effects. If you're treated at once, there should be little or no permanent damage. If the dizziness or imbalance carries on for several months, vestibular rehabilitation exercises can help to retrain your brain's ability to adjust. Full recovery from labyrinthitis may take several weeks.

HOW CAN I HELP MYSELF?

Keep moving around if you can, even if you feel some vertigo and unsteadiness, and despite your natural inclination to remain still.

Epilepsy

Epilepsy is the most common serious brain disorder. About three in 100 people experience a seizure in their lifetime and one in 100 people experience at least two. Treatment with antiepileptic drugs is often extremely effective. Most people with epilepsy have no symptoms between seizures or long-term problems.

HAVE I GOT THE SYMPTOMS?

If you think you have symptoms of either generalized or focal epilepsy, consult your doctor.

Generalized seizures

- Tonic–clonic seizures (formerly known as grand mal): you lose consciousness, become rigid, and collapse; then your limbs move in a jerking rhythm
- Absence seizures (sometimes known as petit mal): a type common in children; the child becomes vacant and appears to be day-dreaming
- Myoclonic seizures: brief, sudden jerking of one or more limbs
- Status epilepticus: repeated tonic–clonic seizures with no regaining of consciousness in between.

Focal (partial) seizures

- Focal sensory seizures: abnormal sensations, such as seeing unexpected colours
- Focal motor seizures: limb twitches
- Temporal lobe epilepsy: starts with odd sensations or a feeling of déjà vu, then detachment from reality, and perhaps repetitive movements.

WHAT IS IT?

An epileptic seizure happens when there's sudden, abnormal, and excessive electrical activity in a group of nerve cells in the cortex (outer region) of the brain. Seizures may either be generalized or focal (partial) in which you remain conscious (see box above).

Some seizures begin in one part of the brain (focally) and then spread and become generalized. Symptoms can range from a mild feeling of detachment to losing consciousness with jerking limbs. Most seizures last for only a few minutes, but occasionally the seizure will not stop spontaneously and you'll need hospital treatment. Status epilepticus (see above) is a serious medical emergency that needs immediate attention.

Seizures can occur without any specific provoking factors, but they can also be triggered by external events. These include:

- Head injury
- Excessive tiredness
- Exposure to either flashing or flickering lights
- Low blood sugar levels
- Alcohol intoxication
- Alcohol withdrawal
- Some recreational drugs.

Sometimes epilepsy arises because there's an underlying structural abnormality in the brain, such as a brain tumour (see p181). Most often, however, the brain appears normal when it's viewed with a scanner, such as an MRI, and no specific structural cause can be found.

WHAT NEXT?

Descriptions of the symptoms, both from the sufferer and from an eyewitness, form a crucial part of the diagnosis. These will help to exclude other potential conditions such as simple fainting episodes and mini-strokes, in which the blood supply to a part of the brain is temporarily blocked. Even types of migraine can sometimes mimic epilepsy.

If your doctor suspects that you have epilepsy, you'll be referred to a neurologist or to a specialist clinic. You'll need to have an electroencephalogram (EEG), in which electrodes are attached all over your scalp and the electrical activity of your brain is recorded. **Driving and epilepsy** If you have had a seizure and lost consciousness, you must not drive

OF SPECIAL CONCERN

Pregnancy and epilepsy

If you have a history of epilepsy and are planning to become pregnant, you should seek specialist advice from your doctor.

- You must take your antiepileptic drugs during pregnancy. Prolonged seizures, or an injury from you falling during a seizure, may damage your unborn child.
- Some medications are safer in pregnancy than others, and you may be able to switch to a drug that is safer for the foetus while still controlling your seizures.
- You should take extra folic acid supplements before conception and throughout your pregnancy.
- The frequency of seizures is not increased during pregnancy or after the birth, but it is important that you eat sensibly, take the appropriate rest and remember to take your medications.
- Although the risk of your child having seizures is slightly higher because of your own history, the absolute risk is low.

Menstruation and epilepsy

In catamenial epilepsy, seizures tend to occur before or during menstruation. Hormonal treatments, in addition to standard drugs, are very effective in preventing such seizures. This type of seizure tends to become less frequent after the menopause.

---

a vehicle and you must inform the DVLA. There are rules for how long you need to be seizure-free before you may drive again.

MY TREATMENT OPTIONS

Medication is the main treatment and your doctor will discuss your options. How long you need to take it depends on the cause of your seizures. If you have an underlying brain abnormality, you may be advised to stay on treatment for life. If the seizures were caused by a specific episode – for example, a head injury – it may be possible to stop medication after a few years and subsequently remain seizure-free.

Antiepileptic drugs (AEDs)

There are many AEDs that act in different ways to reduce the excitability of the brain. Most people are seizure-free on one or two medications taken daily. Modern drugs can be very effective and produce fewer side effects than those used in the past, though many make the oral contraceptive pill less effective. Ask your doctor about potential side effects of your medication.

Surgery This is reserved for people who have severe, frequent seizures that don't respond to drugs. The epileptic focus in the brain may be able to be completely removed, but the operation may cause disability through loss of brain tissue.

HOW CAN I HELP MYSELF?

To reduce your risk of seizures:
Maintain a healthy lifestyle, minimize stress, eat regularly, and get enough sleep (see pp48-69)
Avoid triggers Stay away from flashing or strobe lights if you have photosensitive epilepsy.
Take your AEDs as prescribed Failure to take them correctly is one of the most common causes of uncontrolled seizures.

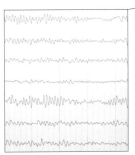

The screen shows different brain wave patterns arising from different areas of the cortex

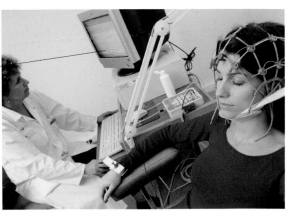

A woman suspected of having epilepsy undergoes an EEG
Electrodes on her scalp painlessly record brain waves. Some forms of epilepsy cause characteristic changes in the normal EEG, even when there is no seizure.

Stroke

Although the incidence of strokes in women and men is about the same, many women still think that stroke is a men's disease. Fortunately, maintaining a healthy lifestyle (see Chapter 3, pp48–69) and preventing or treating risk factors (see below) can help to reduce your risk of stroke in later life.

HAVE I GOT THE SYMPTOMS?

Stroke symptoms appear suddenly and vary greatly, depending on the specific blood vessels and brain regions involved. Strokes often occur at night so you may wake up with symptoms. Severe strokes can cause unconsciousness and may be fatal. **Contact your doctor urgently if** you experience any of the following symptoms:

- Weakness, numbness and tingling in the hand, arm, and maybe the leg on one side of the body
- Drooping of one side of the face
- Slurring of speech, or difficulty finding the correct words
- Poor balance, marked clumsiness
- Impaired vision with inability to see objects in one half of the visual field in each eye.

AM I AT RISK?

Women should take note of these risk factors for stroke:
- High blood pressure
- Diabetes
- Smoking
- Obesity
- A diet high in fat
- Irregular heartbeat
- Oral contraceptive pills, particularly if you also suffer from migraines
- Pregnancy. Strokes in pregnancy are rare. A few specific types, however, are unique to pregnancy
- Age. Strokes are much more common in the over-65s.

WHAT IS IT?

A stroke occurs when a part of the brain loses its function because its blood supply is disturbed by:
- A build-up of fatty tissue, or atheroma, in the blood vessels
- A blockage due to small particles (emboli) lodging in a vessel wall
- Bleeding into the brain tissue
- Reduced blood pressure.

WHAT NEXT?

A CT or MRI scan of the brain may show if you've suffered a stroke and may also reveal the cause. About half of all strokes are caused by blood clots that come from the heart, so you may need an electrocardiogram (see p168) and an echocardiogram (see p169).

MY TREATMENT OPTIONS

One dose of aspirin increases your chance of survival after a stroke and reduces the risk of another stroke in the following days. After that, a daily low dose of aspirin reduces the risk of future strokes.

Other treatments depend on the cause. For example, if your stroke was due to a blocked blood vessel, you may have an injection of a clot-busting drug, ideally within the first three hours. However, as the drug itself can cause excessive bleeding into the brain, the risk needs to be weighed up carefully against any likely benefit.

Your long-term outcome depends on the cause of the stroke. Overall, one in three strokes are fatal, one in three cause some disability, and one in three leave no disability. With rehabilitation, people recover most functions in the first few months, but recovery can take a year.

HOW CAN I HELP MYSELF?

You will receive all kinds of care after suffering a stroke, including nursing, occupational therapy, and physical therapy, but you can also help yourself by establishing a routine of daily exercises and following a healthy diet.

Parkinson's disease

Parkinson's disease is the second most common neurological degenerative disease after Alzheimer's disease. This chronic disease usually affects older people, although in some cases it can occur in younger people. While there is no cure for Parkinson's, there are treatments to control symptoms.

HAVE I GOT THE SYMPTOMS?

Symptoms may be put down to old age, but the stance and gait of people with Parkinson's disease soon becomes obvious. Sufferers often don't swing their arms when walking, are unsteady when they turn, and have reduced facial movements, which make them look depressed.

See your doctor if you have any of these early symptoms:

- Tremor – most marked in the hands (initially on one side). "Pill-rolling" tremor between thumb and index finger
- Stiffness of the limbs
- Rigidity of the body
- Slow, reduced movements – often hesitating when starting a movement, such as walking.

As the disease progresses more symptoms develop:

- Quiet, stumbling speech
- Coughing and choking
- Drooling due to excess saliva
- Disturbed sleep, vivid dreams
- Restless legs
- Depression
- Constipation
- Excessive sweating.

WHAT IS IT?

Nerve cells in the substantia nigra area of the brain secrete dopamine, which fine-tunes muscle control. In Parkinson's disease they degenerate and stop making dopamine.

WHAT NEXT?

Slowness, stiffness, and tremor indicate Parkinson's disease. A brain scan is often unnecessary, although DAT scans can show abnormal dopamine signals in the brain.

MY TREATMENT OPTIONS

Drugs to increase brain dopamine are the mainstay of treatment, but research may offer other options. Ask your doctor about side effects.

Drugs Your doctor will give you one or more drugs, such as levodopa, pramipexole, ropinirole, or selegiline.

Surgery Electrical stimulators in specific parts of the brain can reduce tremor and abnormal movements.

AM I AT RISK?

Most people develop symptoms during their 70s. Other risk factors include:

- Genetic predisposition
- Living in the country
- Exposure to some pesticides
- Exposure to some metals
- Repeated head trauma.

Associated treatment Drugs can help with sleep disturbance, mood disorders, and bladder and bowel problems. Physiotherapy, speech therapy, occupational therapy, and specialist nurses can all help.

HOW CAN I HELP MYSELF?

Stay as active and positive as you can, and work with your doctor to get your medication just right. Join a support group and find out all you can about the disease.

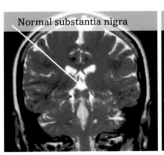

Normal substantia nigra

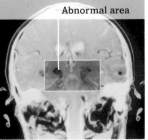

Abnormal area

Diagnosing Parkinson's
A comparison of the scans of a normal brain (far left) and a brain affected by Parkinson's disease (left) can help with diagnosis.

Multiple sclerosis

This complex disorder involves inflammation of the nerve fibres in the brain and spinal cord. Multiple sclerosis (MS) can affect young adults, and is twice as common in women as it is in men. Although there is no cure for MS, many people recover fully between episodes for a number of years.

WHAT IS IT?

MS is caused by inflammation of the myelin (insulating sheath) of nerves in the brain and spinal cord. This occurs when specific white blood cells that normally protect the body from infection become abnormal and attack the body's nervous system. Usually, the body's defences heal the areas of nerve inflammation, but eventually, after many years, this is less effective and sufferers are left with permanent and increasingly severe disabilities. At first, the symptoms (see below) are often vague, but they're real and worrying. Your symptoms may be more marked in hot weather or after you've had a warm bath.

WHAT NEXT?

If your doctor suspects MS, you'll be referred to a neurologist who may make the diagnosis based on a physical examination and your symptoms. MRI scans of the brain and spinal cord often show up characteristic areas of inflammation. A lumbar puncture may reveal abnormal antibodies, which can contribute to making the diagnosis.

MY TREATMENT OPTIONS

Treatment is aimed at symptom relief and speeding recovery during relapses. The following drugs can't halt or slow the progress of MS. Ask your doctor about side effects.
Corticosteroids, intravenously or orally, may help shorten relapses. Because of the risks of long-term treatment, their use is restricted to severe flare-ups.
A selective serotonin reuptake inhibitor (SSRI, see p227) may be prescribed if tiredness and depression are troubling you.
A muscle-relaxant drug may alleviate stiffness.
Injected interferon beta and copolymer 1 can suppress oversensitivity of the immune system, reducing the frequency and severity of relapses.

HOW CAN I HELP MYSELF?

Take gentle exercise regularly to strengthen your muscles, make sure you have plenty of support, and keep stress to a minimum.

HAVE I GOT THE SYMPTOMS?

Symptoms are variable both in type and severity, and tend to occur in "attacks" lasting about a month.
- Visual symptoms such as pain on moving your eyes, blurred vision, and altered colour vision
- Weakness, clumsiness, or stiffness of the limbs
- Numbness, tingling, or tightness in an arm or leg
- Tingling in the face
- Unsteadiness in walking.

After many years, persistent symptoms may include extreme fatigue, depression, cognitive difficulties, and bladder problems.
See your doctor if you notice any of the above symptoms.

AM I AT RISK?

No one yet knows what triggers multiple sclerosis, but there are some pointers:
- The disease is much more common in temperate zones than in countries near the equator. This suggests that an environmental factor, such as a virus that thrives in temperate regions, may be involved
- You're more likely to get MS if one of your parents has the disease, which suggests a genetic link.

Motor neurone disease

This rare degenerative disease affects the nerves that control muscles. Motor neurone disease (MND) usually begins in people over 50 and progresses rapidly. While the muscles become weaker, other brain functions such as memory, personality, and intellect remain unaffected.

WHAT IS IT?

MND is a rare but devastating disease of the motor nerves and pathways that control muscles. It results in muscle weakness in the limbs, difficulty in swallowing, and breathing problems.

This rapidly progressive disease is, understandably, very upsetting for those who have been diagnosed and for their close families and friends. Most people with MND die within a few years of diagnosis.

WHAT NEXT?

No tests specifically diagnose MND. A specialist neurologist will need to perform a clinical examination involving MR imaging and blood tests to exclude other disorders. He or she will arrange electrical tests on your nerves and muscles.

MY TREATMENT OPTIONS

Treatment can't slow or reverse the muscle wasting, only help alleviate symptoms. Ask about the side effects of any medication you're prescribed.

Riluzole This drug can prolong survival on average by a few months.

Antibiotics These are used to treat chest infections.

Muscle relaxants These drugs help to ease stiff muscles.

AM I AT RISK?

The incidence of MND increases with age and is more common among smokers. In around 10 per cent of cases a parent has the disease and a genetic defect is sometimes found.

Artificial aids If swallowing and breathing are difficult, a feeding tube and ventilator can help.

Specialist support Experienced health care professionals and palliative care physicians can help improve your quality of life as you become weaker.

HOW CAN I HELP MYSELF?

Keep your mind active, exercise gently if you can to maintain suppleness, and get plenty of support and counselling.

HAVE I GOT THE SYMPTOMS?

Weakness and muscle wasting develop over a few months, with any of the following symptoms:

- Weakness in the hands or ankles
- Slurred speech or weak voice
- Stiff or floppy limbs
- Involuntary muscle twitching
- Worsening clumsiness affecting arms, legs, and neck.

Over one or two years, there is rapid deterioration leading to:

- Progressive weakness
- Shortness of breath
- Drowsiness
- Visible wasting of the muscles.

See your doctor if you have any of the symptoms described.

DEGENERATION OF MOTOR PATHWAYS

In MND, the motor nerves that make muscles move gradually degenerate, causing progressive wasting and weakness of the muscles.

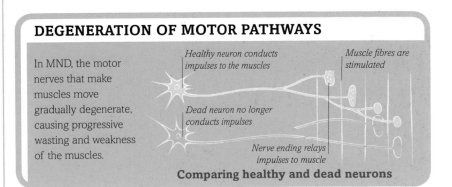

Healthy neuron conducts impulses to the muscles

Muscle fibres are stimulated

Dead neuron no longer conducts impulses

Nerve ending relays impulses to muscle

Comparing healthy and dead neurons

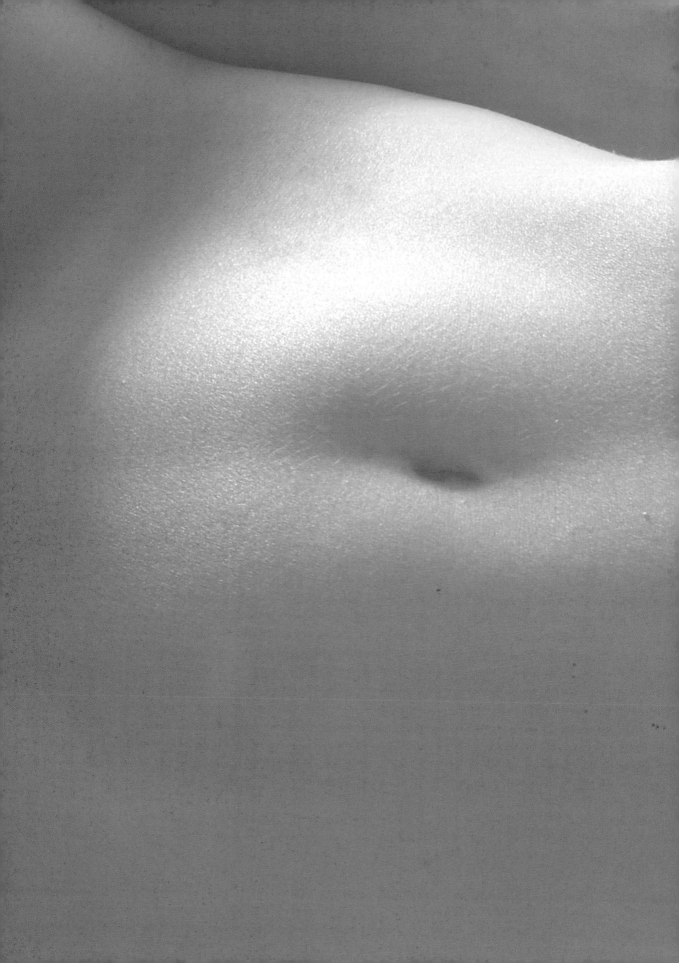

Mental Health

Dr Charlotte Feinmann MD MSc FRCPsych FDS(Hon)

Mental health

In today's world, most women find themselves searching for a balance in their lives. We work hard to integrate the demands of our relationships, families, and careers. We try, often at the very end of the day, to remember to care for ourselves and achieve mental and physical health. While some women are able to juggle these pressures and maintain wellness, there are many and complex reasons why others develop mental health problems. Fortunately, there are effective treatments for many of these problems; the first important step is to ask for help.

SUPERWOMEN

Many modern women feel an expectation from society to be perfect, and today's "superwomen" are expected to be accomplished in all areas, ranging from our beauty and physical wellness, to professional achievement, to happiness in our family and romantic lives. And we're supposed to pull it all off with a feeling of balance and expression of grace. In the post-equal-rights era, we have finally earned the right to do it all, but with these new freedoms have come the burden of new stresses.

MENTAL HEALTH PROBLEMS

All in all, we women tend to be caregivers and feel responsible for other people's needs. Yet many of us tend to overlook our mental wellness until a problem arises and we lose the balance in our lives. We know we can't always be happy and content, and that feelings of frustration, disappointment, sadness, and worry are part of the human condition. However, we can develop a mental health problem, or symptom, when these emotions become significantly distressing and impair our ability to function. Some psychological

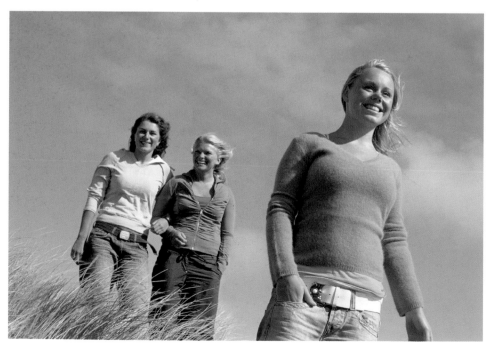

A good enough balance
What does achieving a healthy balance in life involve? Experts agree that a healthy approach is to find a *good enough* balance between work, play, and love. The balance doesn't have to be perfect — but it should be meaningful and satisfying to you.

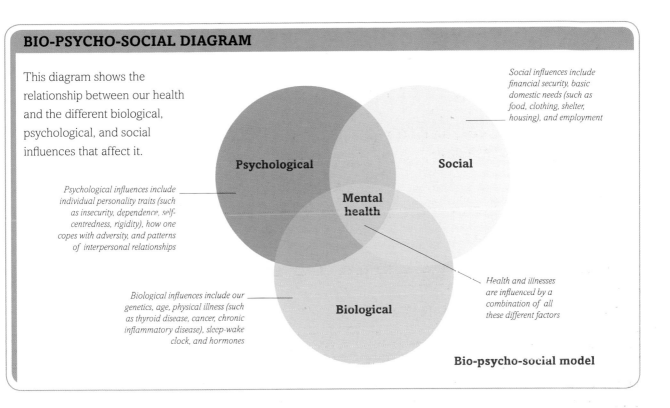

BIO-PSYCHO-SOCIAL DIAGRAM

This diagram shows the relationship between our health and the different biological, psychological, and social influences that affect it.

Social influences include financial security, basic domestic needs (such as food, clothing, shelter, housing), and employment

Psychological

Social

Mental health

Psychological influences include individual personality traits (such as insecurity, dependence, self-centredness, rigidity), how one copes with adversity, and patterns of interpersonal relationships

Biological

Biological influences include our genetics, age, physical illness (such as thyroid disease, cancer, chronic inflammatory disease), sleep-wake clock, and hormones

Health and illnesses are influenced by a combination of all these different factors

Bio-psycho-social model

symptoms may be expected for a given age group – many women experience a brief but manageable period of anxiety surrounding transitions, such as moving out of their childhood home, getting married, being pregnant or going through the menopause. Other emotions may be linked with hormonal changes as our bodies develop and change from menstruation through menopause.

This chapter addresses some of the mental health problems that women experience, from anxieties and depression to eating disorders and sexual dysfunction. Unfortunately, the history of psychiatric research has not always reflected gender differences, as women have frequently been excluded from studies. More recently, it has been recognized that women, due to their physiology, may have a different experience

> "Modern women have earned the right to do it all, but with these freedoms have come the burden of new stresses."

from men in their symptoms and treatment of mental health problems.

THE BIO-PSYCHO-SOCIAL MODEL

Despite significant progress identifying and treating mental health problems, their causes are still not fully understood. Many mental health problems, including depression, may be influenced by a number of different sources. In an attempt to explain these sources, and why some people develop psychological symptoms while others don't, scientists have developed a framework called the "bio-psycho-social" model. This combines the biological, psychological, and social influences (see box above), which all work together on the brain to alter the way neurotransmitters – chemicals in the brain – such as serotonin and dopamine, produce changes in our emotional states.

The following pages outline the mental illnesses that affect women the most. Specific treatments are mentioned in each article but refer to pp224–7 for a general discussion of treatment.

Anxiety disorders

Feelings of anxiety and panic, and the physical signs of sweating, palpitations, and breathlessness, can be a common response to stress. However, if you get these reactions frequently and they disrupt your everyday activities, you may have an anxiety disorder.

Anxiety disorders, like other mental health disorders, are caused by a combination of biological, psychological, and social factors (see pp202–3). If you have a family history of an anxiety disorder, you may be more vulnerable to stress, and this may increase your risk of developing an anxiety disorder.

Sometimes there may be a medical factor that is responsible for your anxiety, such as thyroid disease or substance abuse, and any such possible medical causes must be ruled out before your doctor can diagnose anxiety as a mental health condition.

Generalized anxiety disorder

If you have generalized anxiety disorder (GAD), you worry excessively about anything and everything, although you might not know exactly why you feel so anxious. GAD affects more women than men and is most common during the early adult years.

WHAT IS IT?

Most people get nervous when they are stressed, but what makes someone with GAD different is that they are worried most or all of the time. Although to many people this may seem to be a minor problem, in fact it can seriously interfere with daily life.

If you have GAD, you may also have other mental health problems, such as major depressive disorder (see pp210–11), another anxiety disorder, or substance abuse (see pp220–1).

WHAT NEXT?

Your doctor will do a thorough evaluation and make a diagnosis based on your symptoms.

MY TREATMENT OPTIONS

Depending on your particular symptoms, your doctor may advise therapy, medication, or both.

Therapies Cognitive-behavioural therapy is effective for many people with GAD, although behaviour therapy may also be recommended (see p225).

Medication The most common medication is either an SSRI or SNRI antidepressant (see p227). Ask your doctor about side effects.

HOW CAN I HELP MYSELF?

Symptoms may be alleviated by regular exercise, relaxation methods, avoiding caffeine, not drinking excessively, and not smoking,

HAVE I GOT THE SYMPTOMS?

To be diagnosed with generalized anxiety disorder, you must be unrealistically anxious about two or more life circumstances for at least six months. You must also have at least three of the following symptoms:

- Problems sleeping
- Fatigue
- Muscle tension
- Restlessness
- Inability to concentrate
- Irritability.

See your doctor if you have symptoms that cause you distress in your daily life.

For your doctor to diagnose generalized anxiety disorder, your symptoms must not be caused by a medical condition or by another type of mental health disorder.

Panic disorder

Panic disorder is a condition in which a person experiences unexpected episodes of intense fear accompanied by physical symptoms. Panic disorder is roughly twice as common in women as in men and you can get it at any time in life, but women in their 20s–40s are at greatest risk.

WHAT IS IT?

If you have a panic attack it doesn't necessarily mean that you have panic disorder. That diagnosis is only made if you also have anticipatory anxiety (anxiety about future panic attacks) on a regular basis for at least a month. Your attacks may be caused by specific triggers or situations, such as agoraphobia (the fear of being in

crowds and public places) or you may get them more randomly.

Panic attacks also give you physical symptoms, and it's common for people to go to an accident and emergency department because they think they are having a heart attack.

Panic disorder hardly ever gets better on its own, and so it's important that you see your doctor if you think you may be suffering from it. In about 20 per cent of the most severely affected people it can lead to attempted suicide, especially where it's coupled with major depressive disorder (see pp210–11).

WHAT NEXT?

Your doctor will do a thorough evaluation and make a diagnosis based on your symptoms.

MY TREATMENT OPTIONS

The two main treatment choices are therapy and medication.

Therapies Cognitive-behavioural therapy or behaviour therapy (see p225) are often effective.

Medication Your doctor may prescribe antidepressants (see p227), including an SSRI, SNRI or tricyclic antidepressant. Benzodiazepines may also be used in some cases. Ask your doctor about any possible side effects.

HOW CAN I HELP MYSELF?

Creative visualization of a peaceful scene or situation, relaxation techniques, and regular exercise can all help to relieve symptoms.

HAVE I GOT THE SYMPTOMS?

Panic attacks occur in discrete episodes peaking within 10 minutes. To be classed as panic disorder, you must have four or more symptoms featured in the box right, and accompanied by intense fear. You must also have:

● One month (or more) of worry about future panic attacks, worry about the implications of an attack, or changed behaviour due to the attacks.

See your doctor if any of these features apply to you.

THE SIGNS OF A PANIC ATTACK

As well as feelings of anxiety, panic attacks also produce physical symptoms, at least four of which must be present for an attack to be classed as a panic attack, together with a feeling of unreality, fear of losing control, and fear of dying.

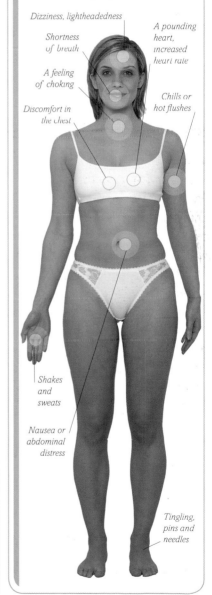

Dizziness, lightheadedness

Shortness of breath

A feeling of choking

Discomfort in the chest

A pounding heart, increased heart rate

Chills or hot flushes

Shakes and sweats

Nausea or abdominal distress

Tingling, pins and needles

Social anxiety disorder

At one time or another most of us have felt shy, lacking in confidence, or anxious in social situations, but these feelings are usually fairly mild and we manage to overcome them. However, if the distress is so severe that it affects your personal and work life, you may have social anxiety disorder.

WHAT IS IT?

Sometimes known as social phobia, social anxiety disorder makes you feel intensely anxious about being humiliated or embarrassed when you are in a social situation. You then become self-conscious and suffer from symptoms of anxiety, which may include blushing, a pounding heart, and sweating. As you become anxious, your symptoms cause more stress and this makes you even more anxious, so you find yourself in a vicious cycle. Eventually, these reactions may become your normal conditioned response to social situations. Such severe anxiety can have a negative impact on both your personal and your work life.

Common problems for people with social anxiety disorder are a fear of public speaking and other situations involving performance. Other symptoms may include fear of eating or drinking in public, and a fear of using public toilets. Associated personality features seen in people with social anxiety disorder include low self esteem, over-sensitivity to criticism, and difficulty being assertive.

Social anxiety disorder is a relatively common problem. About 7 per cent of the population experience social anxiety in adulthood, and it is more common in women than men. The exact cause isn't known, but it probably has bio-psycho-social roots (see p203). It's likely that the chemistry of the brain and the functioning of the amygdala (a part of the brain concerned with emotions and feeling, including fear) are involved.

Many people with social anxiety disorder also suffer from depression (see pp210–11). Some also turn to substance abuse, possibly in an unconscious attempt to reduce their social anxiety by self-medication.

WHAT NEXT?

Your doctor will do a thorough evaluation and make a diagnosis based on your symptoms.

MY TREATMENT OPTIONS

Your doctor may advise talk therapy, medication, or both.
Therapy Behavioural therapy and cognitive-behavioural therapy (CBT, see p225) may help. CBT, in particular, has proved to work for many women.
Medication Your doctor may prescribe an antidepressant (see p227), such as an SSRI (e.g. Prozac) or an SNRI (e.g. venlafaxine). Benzodiazepines may also be used in some cases.

HOW CAN I HELP MYSELF?

The most important thing is to persevere with treatment, even if it does not seem to be working at first. Both medication and therapy may take time to produce noticeable benefits.

HAVE I GOT THE SYMPTOMS?

If you have social anxiety disorder, you will fear situations in which you may be exposed to scrutiny by others. This response must not be due to another medical or mental health condition and must last for at least six months. Symptoms of social anxiety disorder include:

- Fear of behaving in a way that is embarrassing
- Severe anxiety in social situations or situations in which you have to perform (e.g. speaking in public)
- A recognition that your anxiety is unreasonable
- Avoidance of stress-producing situations.

See your doctor if these symptoms interfere with your normal daily life.

"Although social anxiety disorder can feel overwhelming, it can often be treated effectively."

Obsessive compulsive disorder

In obsessive compulsive disorder (OCD), you are bothered by unwanted and intrusive thoughts and/or overwhelming urges – compulsions – to repeatedly carry out particular actions. This obsessive-compulsive cycle may become so time-consuming that it disrupts your daily life.

WHAT IS IT?

If you suffer from OCD, you have thoughts or worries that keep coming into your mind. Although you may realize these obsessions are irrational, they still make you anxious. For example, you may

have such a powerful fear of germs that you can't go out because of your worry about contamination.

You may also feel compelled to perform specific rituals to reduce anxiety. Although these compulsions are intended to be reassuring, they may actually prevent you from functioning normally in everyday life. A classic example is repeatedly checking that a door is locked even though you know you've already locked it.

As with other mental disorders, OCD probably has bio-psycho-social causes (see p203).

About 1 per cent of adults have OCD. In women it tends to appear in adolescence or early adulthood. Women may have a new onset of OCD symptoms when they are pregnant. Women with OCD may also find their symptoms are more severe before a period.

WHAT NEXT?

OCD is a long-term disorder that won't get completely better unless you have treatment, so if you're concerned that you have OCD, see your doctor. He or she will make a diagnosis based on your obsessions

or your compulsions, though it's common to have both. For OCD to be diagnosed, your obsessions or compulsions must be distressing and disrupt daily activities.

MY TREATMENT OPTIONS

Your doctor will do a thorough evaluation and discuss the most appropriate therapies and medication with you.

Therapies Exposure and response prevention (ERP) is a specific behavioural therapy for OCD in which you are exposed to situations that make you fearful but are prevented from performing your usual rituals. This can be difficult at first but may be effective over time. Alternatively, cognitive-behavioural therapy (see p225) may be helpful.

Medication Your doctor may also prescribe an SSRI antidepressant (see p227) or the tricyclic antidepressant clomipramine.

HOW CAN I HELP MYSELF?

Treatment may take time to produce noticeable benefit, so the best way you can help yourself is to persist with it.

HAVE I GOT THE SYMPTOMS?

You may have OCD if you have obsessions and/or compulsions which you recognize are unreasonable but which still interfere with daily life. Your symptoms must not be due to another medical or mental health condition. Symptoms include:

- Obsessions – recurrent thoughts, impulses, or images that you know are a product of your own mind but which still cause anxiety
- Compulsions – repetitive behaviours in response to obsessions that are aimed, unrealistically, at preventing distress.

See your doctor if any of these symptoms impair normal life.

Post-traumatic stress disorder

Any of us can witness or experience a distressing or life-threatening event and most of us recover without needing help. But for some people, and women being particularly at risk, such an event is experienced as a trauma that haunts them over time and, as a result, they suffer various symptoms that disrupt daily life.

HAVE I GOT THE SYMPTOMS?

The symptoms of PTSD occur after a person has been exposed to a traumatic event. The symptoms must last for at least one month and must impair your daily functioning or cause distress. The memory of the event haunts you, recurring in flashbacks or nightmares that trigger the same intense fear that you originally felt. In addition, you will have three or more of the following:

- Emotional numbness
- Loss of pleasure in activities you usually enjoy
- Memory loss
- Active avoidance of reminders of the event.

You will also be constantly "on edge" (hyperaroused) with two or more of the following:

- Poor concentration
- Hypervigilance
- Insomnia
- Irritability
- Exaggerated startle response.

Consult your doctor if your symptoms are distressing and interfering with your daily life.

WHAT IS IT?

Post-traumatic stress disorder (PTSD) is a severe anxiety response that you can develop after you have been involved in or witnessed a psychologically stressful or life-threatening event. It can affect anybody, including children, and the symptoms (see Have I got the symptoms?) may develop immediately or may not appear until months after the traumatic event. Initially, it may be difficult to distinguish PTSD from acute stress disorder, which has the same features as PTSD. However, with acute stress disorder the symptoms always develop immediately after the traumatic event and usually get better within a month.

PTSD is about twice as common in women as in men; it's estimated that about 10 per cent of women will suffer from PTSD at some time in their lives. More than half of rape victims are diagnosed with PTSD.

As well as causing unpleasant, life-disrupting symptoms, PTSD also puts you at increased risk for suicide and impulsive behaviours,

AM I AT RISK?

A number of factors make you more at risk of having PTSD:

- Directly experiencing or witnessing a violent personal assault, an accident, a violent terrorist incident, a natural or human-caused disaster, or war.
- Women are at higher risk of PTSD because they are more likely to be the victims of a sexual assault or of physical, sexual, or emotional abuse from their partner (known as intimate partner violence).

- Women who are pregnant, especially if the pregnancy was not planned, are at increased risk of being the victim of intimate partner violence and therefore of developing PTSD.
- People who have suffered from anxiety or depression in the past are at greater risk of suffering from PTSD.
- Children who have been exposed to a traumatic event are at greater risk of developing PTSD as adults.

especially if you have also been sexually assaulted. In addition to suffering from PTSD, victims of intimate partner violence may also experience anxiety and depression. They also often have a diminished sense of self-worth, and frequently feel socially isolated.

Although the various external factors that can result in PTSD are well known, the entire causative mechanisms and processes are unclear, and it is not known why some people who experience traumatic events develop PTSD while others don't.

Like many other psychiatric conditions, PTSD is thought to be due to a combination of biological, psychological, and social factors (see p203). On the biological side, it is thought that part of the brain called the amygdala may play a central role. The amygdala is part of the brain's limbic system (see box, right) and is considered by many scientists to be the place where we store our fears and the memories of our emotions. Other areas of the brain that play a part in the formation of memories and in the body's response to stress are also thought to be involved, notably the medial prefontal cortex, the hippocampus, the hypothalamus, and the thalamus (see Areas of the brain affected in PTSD, right).

WHAT NEXT?
Your doctor will do a thorough evaluation and be able to diagnose PTSD from your description of the symptoms. He or she will probably refer you to a psychologist or psychiatrist for treatment.

MY TREATMENT OPTIONS
You may be offered therapy, medication, or a combination of the two, and the treatment will be tailored specifically for you.

Cognitive-behavioural therapy (CBT) This form of therapy is often used for PTSD and is usually very effective (see p225).

Eye movement desensitization and reprocessing (EMDR) This therapy involves you rhythmically moving your eyes to help you relax (see p225). Your therapist then asks you to talk about the trauma. The goal of this therapy is to break the link between your memories and your anxiety symptoms.

Supportive therapy This is an important part of treatment for victims of violence. It is particularly valuable for rape victims, as it can help them to regain their sense of self-worth.

Medications Antidepressants such as SSRIs (see p227) may also be helpful. Ask your doctor about potential side effects.

HOW CAN I HELP MYSELF?
You can best help yourself by seeing a doctor as soon as possible and then by following your treatment plan. It's never too late to seek treatment – PTSD can be treated even years after the trauma.

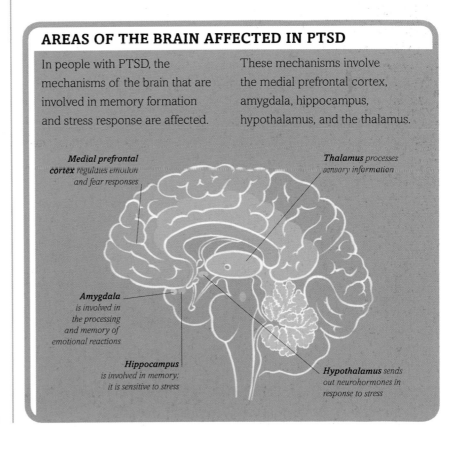

AREAS OF THE BRAIN AFFECTED IN PTSD

In people with PTSD, the mechanisms of the brain that are involved in memory formation and stress response are affected.

These mechanisms involve the medial prefrontal cortex, amygdala, hippocampus, hypothalamus, and the thalamus.

Medial prefrontal cortex regulates emotion and fear responses

Thalamus processes sensory information

Amygdala is involved in the processing and memory of emotional reactions

Hippocampus is involved in memory; it is sensitive to stress

Hypothalamus sends out neurohormones in response to stress

Depression

We all feel down or sad sometimes, but if "the blues" persists and becomes so bad that it interferes with daily life, this may be a sign of depression. Roughly 15 per cent of people become clinically depressed at some point in their lives and, compared to men, women are twice as likely to develop depression.

WHAT IS IT?

In everyday life, when people say they are "depressed" they are often referring to feelings of sadness that will pass after a relatively short time. But in clinical depression, feelings of intense sadness, hopelessness, worthlessness, and loss of interest in life last for weeks or months and have a significant negative impact on your life. These feeling are deeper, more disruptive, and last longer than transient unhappiness. If you are depressed, you may also suffer from various physical symptoms, such as disrupted sleep, fatigue, aches and pains, and weight loss or gain, In the worst cases, people with untreated depression may even take their own lives. In addition, untreated depression can have secondhand effects on other family members and friends, and is a leading cause of disability. In the longer term, depression can also increase your risk of heart disease.

It is important to distinguish between depression, which is an illness, and grief, which is a natural reaction to loss. Both share many of the same features but, unlike depression, grief is a healing process that typically resolves itself in five stages and does not require treatment. The first stage is shock and denial. Then there is anger and guilt, followed by an urge to bargain to get back what you have lost. The fourth stage is deep sadness or despair. Finally there is acceptance, when you come to terms with the loss and are able to move forwards. However, for some people the process does not resolve itself in acceptance; this is known as complicated grieving and requires professional help.

There are various types of depression and the causes are still unknown, but bio-psycho-social factors (see p203) may play a part. Women and men are different, and the anatomy and physiology of the female brain affect women in unique, specific ways.

Psychologically, we experience specific sources of stress, including worries about fertility, pregnancy, motherhood, and single parenthood. And socially, women have historically suffered more than men

HAVE I GOT THE SYMPTOMS?

You may meet the criteria for a major depressive episode if you have at least five of the symptoms listed here (one of the first two symptoms must be present) during the same two-week period. These symptoms must be abnormal for you personally and must not be due to a physical illness, medications, or to substance use. They must also cause severe distress or impair your everyday life, and they must not be accompanied by symptoms of bipolar disorder (see p212) or be due to grief.

- Low mood
- Diminished interest or pleasure in activities you used to enjoy
- Significant weight loss or gain
- Inability to sleep or dramatically increased sleep
- Feeling as if your body is slowed down or feeling agitated
- Loss of energy
- Feelings of worthlessness or guilt
- Poor concentration
- Recurrent thoughts of death or suicide, or a suicide attempt.

See your doctor if you have a number of these symptoms. If you are suicidal, get help urgently.

from challenges such as juggling domestic and career duties, job discrimination, and abuse.

Each of the many different types of depression has different symptoms and different degrees of severity. The main types and their features are outlined below.

Major depressive disorder (MDD) Previously called unipolar depression, MDD is when episodes of depression are severe and involve a particular combination of features (see Have I got the symptoms?). For a diagnosis of MDD you must have one or more depressive episodes in the absence of manic, hypomanic, or mixed episodes. (Mania is a feeling of extreme elation; hypomania is similar to mania but milder; a mixed episode is when symptoms of both depression and mania are present at the same time.)

Minor depression This is diagnosed when you have some of the symptoms of depression but not all of the elements necessary for a major depressive episode (see Have I got the symptoms?).

Dysthymia This is characterized by symptoms that are relatively mild but long-lasting. If you have at least two of the symptoms of a major depressive episode but generally feel depressed in everyday life, then you may have this disorder.

Adjustment disorder with depressed mood This is diagnosed when you have the same symptoms as those of a major depressive episode (see Have I got the symptoms?), but

symptoms begin only after you've suffered a specific stressful event within the past three months.

Premenstrual dysphoric disorder (PMDD) A diagnosis of PMDD may be made when you have the same symptoms as those of a major depressive episode but the symptoms only occur during your premenstrual period and then clear up during the first few days of your period (see also p93).

WHAT NEXT?

Your doctor will do a thorough evaluation and will be able to diagnose your specific type of depression from your symptoms.

MY TREATMENT OPTIONS

Modern treatments for depression are highly effective, so the sooner you seek help from your doctor, the sooner you'll be on the road to recovery. Your doctor may advise one or more of the following:

Talk therapies Commonly used talk therapies include cognitive–behavioural therapy, interpersonal therapy, and psychodynamic therapy (see pp224–5).

Medications There are several types of antidepressants but your doctor will probably prescribe an SSRI or an SNRI (see p227). Ask your doctor about any side effects.

Electroconvulsive therapy (ECT) This is usually reserved for severe depression that cannot be cured by therapy and medications. It is carried out under carefully controlled conditions and involves passing an electric current through

AM I AT RISK?

The following risk factors may increase your chance of developing the symptoms that may be diagnosed as one of the types of depression:

- Family history of depression
- Prior episodes of depression
- Having another mental health disorder
- Aged between 20 and 40
- Recent stressful life events
- History of childhood abuse and/or sexual abuse
- Poor sleeping habits
- Smoking
- Alcohol or substance abuse
- Relationship stress
- Parenting stress.

the brain to change the chemistry of the part of the brain that is causing the depression.

HOW CAN I HELP MYSELF?

The main way to help yourself is to follow your treatment plan. There are also self-help measures you can try, although you should discuss them with your doctor first.

Alternatives Many women have found that regular exercise (see pp56–7) and a healthy diet (see pp52–5) are helpful. Daily exposure to light, acupuncture, the herbal remedy St. John's Wort, and the dietary supplement SAMe (S-adenosylmethionine) might also be useful. A word of caution: these last two may react with medications, so it is vital to talk to your doctor first.

Bipolar disorder

Most of us have periods when our mood fluctuates but people with bipolar disorder experience extreme mood swings: they have episodes of depression followed by periods of feeling elated. These low and high phases are so extreme that they can have a major impact on every aspect of life.

WHAT IS IT?

A form of depression, bipolar disorder is probably caused by a chemical imbalance in the brain that is likely to be related to genes – having a parent with the disorder puts you at greater risk. It is categorized into two types.

Bipolar disorder I Once known as manic depression, this is characterized by alternating episodes of major depression (see pp210–11) and mania – a period in which you feel extremely high (see Have I got the symptoms?). These episodes last for a week or more. Most people with bipolar I spend more time in a state of depression than in a state of mania, although some people have only manic episodes. You must have at least one manic episode to be diagnosed with bipolar I.

Bipolar disorder II This is more common than bipolar I and is similar to it. The main difference is that the high periods (known as hypomanic episodes) are shorter – but still last for at least four days – and less extreme. Bipolar II may not adversely affect your social or work life and may not require hospitalization. If you suffer from bipolar II, you will have at least one hypomanic episode and at least one episode of major depression.

In both types, the occurrence of symptoms varies widely. Some people have only a few episodes while others have many.

WHAT NEXT?

You doctor will do a thorough evaluation and make a diagnosis from your symptoms. If you have bipolar I or II you will be closely monitored by your doctor because episodes of illness are likely to recur over the course of your life.

MY TREATMENT OPTIONS

If you have severe bipolar disorder, you probably need medication and treatment for the rest of your life.

Medication After a manic episode, you will require long-term medication. You will probably be treated with lithium or other mood-stabilizers (see pp226–7). Ask your doctor about side effects.

Monitoring Your doctor will make sure that you are monitored as an outpatient. You may have to be admitted to hospital during a manic or depressive episode for safety and treatment.

HOW CAN I HELP MYSELF?

You should follow the treatment plan set out for you by your doctor.

HAVE I GOT THE SYMPTOMS?

A manic episode is a period of abnormally elevated or irritable mood. It must impair daily life and must not be due to a medical condition, medications, or drugs. It must last for at least a week (but may be shorter if hospitalization is required) and include at least three of the following (at least four if your mood is irritable):

- Increased energy/activity
- Talking fast and emphatically
- Racing thoughts
- Poor concentration
- Decreased need for sleep
- Grandiosity/inflated self-esteem
- Distractability
- Excessive indulgence in pleasurable but dangerous activities (e.g. spending, sexual activity)
- Increased goal-directed activity or physical agitation.

See your doctor if you have these symptoms.

Seasonal affective disorder

During the dark winter months many of us feel lethargic, less sociable, and generally a bit low. But for people with seasonal affective disorder these symptoms are more severe; sometimes, they can be bad enough to cause significant problems with everyday activities.

WHAT IS IT?

Seasonal affective disorder (SAD) is a type of depression whose symptoms are linked to the changing patterns of sunlight during the year. The change in light levels causes alterations in brain chemistry that affect your mood, energy levels, and even sex drive. Most people suffer from SAD during the winter but some people experience symptoms during the summer. As with other mental health conditions, SAD is likely to be caused by bio-psycho-social factors (see p203). In some people, it may be inherited.

WHAT NEXT?

Your doctor will diagnose SAD only if you have had symptoms during the same season (usually autumn–winter) in two consecutive years and are not suffering from major depressive illness (see pp210–11).

MY TREATMENT OPTIONS

SAD can usually be treated effectively with light therapy, antidepressants, or talk therapy.
Light therapy With this therapy, you sit in front of a special light box that produces bright light similar to outdoor light.

HAVE I GOT THE SYMPTOMS?

Most people with SAD have symptoms of depression during the winter months. Symptoms of winter SAD may include:

- Lethargy and tiredness
- Food cravings for sugar, starch, and alcohol, and weight gain
- Irritability and anxiety
- Avoidance of social activities.

Symptoms of the less common summer SAD include:

- Insomnia
- Loss of appetite and weight loss
- Irritability and anxiety
- Increased sex drive
- Agitation.

See you doctor if you have any of these symptoms.

Therapies Psychotherapy or counselling (see pp224–5) may be helpful for some people.
Medication Your doctor may prescribe an antidepressant (see pp226–7). Ask your doctor about any side effects.

HOW CAN I HELP MYSELF?

The main way to help yourself is to increase your exposure to light, ideally by spending at least 30 minutes outside every day. It is also worthwhile making your home and workplace are as light as possible.

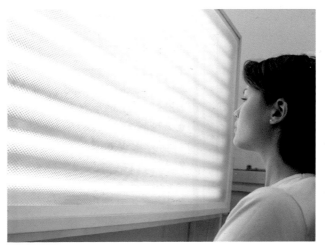

Light therapy for winter SAD
This involves sitting in front of a special light box every day (ideally in the morning) for between 30 minutes and two hours, depending on the strength of the light it gives out.

Mental health treatment options

If you are suffering from a mental health problem you should first visit your doctor, who will try to find the right kind of treatment for you. There is a wide range of different therapies and medications available, and the main ones are summarized and explained in the next few pages.

After talking with you and listening to your troubles, your doctor will assess the kind of treatment you might need. He or she may be able to treat any of your symptoms that are mild or straightforward, but for more complicated problems your doctor will refer you to a specialist in "talk therapies" (see Therapies) or to someone who also specializes in prescribing medication (a psychiatrist). Throughout the process towards treatment you will undergo the crucial steps of screening and diagnosis.

The next four pages explain the "menu" of treatment options that are available. The two main approaches to reducing symptoms are psychotherapies (where you talk to a professional about your thoughts and feelings) and medications (drugs that change the chemistry in your brain to regulate your mood and behaviour). Your doctor will recommend if you need one or the other, choosing from the range of options outlined here. Most people do best with a combination of both.

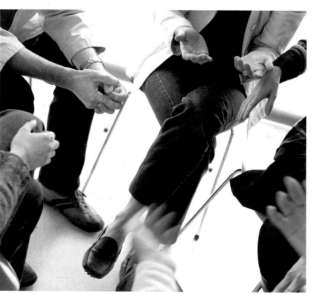

Talk therapies
Another term for psychotherapies, talk therapies come in many forms. They can involve anything from two people – the therapist and the person who is looking for help – talking together, to a group of people who come together to work on a shared problem.

Therapies

There are many different approaches to psychotherapy, and all of them involve some kind of talking, which is why they are often called "talk therapies." Ideally, you will meet face to face with a therapist, although some therapists offer the chance to talk things through over the phone or on the internet. Therapy can be either one-on-one, with a whole family, as a couple, or with a group who share the same symptoms or problem. Many different mental health professionals are trained as therapists (psychiatrists, social workers, nurse practitioners, psychologists, counsellors, coaches), but only psychiatrists are licensed to prescribe medications.

PSYCHODYNAMIC THERAPY
This therapy is based on the idea that painful emotions and feelings buried in your unconscious need to come to the surface so you can experience and understand them. Often these hidden feelings stem from past experiences, so your therapist may want to explore your

childhood memories; your dreams which may give clues to your innermost fears, as well as your conflicts in daily life.

PSYCHOANALYSIS

This is an intensive "talk therapy" that is similar to, but more intense than, psychodynamic therapy. It is a long-term therapy, taking several years, and may involve 3–5 sessions a week. Usually you lie on a couch while your analyst helps you become more self-aware, often pointing out how patterns in your life are played out in your relationship with your therapist.

COGNITIVE-BEHAVIOURAL THERAPY (CBT)

Consisting of a programme that lasts for 16–20 weeks, CBT focuses on specific patterns of thinking or behaviour that give you problems and shows you how you can change these irrational or unhelpful patterns. You are given homework assignments, such as keeping a diary of events that upset, so you can explore your thoughts and feelings with your therapist.

BRIEF DYNAMIC THERAPY

This focused, short-term treatment, based on psychodynamic techniques, is tailored to a specific problem in your life rather than looking into other larger issues.

BEHAVIOURAL THERAPY

The aim of this therapy is to change your dysfunctional patterns of behaviour by teaching you how to respond to things differently; the focus is on outward behaviour, not internal states, with the emphasis on rewards and not punishments. Behavioural therapy often includes exercises such as relaxation training, stress management, and biofeedback (see right). The latter uses physical signs from your body, such as heart rate, to get information about and control your mental state in a stressful setting.

DIALECTICAL BEHAVIOUR THERAPY (DBT)

This is a specific type of therapy that was originally designed for borderline personality disorder (see p218), although it may be useful for other problems, too. Its techniques are similar to those used in CBT. The goal of DBT is to teach you self-awareness, how to get on with other people, control your emotions, how to avoid acting impulsively, and how to calm yourself down.

EXPOSURE THERAPY AND DESENSITIZATION (EDT)

Often known simply as EDT, this is a specific branch of behavioural therapy and CBT in which you must face your particular fear, either virtually, in the safety of the therapy room, or in reality. For example, if you have a fear of heights, your therapist will actually go with you to a bridge. This form of therapy may take you either gradually or suddenly through the process of exposure and desensitization.

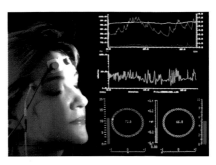

Biofeedback machine
This apparatus monitors the physical signs that accompany different moods.

EYE MOVEMENT DESENSITIZATION AND REPROCESSING (EMDR)

This may be used to treat disorders such as post-traumatic stress disorder. It involves rhythmically moving your eyes to help you relax then talking about your trauma with the therapist. Its aim is to break the link between your memories and anxiety symptoms.

SUPPORTIVE PSYCHOTHERAPY

This therapy is widely used to bolster self-esteem and coping mechanisms, and to help you become more successful in daily life. You may have a number of brief therapy sessions over a long period or a few extended sessions over a shorter period.

INTERPERSONAL THERAPY (IPT)

A short-term therapy often used to treat depression, IPT focuses on how the stresses of everyday life can trigger symptoms, and how emotional difficulties can lead to problematic behaviours. It is based

Breathing and respiration

Dr Lisa Davies BM BCh BA(Oxon) FRCP FRCP(E)

Breathing and respiration

From the moment we emerge into this world, we breathe completely automatically and unconsciously. Breathing in is just the first step in a complex process that uses gas exchange to supply the oxygen we need to power our bodies; breathing out takes away the carbon dioxide waste product that is produced. Just like other body systems, such as your heart or muscles, your entire respiratory system is capable of responding to all the various demands you place on it – from running for a bus to doing a marathon.

WHAT IS THE RESPIRATORY SYSTEM?

You can think of your respiratory system as being made of two fundamental parts: an upper and a lower respiratory tract. The upper respiratory tract consists of your nose, sinuses, mouth, throat (pharynx), and voice box (larynx); the lower respiratory tract consists of the windpipe (trachea) and the tubes that branch from that in ever-decreasing sizes (bronchi and bronchioles), ending in millions of tiny balloon-like sacs called alveoli, within the lungs.

The main function of the respiratory system is to supply oxygen to the blood, which absorbs it and carries

WHAT HAPPENS WHEN YOU BREATHE

When you breathe, air flows down the trachea, into the bronchi and through smaller and smaller bronchioles until it reaches tiny, gas-permeable air sacs, the alveoli. In the alveoli, oxygen from the air diffuses into the blood stream, to be transported to all the cells of your body. At the same time, carbon dioxide waste produced by your body diffuses from the blood into the alveoli, to be breathed out.

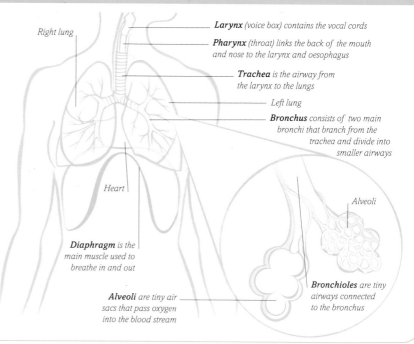

Right lung

Larynx (voice box) contains the vocal cords

Pharynx (throat) links the back of the mouth and nose to the larynx and oesophagus

Trachea is the airway from the larynx to the lungs

Left lung

Bronchus consists of two main bronchi that branch from the trachea and divide into smaller airways

Heart

Alveoli

Diaphragm is the main muscle used to breathe in and out

Bronchioles are tiny airways connected to the bronchus

Alveoli are tiny air sacs that pass oxygen into the blood stream

it to all parts of the body, and to remove the waste product carbon dioxide from it. Oxygen is required by every cell in the body and because it cannot be stored, we need a continuous supply from the outside air.

A healthy person breathes between 12 and 20 times per minute at rest. How fast and how deeply we breathe depends on our size and on how fit we are. Generally, an adult woman inhales about 450–500ml (16–18fl oz) of air – about the size of a pint bottle of milk – in a normal breath, and can take in about 4 litres (7 pints) with a maximal breath. On average, lung capacity in men is 25 to 30 per cent higher.

Breathing is one of the few automatic bodily functions that we can consciously control. Taking slow deep breaths can help us handle stress, as demonstrated by the techniques taught to women in labor through the Lamaze method.

BREATHING AND EXERCISE
As we get older, the amount of air we can breathe (lung capacity) and the amount of oxygen we can extract from each breath declines, but this doesn't mean an inevitable decline in fitness. Women of all ages should be able to exercise for 30 to 60 minutes and not get out of breath. If you are 35 years old, then you should be able to cycle at 24kph (15mph), play vigorous singles tennis, or jog 1.6km (1 mile) in 10 minutes. If you are 50, then you should be able to jog 1.6km (1 mile) in 12 minutes, and swim or walk vigorously. If you are 65 years old you should be able to cycle at 16kph (10mph), dance, or play doubles tennis. Even if you are 80, you should still be able to walk 1.6km (1 mile) in less than 20 minutes, play golf (but no club carrying), or do water aerobics.

THE EFFECTS OF SMOKING
There is one huge threat to breathing (and health) that affects all parts of the respiratory system – cigarette

> **"Breathing is one of the few bodily functions that can be controlled consciously and unconsciously."**

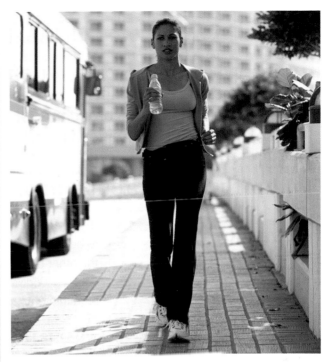

Benefits of exercise
Any vigorous exercise, such as power walking or jogging, will make you breathe harder and deeper, strengthening your lungs and delivering more oxygen to your body.

smoking. Smokers run a higher risk of developing each and every respiratory illness from coughs and colds (see p232) and laryngitis (see p236) to asthma (see pp238–9) and lung cancer (see pp242–3).

As a smoker you not only affect your own health but also the health of those around you, including your children and grandchildren. Living with a smoker puts children at higher risk of developing asthma and allergies, and of missing school with colds and other respiratory infections. If the smoker in the family is the father, the risk rises by about one-third; but if mummy smokes, the risk goes up by a massive three-quarters.

People who grow up in a household with smokers are three times more likely to get lung cancer than people who grow up in non-smoking households, even if they don't smoke themselves. So, if you smoke, try to stop now (see pp64–5); if you get enough support from family and friends as well as a smoking cessation clinic you can make it the last time you quit. You want to be playing golf and swimming at 80, don't you?

Chronic obstructive pulmonary disease

Historically, chronic obstructive pulmonary disease (COPD) was more common in men, but it is now more common in women. The reason may be linked to the fact that more women smoke, and also because many industries where men worked that contributed to the disease are in decline in the developed world.

COPD is a combination of two lung diseases – chronic bronchitis and emphysema – where the airways and tissues of the lungs gradually become damaged over time, causing increasing shortness of breath. Although there is no cure, and the symptoms may worsen over time if they aren't treated, with an early diagnosis the decline can be slowed down.

WHAT IS IT?

In chronic bronchitis, the airways (bronchi and bronchioles) that carry air to the tiny air sacs (alveoli) embedded in the lung tissue become inflamed and blocked, making it harder for air to flow through them. In emphysema, the air sacs become damaged or destroyed, and the exchange of oxygen and carbon dioxide within the air sacs becomes more difficult. The main cause of both chronic bronchitis and emphysema, and therefore COPD, is smoking.

COPD symptoms typically begin in people aged over 40 who have usually smoked for 20 years or more.

In the early stages, COPD may produce minimal or no symptoms, and as the disease progresses the symptoms in individual patients may vary (see opposite).

The prevention and early recognition of COPD in women is vital, as the following facts and figures show:

- COPD affects more women than men, and kills more women than men. The mortality rate in women has doubled since 1980
- Chronic bronchitis afflicts twice as many women as men, and

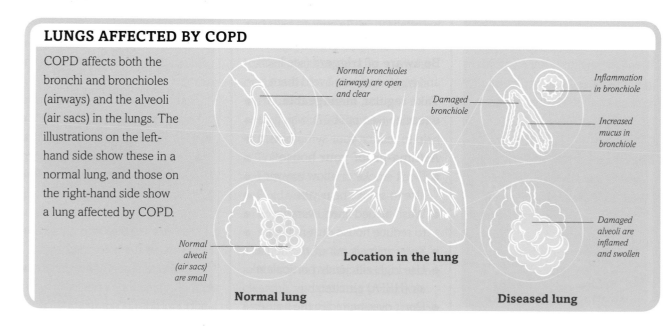

LUNGS AFFECTED BY COPD

COPD affects both the bronchi and bronchioles (airways) and the alveoli (air sacs) in the lungs. The illustrations on the left-hand side show these in a normal lung, and those on the right-hand side show a lung affected by COPD.

Normal bronchioles (airways) are open and clear

Damaged bronchiole

Inflammation in bronchiole

Increased mucus in bronchiole

Normal alveoli (air sacs) are small

Location in the lung

Damaged alveoli are inflamed and swollen

Normal lung

Diseased lung

As COPD progresses, your symptoms will gradually get worse:

- A cough is usually the first symptom to develop, and tends to come and go at first and then gradually become more persistent, with phlegm lasting for months
- Frequent coughs of any kind, especially in the morning
- Increased mucus
- Frequent clearing of your throat
- Shortness of breath when you exercise. Often the first sign is noticing that you need to rest more often while exercising
- More frequent colds, which last longer than in the past.

See your doctor if you have two or more of the above symptoms.

emphysema is almost as common in women as men

- Women with COPD are on the rise, while the number of men with the disease is decreasing
- Women who smoke are more likely to get COPD, and die from COPD, than men who smoke.

WHAT NEXT?

Your doctor can diagnose COPD in a similar way as he or she would diagnose asthma (see p238). If your doctor suspects that you may have COPD, you will be referred to

There are a few definite risk factors for developing COPD:

- The disease is rare in women under 40, and most common in women over the age of 60
- It's usually seen in smokers
- Exposure to dust and/or chemicals at work may contribute to 10–15 per cent of cases of COPD in the UK.

a specialist for lung function tests. One test is spirometry, which shows how much air you can exhale after a deep breath in.

After your diagnosis, the first goal is to prevent further damage to your lungs. If you smoke, you must stop (see p64). Infections can worsen your lung damage and to prevent them make sure that you receive the following:

- An annual flu vaccination at the beginning of the winter
- A pneumonia vaccination, or "pneumovax", every 10 years.

The next goal is to control the symptoms of COPD.

MY TREATMENT OPTIONS

COPD treatments aim to ease the symptoms rather than cure them. Ask your doctor about side effects. **Drug therapy** and preventative methods, such as those listed below, are the main treatments:

- Inhaled bronchodilators
- Inhaled corticosteroids
- Vaccinations against flu and pneumonia

- Antibiotics and/or steroid tablets may be needed when you have an "exacerbation", or acute worsening of the symptoms.

Medications such as bronchodilators relax the muscles of the airways and relieve shortness of breath. Anti-inflammatory drugs – mainly inhaled corticosteroids – reduce inflammation within the airways (see p239). When the disease is advanced, you may need oxygen therapy at home – breathing oxygen through tubes in your nostrils. Before this can be decided, a chest specialist will measure your oxygen levels with a blood test.

Pulmonary rehabilitation programmes educate you about your condition and how to manage the symptoms better. This will include exercise training, disease management, and support. The aim is to increase your tolerance to exercise so you can get around without shortness of breath, and encourage you to be more independent and less anxious.

HOW CAN I HELP MYSELF?

We all cough sometimes and get short of breath when we exercise more than usual. It's easy to dismiss early signs of COPD.
Pay attention to your body Get help if you think you have COPD symptoms.
Don't smoke, and if you do, get help to stop (see p64).
Stay active Exercise, including walking, helps keep your lungs and muscles as healthy as possible.

Blood disorders

Dr Nina Salooja DM MSc (Ed) FRCP FRCPath

Blood disorders

Although we're aware of blood as a life-sustaining substance, we're not always so familiar with its many functions. The blood circulating around your body in the arteries and veins is an extremely efficient transport system, carrying substances essential for your survival such as oxygen, nutrients, and hormones to all your organs and tissues, and picking up waste products to process and eliminate from the body. In addition, your blood is vital to your body's defence system, containing cells that identify and fight invading organisms.

THE STRUCTURE AND FUNCTION OF BLOOD

Blood is made up of a fluid called plasma, which contains three different types of cell – red blood cells, white blood cells, and platelets. Plasma contains many essential substances, including glucose, proteins, fats, vitamins, and minerals, which it delivers to every tissue as it travels around the body. Plasma also collects waste products, such as urea and carbon dioxide, from the body's cells and carries them away for disposal – the carbon dioxide is removed from the body via the lungs, and other waste products are broken down and expelled via the liver and kidneys.

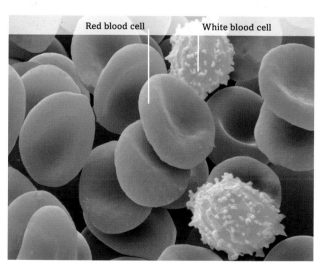

Red and white blood cells
Red blood cells have a distinctive disc shape and contain the red pigment haemoglobin. There are fewer white blood cells, but they play a vital role in defending the body against infection.

The red blood cells contain an important protein called haemoglobin, which has the crucial job of carrying oxygen from your lungs to every cell in the body's tissues and organs.

The white blood cells, of which there are various kinds, are part of the immune system (see p259). They fight infection, either by engulfing and destroying unwanted organisms, or by multiplying and producing antibodies that destroy invading bacteria.

The platelets are the smallest blood cells and come into their own when a blood vessel is damaged or cut. They work together with various coagulation proteins (see p250) in the plasma to form a blood clot at the site of the damage. This quickly stems the bleeding.

HOW BLOOD CIRCULATES

Blood is transported around the body by a dense, branching network of arteries, veins, and capillaries. The blood absorbs oxygen in the lungs (see Breathing and Respiration, p230) and passes to the heart (see Your Heart, p160) via the pulmonary vein.

Arteries, which have thick muscular walls and carry blood under high pressure, carry the oxygenated blood around the body to the organs and tissues. Here, they branch into smaller and smaller vessels until they form tiny capillaries that release the oxygen and nutrients to individual cells. Tiny veins that gradually become large veins return the deoxygenated blood to the heart and to the lungs, where the carbon dioxide is exhaled and fresh oxygen is collected.

WHAT IS IN YOUR BLOOD

This cross-section through a blood vessel shows the composition of the blood flowing through it. The plasma, which carries many essential substances (see opposite) accounts for about 55 per cent of your total blood volume. Ninety per cent of that is water.

Red blood cells contain the protein haemoglobin

White blood cells fight infection

Plasma delivers vital substances

Platelets help blood to clot after injury

HOW WOMEN ARE DIFFERENT

There are relatively few differences between the blood of men and women, but a man, since he is normally larger than a woman, will have a greater volume of blood in his body. However, when a woman is pregnant, the volume of blood in her body increases and this ensures that the developing fetus will have all it needs in the way of blood, oxygen and nutrients. A additional key difference is that men have more red blood cells than women, and they also have a higher concentration of haemoglobin.

Because they menstruate, women are more prone than men to iron-deficiency anaemia (see pp248–9). During menstruation they lose a small amount of blood (usually between 10 and 80 ml). If they lose more than this over a sustained period of time, they may become deficient in iron, which can then lead to that type of anaemia. Women are also more likely than men to experience bruising (see p251).

WHAT BLOOD REVEALS

When we talk about blood disorders we are referring to illnesses that affect blood cells rather than changes within the plasma component. Simple laboratory tests on blood samples provide a great deal of information about these disorders and illnesses. If you are unwell or need an operation, you will probably have a routine investigation to see the number of red and white blood cells and platelets in your blood. The analysis will also look at the size of your red blood cells and measure your total haemoglobin concentration. If your blood shows an abnormal number of cells, then the appearance of the blood cells is studied under a microscope.

BONE MARROW TEST

Red blood cells, white blood cells, and platelets are all produced in the bone marrow from cells known as precursor cells. In adults, bone marrow is located in the bones of the central skeleton, such as the pelvic bone, the sternum, and the long bones.

If there is no obvious explanation why your blood count is too high or too low, or your blood cells have an abnormal appearance, then you may be given a bone marrow test. This might reveal some abnormalities in the precursor cells or it may indicate the existence of another disease affecting the bone marrow. This may, for example, be an infection or a cancer that is not related to the blood itself.

> "Due to menstruation, women are more prone to iron-deficiency anaemia than men."

Bleeding disorders

Having monthly periods means that women are used to bleeding, and if the bleeding is heavy or prolonged, it may not occur to them that there is something wrong with the way their blood is clotting. Bleeding disorders are quite common in women, but they are not always that easy to detect.

WHAT IS IT?

When you damage a blood vessel, the clotting process in your blood immediately seals the wound. In this process, known as coagulation, the platelets in your blood (see p246) clump together and interact with proteins called clotting factors to stop the bleeding.

There are two types of clotting factor: "procoagulants" help the blood to clot, and "anticoagulants" prevent it from clotting too readily. If your body's procoagulant and anticoagulant proteins aren't in balance, or if there's a problem with the number or the function of platelets, your blood can become either too runny or too sticky, and this can lead to a bleeding disorder.

Occasionally, a person has the normal numbers of platelets, but they don't work properly. This can be an inherited condition or, more commonly, the result of taking anti-inflammatory drugs, such as aspirin, which can affect the way the platelets function.

Thrombocytopenia This is a reduction in the number of platelets. It can occur if they aren't being produced in sufficient numbers (for example, as with leukaemia or after chemotherapy). It can also occur if the platelets are being destroyed too quickly, as when they are attacked by the body's immune system.

Hypercoagulability This occurs if there are too many platelets or coagulation factors. Some patients inherit extra-sticky clotting factors, and others, low levels of anticoagulant. These increase the tendency to form blood clots (or thrombosis). If a thrombus starts to move freely in the circulation, it is called an embolism. If it gets stuck within the circulation of the lung, it can have potentially fatal consequences (see pp252–5).

HAVE I GOT THE SYMPTOMS?

The following symptoms may indicate a bleeding disorder:

- Easy or spontaneous bruising that is unexplained
- Recurrent severe nose bleeds
- Heavy periods from the menarche (the time that periods started)
- Prolonged or major bleeding after surgery or dentistry.

See your doctor if you suffer with any of the above.

AM I AT RISK?

The risk factors for a particular bleeding disorder depend on its cause. For example, you may have an increased risk of a bleeding if you:

- Have a family history of bleeding disorders
- Are taking drugs such as warfarin or aspirin.

Von Willebrand's disease is named after the Finnish doctor who discovered that some people lacked a key clotting factor, which then became known as von Willebrand's factor. This inherited disease is the most common bleeding disorder – between one and two per cent of the population have it – and it affects men and women equally. Bleeding is excessive or prolonged.

Haemophilia is an inherited disease that involves excessive bleeding that can go on for hours or even days. Sometimes bleeding starts spontaneously. Haemophilia really only affects men (see p17), although some women can have mild symptoms. It is caused by a reduction in the level of a blood protein known as Factor VIII.

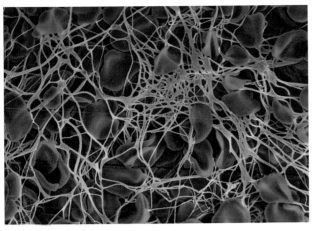

What happens when blood clots

When a blood vessel is damaged, a mesh of a protein called fibrin (coloured green in this scan) develops to bind the blood cells together. The result is a blood clot, that prevents you from losing too much blood.

WHAT NEXT?

If your symptoms seem to suggest a bleeding disorder, your doctor will arrange a test to measure your full blood count, check the number of platelets, establish the presence of the clotting proteins, and measure your blood's clotting time. You may need further tests to measure the levels of specific proteins, such as Factor VIII and von Willebrand's factor. Platelet function tests may also be carried out in a specialized haematology centre. Sometimes, test results are affected by stress, exercise, or medications, and the test may need to be repeated.

MY TREATMENT OPTIONS

There's no cure for bleeding disorders, but treatment can enable women to lead normal, active lives. Treatment is either via medications or injection, and will depend on what causes the disorder. For mild disorders, medication is not really needed, other than after an injury, and before or after surgical or dental treatment. However, if the disorder is severe, you may need to take medication every day.

Desmopressin acetate helps to release clotting factors that are stored in the body. You can take it as an injection or via a nasal spray to combat heavy periods and stop nose bleeds.

Antifibrinolytic medications help to prolong the life of a blood clot by preventing it from breaking down. They can be used before dental treatment, to stop nose bleeds, and to control mild bleeding in the intestine.

Intravenous injections of immunoglobulin or steroids can boost platelet numbers if your platelets are being broken down because you have an autoimmune disease. You can also have injections of plasma containing specific clotting factors, such as von Willebrand's factor or Factor VIII.

Changing medication If a bleeding disorder is caused by a medication, your doctor will suggest an alternative. If you are taking warfarin and need surgery, you may have to stop the warfarin

HOW CAN I HELP MYSELF?

Follow your doctor's advice with regard to your treatment and make sure your lifestyle is healthy (see Chapter 3, pp48–69).

EASILY BRUISED?

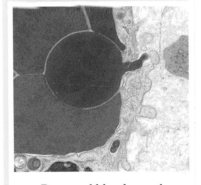

Damaged blood vessel
When the wall of a blood vessel (here shown in green) is damaged, red blood cells leak through into surrounding tissues, causing bruising.

Women seem to bruise more easily than men. Sometimes this bruising is unexplained and may indicate a bleeding disorder, particularly when it is accompanied by a bleeding nose or gums, and heavy or prolonged periods. If you have bruises that take a long time to disappear, consult your doctor.

"Von Willebrand's disease is the most common inherited blood disorder in women, affecting about 1 in 100 women."

Venous thrombosis

We know that long-haul flights and surgery can encourage a venous thrombosis, but some women are particularly at risk – for example, if you're pregnant or are taking the combined oral contraceptive pill. Simple measures to keep your circulation healthy can reduce your chances of developing blood clots.

WHAT IS IT?

A thrombosis occurs when the flow of blood in a vein or artery is blocked for some reason. Fatty deposits on the inside of an artery, caused by a condition called atherosclerosis, are prime sites for thromboses. A venous thrombosis is a specific type of blood clot that occurs in a vein. In the case of the veins in your limbs, these are either near the surface (superficial) or deep. You can get a venous thrombosis in either of these. When a clot occurs in a deep vein, it is known as a deep vein thrombosis (DVT).

Up to 50 per cent of thromboses in the veins may be linked to hormonal or biochemical changes in the composition of the blood. Veins may also develop thromboses after you have been immobile for a long period of time – for example, sitting in an aircraft. If you get a clot in a superficial vein it may be painful, but it's unlikely to be dangerous.

Likewise, a DVT is not necessarily dangerous in itself, but it may break away from the place where it forms and become an embolus (abnormal blood clot) that travels in the blood to the lung. Once it reaches the lung, it can then block a pulmonary (relating to the lungs) blood vessel. This is known as a pulmonary embolism (PE) and can lead to permanent loss of lung tissue that is potentially fatal. A PE may occasionally develop on its own.

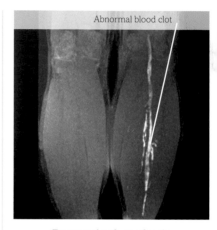

Abnormal blood clot

Deep vein thrombosis
This magnetic resonance imaging (MRI) scan shows a patient suffering from a DVT in a vein in the leg. The clot shows up as the white area.

WHAT NEXT?

It's important to diagnose and treat a DVT or a PE promptly. If your doctor suspects you have a DVT, he or she will first take a detailed medical history and will arrange for you to have a blood test to identify whether you are at a high or low risk of a venous thrombosis. Depending on your symptoms, you may have an X-ray to establish whether a thrombosis has occurred.

HAVE I GOT THE SYMPTOMS?

If a clot forms in one of your deep veins you may have the following symptoms:
- Pain or tenderness in a limb
- A feeling of cramp that doesn't go away
- Swelling of the affected limb.

In rare cases, when a clot travels to the lungs, the following symptoms can occur:
- Chest pain
- Shortness of breath
- A cough.

See your doctor as soon as possible if you suspect you have a DVT. If you have the symptoms of a pulmonary embolism, treat it as a medical emergency.

"Although taking the pill or HRT has been linked to deep vein thrombosis (DVT), the actual risk of hormone-induced DVT is still very small."

AM I AT RISK?

The following factors can increase your risk of thrombosis:

- A family history of thrombosis
- The combined oral contraceptive pill
- Pregnancy
- Hormone replacement therapy (HRT)
- Recent hip or knee surgery
- Other major surgical procedures and a period of hospitalization
- Wearing a plaster cast
- Long-haul flights and prolonged travel by road
- A prolonged period of immobility
- Cancer
- Inherited and acquired factors in the blood.

If a DVT is suspected, you may have a Doppler ultrasound scan to measure the blood flow within your veins and to establish whether a deep vein is blocked. If you have a suspected PE, you may have a scan to check the flow of blood and air in your lungs. Alternatively, you may have a computerized tomography (CT) scan, which involves taking a series of X-rays to build up a detailed picture of your chest. If these tests don't give a clear diagnosis, you may need to repeat them a week or so later, or other tests may be carried out. If there is a wait of several hours or days for further tests, your doctor may decide to start treatment before the results are available.

MY TREATMENT OPTIONS

Venous thrombosis is commonly treated with anticoagulant drugs that thin the blood.

Anticoagulant drugs include warfarin. This takes a few days to become effective so, during the first week, you may also have injections of the anticoagulant drug heparin (which works immediately). Occasionally, a person with a large thrombosis in the lung that isn't linked with a DVT may need to take warfarin on a long-term basis.

Preventive measures "Post-thrombotic syndrome" can occur after a DVT. This causes pain and ulceration in the affected limb. If you wear compression stockings for the two years immediately following the DVT, it can help to reduce the risk of post-thrombotic syndrome in the future.

Blood tests can help find an underlying cause for an episode of thrombosis, but anticoagulants such as warfarin can affect the results. Repeat tests may be needed or tests may be delayed until you stop taking warfarin.

HOW CAN I HELP MYSELF?

Several preventive measures can help you to avoid DVT or a reoccurrence of the condition.

If you've had a thrombosis tell your doctor if you become pregnant, need surgery, or are admitted to hospital for any reason.

If you're high risk and due to have surgery, talk to the surgeon about the possibility of having heparin injections around the time of the operation.

Keep your weight down You need to maintain a healthy weight to help you reduce your risk of developing a DVT (see p58–9).

When travelling, avoid alcohol and sleeping tablets; try to walk around on long plane journeys, wear compression stockings and practise ankle exercises to help your circulation. Drinking plenty of water can help, too.

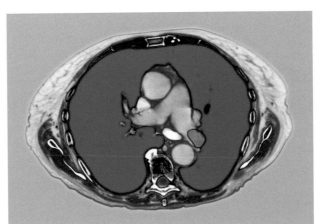

Pulmonary embolism

A computerized tomography (CT) scan of the lungs reveals a pulmonary embolism (green patch) in the left pulmonary artery.

Blood cancers

Cancers of the white cells in the blood and lymph system appear to affect men and women equally, and even though they are quite common, they are poorly understood. However, many types of blood cancer now have a good outcome – for example, some types of leukaemia.

WHAT ARE THEY?

White blood cells are on the front line of our defences, protecting us from illness by destroying invading organisms. The two main types of white blood cells, granulocytes and lymphocytes, work in different ways. Granulocytes engulf and destroy bacteria, while lymphocytes destroy organisms with antibodies. These two types of white cells are the ones affected when we talk about blood (haematological) cancers. There are several different types of blood cancer, each with its own characteristics.

Leukaemia occurs when there is an increased number of abnormal white cells in the bone marrow. There are two main types: acute leukaemia, which develops rapidly, and chronic leukaemia, which can take years to develop and is more common among the middle aged and elderly. There are two types of acute leukaemia: acute lymphoid leukaemia (ALL) is more common in childhood, while acute myeloid leukaemia (AML) can occur at any age. There are also two types of chronic leukaemia: chronic myeloid (CML) and chronic lymphocytic (CLL). Both types can cause bone marrow failure.

Lymphomas are cancers in which malignant lymphoid cells build up in the lymph nodes, liver, and spleen. There are two types of lymphoma: Hodgkins and non-Hodgkins lymphoma.

Myeloma occurs when plasma cells (see p246) become malignant, often in bone marrow. This impairs the production of normal blood cells, causing anaemia (see p248) and other related conditions. The malignant plasma cells also produce massive quantities of an antibody known as "paraprotein", which can be toxic to the kidneys and lead to kidney failure.

Increased abnormal white blood cells

Red blood cell

Leukaemia
In chronic lymphocytic leukaemia, there is an increased number of abnormal white blood cells in the bone marrow.

HAVE I GOT THE SYMPTOMS?

The following are some of the general symptoms of chronic leukaemia:

- Fatigue and shortness of breath, caused by anaemia (see p248)
- Nose bleeds and bruising (see p250) caused by low platelet levels
- Fevers and infections, caused by low levels of white blood cells.

Chronic leukaemia may initially have no symptoms, but in the later stages there may be:

- Anaemia
- Easy bruising (see p251), bleeding
- A tendency to develop infections.

Symptoms of lymphomas include:

- Enlarged lymph glands in the neck, armpits, or groin
- Weight loss
- Raised temperature
- Drenching sweats at night
- Symptoms of anaemia, such as tiredness and shortness of breath.

See your doctor if you have one or more of these symptoms.

AM I AT RISK?

The following factors increase the risk of developing the acute form of leukaemia:

- Previous exposure to chemotherapy
- Exposure to radiation
- Down's syndrome.

Other cancers of the blood are more common in middle-aged and elderly people. CML (see below) is sometimes linked to an abnormal chromosome, but otherwise this group of cancers has no significant risk factors.

WHAT NEXT?

The diagnostic tests your doctor may recommend vary according to the type of blood cancer.

Acute leukaemia needs to be diagnosed and dealt with quickly. Your doctor will arrange an urgent full blood count, which may reveal low numbers of red and white cells and/or platelets. If your blood count is abnormal, the laboratory will look for leukaemia cells in a blood sample. If there are only a few circulating abnormal cells, you may be given a bone marrow test.

Chronic leukaemia (CML) is identified by blood tests and confirmed by further specialized tests. An abnormal chromosome, known as the Philadelphia chromosome, is usually present.

Lymphoma requires specialist scans to assess the extent of the condition. You may also have a gland removed for examination.

Myeloma requires tests to identify two or more of the following: a significant number of plasma cells in the bone marrow; bone problems identified through a skeletal X-ray; and the presence of "paraprotein" antibodies in the blood or urine.

MY TREATMENT OPTIONS

Chemotherapy, radiotherapy, and medications are used in the treatment of blood cancers.

Chemotherapy/radiotherapy

Acute leukaemia is potentially curable, particularly in children and young adults. Chemotherapy drugs are usually given in hospital; you will probably go into isolation to reduce your exposure to infection.

Chemotherapy can reduce the number of malignant cells in CLL but it doesn't cure. Treatment is only started if you have particular symptoms or signs of bone marrow failure, such as anaemia, a low platelet count, or too few neutrophils (a type of white blood cell).

Some lymphomas, such as Hodgkins lymphoma, are curable with chemotherapy and/or radiotherapy. In younger myeloma patients, chemotherapy can lead to remission but not to a cure. However, high doses can improve the length and quality of survival. Older patients are usually treated with chemotherapy tablets and/or radiotherapy to help symptoms.

Other medications The most popular form of treatment for CML is a drug called imatinib, which is designed to reverse the process of leukaemia in CML without affecting other tissues.

HOW CAN I HELP MYSELF?

It is essential to follow your doctor's advice carefully and to lead a healthy lifestyle (see Chapter 3, pp48–69).

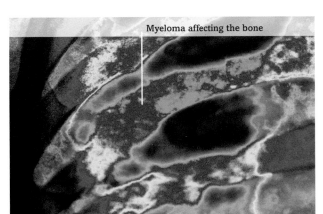

Myeloma affecting the bone

Myeloma
This coloured X-ray of a patient's ribs shows myeloma affecting the bones on one side of the chest. An X-ray will help in the diagnosis of the condition.

Bones and joints

Dr Nurhan Sutcliffe MD FRCP
Chronic fatigue syndrome Donnica Moore MD

Your bones and joints

Your skeleton is the bony, rigid framework that supports your body, gives it shape, protects some of the delicate internal organs, and allows you to move about. A complex system of overlying muscles, tendons, ligaments, cartilage, and other connective tissues works alongside your bones, allowing you to perform almost any movement you want. Your joints are the meeting points between two bones and are designed to help you make smooth, fluid movements, as well as cushion sudden jumps or falls.

HOW JOINTS WORK

In a healthy joint that is mobile, the end of each bone is covered with smooth cartilage, which allows movement at the joint, reduces friction, and acts as a cushion. A membrane called the synovium lines the joint and produces synovial fluid to lubricate the joint. The outer layer of the synovium is called the capsule. Tough bands called ligaments help to hold the joint together by attaching one bone to another. Fibrous tendons attach muscles to the bones.

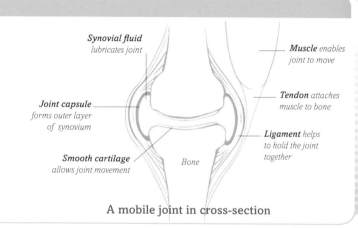

Synovial fluid lubricates joint

Muscle enables joint to move

Tendon attaches muscle to bone

Joint capsule forms outer layer of synovium

Ligament helps to hold the joint together

Smooth cartilage allows joint movement

Bone

A mobile joint in cross-section

BONE REMODELLING

Throughout your life your bones are continuously broken down (bone resorption) and rebuilt (bone formation). This so-called "bone remodelling" is essential for the growth and maintenance of healthy bones. During childhood, bone is built up more rapidly than it is broken down – which is how you grow to be an adult – and so your bones become denser. Your bone density (also called bone mineral density or BMD) continues to increase until young adulthood (25–30 years), when it peaks. Bone resorption and bone formation are tightly coupled so that bone density remains pretty constant during this period.

After the age of 30, though, your bone density gradually declines year on year – between her 30s and 50s, the average woman loses 0.5 per cent of bone density each year – so regular weight-bearing exercise (which promotes bone formation) is needed in order

to maintain bone density. If the processes of resorption and formation become uncoupled, as with the condition osteoporosis (see p260), there's an increase in bone resorption without a matching rise in formation. The result of this disparity is lighter, less-

BONE DENSITY OVER A LIFETIME

Bone mineral density (BMD) peaks between the ages of 25 and 30. After this, BMD gradually declines as more bone is lost than is made.

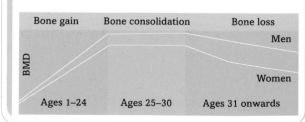

Bone gain	Bone consolidation	Bone loss
		Men
Ages 1–24	Ages 25–30	Women
		Ages 31 onwards

BMD

dense, and more fragile bones. Oestrogen provides women with added protection against bone resorption, but as oestrogen levels decline after the menopause, the rate of bone loss accelerates.

HOW ARE WOMEN DIFFERENT?

In addition to the anatomical differences between women and men (women have a flatter, more rounded pelvis; they are normally shorter than men; and they have narrower ribcages, to name but a few), women suffer much more from autoimmune diseases, such as rheumatoid arthritis (see p266 and below).

The hormones our bodies produce may actually put us at risk of developing autoimmune diseases. Doctors think that female hormones influence the immune system, which is backed up by the fact that at times of hormonal flux, such as pregnancy or the menopause, some autoimmune diseases can flare up or subside.

JOINTS, MUSCLES, AND CONNECTIVE TISSUES AND YOUR IMMUNE SYSTEM

Discomfort you experience in your joints, muscles, and connective tissues can be linked to problems in your immune system. Inflammation is the way in which your body defends itself against infection or injury and fights off bacteria and viruses. If there is a breach of your body's defences, your body increases blood supply to the affected site, which brings in elements of your immune system and raises your temperature (giving you a fever). Blood vessels become leaky, allowing other cells to join the assault. These cells make chemicals and antibodies to attack the foreign invaders. This response is how your body staves off disease and keeps healthy.

If you have an autoimmune disease, your body's immune system triggers such a response when there are no foreign invaders. Instead, it produces an immune response against itself, damaging its own tissues in the process. If you have an autoimmune disease, it is highly likely that your blood contains autoantibodies – antibodies made against yourself. The damage such a disease can do can be wide ranging: on the joints in rheumatoid arthritis (see pp266–8); and on joints, skin, heart and nerves in lupus (see p269).

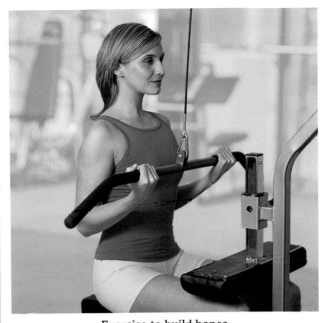

Exercise to build bones
Lifting weights not only boosts muscle strength but the action of the tendons pulling on bones promotes bone density too.

THE INFLAMMATORY RESPONSE

When invaders such as bacteria get into your body (in this example into your skin), your body triggers an inflammatory response that helps fight them off.

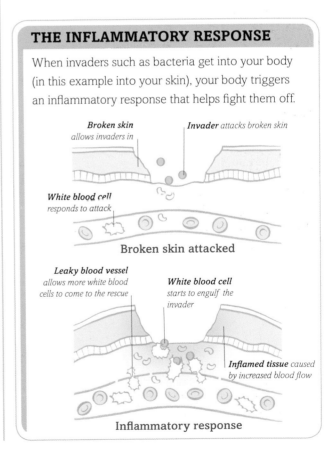

Broken skin allows invaders in

Invader attacks broken skin

White blood cell responds to attack

Broken skin attacked

Leaky blood vessel allows more white blood cells to come to the rescue

White blood cell starts to engulf the invader

Inflamed tissue caused by increased blood flow

Inflammatory response

Osteoporosis

Your bones are strongest in your late 20s, but as you age they become thinner and lighter. Oestrogen helps to keep bones strong, so after the menopause (when oestrogen levels fall) your built-in protection subsides and it's more important than ever to have a bone-conscious lifestyle to prevent osteoporosis.

WHAT IS IT?

Osteoporosis, which literally means "porous bones", results in weaker bones that are more brittle and so can break more easily. In fact, bones can be so brittle that even mild exertions, such as coughing or lifting a heavy bag of shopping, can cause a fracture.

Anyone can develop this condition as they get older; though some people have a higher than normal risk of osteoporosis (see Am I at risk?, opposite).

With age, we gradually lose some height as our backs become

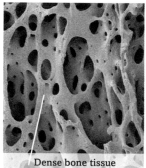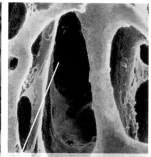

Dense bone tissue   Larger holes develop

Normal and osteoporotic bone
Younger bones have a strong, dense structure with a small "honeycomb" effect (far left). With age the bone becomes less dense and larger holes appear as bone material is lost (left).

more curved than in our youth. These physical changes may well be related to the effects of osteoporosis on the spine. Amazingly, you can have a spinal fracture without any symptoms at all, but some fractures may cause persistent back pain and restrict what you can comfortably do.

WHAT NEXT?

Osteoporosis is often first diagnosed when you break a bone after a minor bump or fall. If your doctor suspects that you have osteoporosis, he or she may ask you questions to see how many of the risk factors (see box, opposite) might apply to you.

Then, it's likely you'll be sent for a bone density scan (dual-energy X-ray absorptiometry scan or DEXA scan for short). This procedure is quick, simple, and

accurate. It measures the density of bones in your spine, hip, and wrist (those areas most likely to be affected by osteoporosis).

You may also have to give a blood sample for tests to detect or rule out any underlying conditions.

MY TREATMENT OPTIONS

Obviously, you need to prevent any future fractures and also reduce the symptoms related to any existing fractures. The medications listed below are long-term treatments, and work by reducing bone loss and/or by helping to build new bone. Ask about the potential side effects of any medication when discussing these with your doctor.
Calcium and vitamin D dietary supplements You may benefit from taking small daily amounts of vitamin D and calcium. Women who have been diagnosed with

HAVE I GOT THE SYMPTOMS?

Osteoporosis does not have any symptoms, but you may have the condition if:

- You suffer any hip, wrist, or spine fracture
- You are aged between 45 and 65 and you fracture your wrist in a fall
- You are over 70 years old and frail, and you fracture your hip in a fall.

Your doctor may then decide you have this condition.

osteoporosis should consume 1,200mg calcium per day (see p262), and consume 800IU of vitamin D a day. The body requires plenty of calcium and vitamin D to make bone.

Bisphosphonates These drugs slow bone loss. Your doctor is likely to prescribe alendronate or risedronate, which are taken daily or weekly, to reduce the risk of further hip and spine fractures (though these drugs can irritate your oesophagus).

Hormone replacement therapy If you have had an early menopause, your doctor may prescribe hormone replacement therapy (HRT, see pp137–8). Although HRT contains oestrogen, which is good for bones, it does come with side effects.

Selective oestrogen-receptor modulators You may be prescribed raloxifene, which has a similar effect to oestrogen and reduces spine fractures. It may give you hot flushes, however, and it can increase your risk of blood clots.

Strontium This newer treatment slows bone loss, helps to build new bone, and reduces the incidence of spine and hip fractures.

Calcitonin is a hormone that is naturally produced in your body to help keep your bones strong. Doctors can give calcitonin as an injection or as a nasal spray.

Teriparatide This new drug helps to build new bone as well as reduce your risk of fractures. You'll need daily injections for up to 18 months. Currently, it's mainly given to people who continue to have fractures despite using other treatments or to those who can't tolerate other treatments.

HOW CAN I HELP MYSELF?

Did you know that 1 in 2 women over the age of 50 in the UK will break a bone mainly because of osteoporosis? Well, that statistic may be enough to spur you on to do something about your bone density – it's never too early or too late to start. You can help to prevent osteoporosis by leading an active life and eating a diet rich in calcium and vitamin D (see p262).

Reduce the risk of falling Make sure that there's nothing you can trip over at home, wear robust shoes, and be careful when you go outdoors during the winter. Use a walking stick if you have problems or need some extra assistance. If you're prone to falling, it may be worth looking into getting some hip protectors (specially padded underwear that cushions the hips). If your osteoporosis is severe, you need to take care when carrying or lifting things, as sudden stresses can easily cause a spine fracture.

Eat foods that build bones It's easy to eat bone-building foods, just look at the variety of good sources of calcium (see p262).

Exercise for strong bones Weight bearing exercise like walking and running help to keep your bones strong. Lifting weights can also promote bone density but should be avoided in those with osteoporosis. Women with osteoporosis should walk briskly for 30 minutes three to four days a week. Keeping physically active may reduce your risk of falls and improve your nerve and muscle responses if you do fall.

Stop smoking Chemicals from tobacco worsen bone loss and interfere in calcium absorption.

AM I AT RISK?

Osteoporosis affects everyone to some degree as they age, but your risk of the disease increases if:

- You have had an early menopause (before the age of 45)
- You take steroid drugs for a long period of time
- You have a family history of osteoporosis (especially if your mother broke a hip)
- You eat a diet that's low in both calcium and vitamin D
- You live, or have lived (particularly in your teenage years), a sedentary lifestyle, or you can't exercise for some reason
- You smoke
- You drink too much alcohol (see p65)
- You have certain conditions, such as coeliac disease (see p301) or hyperthyroidism (see pp328–9)
- You're underweight, or have suffered from an eating disorder (see pp216–17) in the past.

How to get your daily calcium

For healthy, strong bones you need plenty of calcium, and you need vitamin D to be able to absorb the calcium from your food. Your skin makes vitamin D from sunshine – 10–15 minutes outside without sunscreen at the hottest time of every day in summer (not enough to burn your skin) will usually give you enough vitamin D to last you all year round.

Recommended daily allowance (RDA) of calcium is 800mg

Increase to **1,200mg** calcium a day if you've been diagnosed with osteoporosis

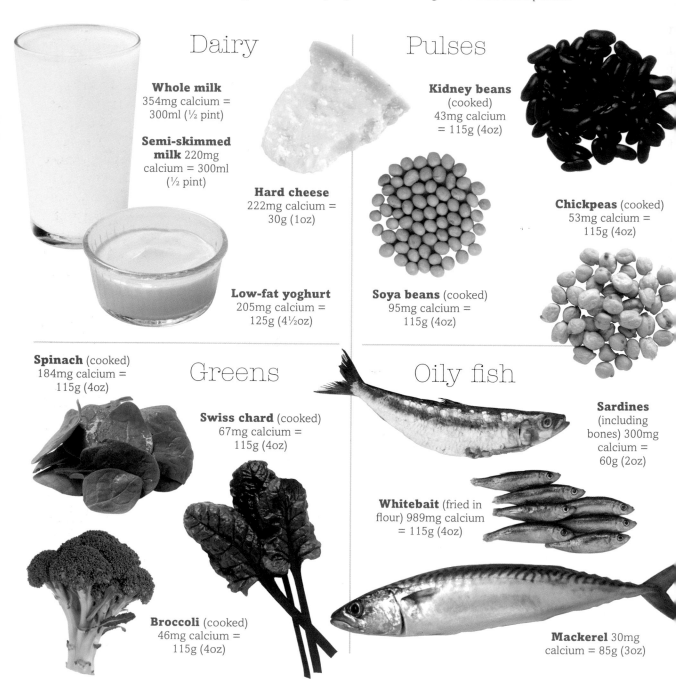

Dairy

Whole milk
354mg calcium =
300ml (½ pint)

Semi-skimmed milk 220mg calcium = 300ml (½ pint)

Hard cheese
222mg calcium =
30g (1oz)

Low-fat yoghurt
205mg calcium =
125g (4½oz)

Pulses

Kidney beans
(cooked)
43mg calcium
= 115g (4oz)

Chickpeas (cooked)
53mg calcium =
115g (4oz)

Soya beans (cooked)
95mg calcium =
115g (4oz)

Greens

Spinach (cooked)
184mg calcium =
115g (4oz)

Swiss chard (cooked)
67mg calcium =
115g (4oz)

Broccoli (cooked)
46mg calcium =
115g (4oz)

Oily fish

Sardines
(including
bones) 300mg
calcium =
60g (2oz)

Whitebait (fried in flour) 989mg calcium = 115g (4oz)

Mackerel 30mg
calcium = 85g (3oz)

Osteoarthritis

It's normal to have the odd creaky or stiff joint as you get older; none of us is the bionic woman. But if you notice a hip or knee, for example, that is becoming troublesome then it might be suffering the effects of osteoarthritis – a "wear and tear arthritis" – that develops slowly over many years.

WHAT IS IT?

In a joint affected by osteoarthritis, the surface of the cartilage on the end of the bones becomes rougher and thinner, and the bone beneath thickens and grows outwards, forming bony spurs. Movements are no longer smooth and fluid; joints become swollen, painful, and creaky as you try to move.

It's unclear why osteoarthritis can affect one joint but not another, and why, for example, one hip is affected more than the other.

Osteoarthritis is most common in the weight-bearing joints of the knees and hips, and in the spine (see Back and neck pain, p272). In women, it also affects the hands (especially the fingers and the base of the thumb) and the big toes (see Bunions, p265).

WHAT NEXT?

After going through your medical history your doctor will want to know about your symptoms. Tell him or her about any joints that are tender, swollen, or unstable. Before you visit your doctor try to pin down the times when your pain or stiffness is worst and what, if anything, makes it better or worse.

Your doctor will then want to examine you. He or she may be able to feel bony swellings and any creaking of an affected joint, as well as discover if there is any restricted movement at that joint.

You will probably have to give some blood, which will be sent for laboratory testing. Blood tests are

HAVE I GOT THE SYMPTOMS?

Symptoms of osteoarthritis can come and go, but they gradually worsen over time. You may find that there is:
- Pain after moving the joint
- Stiffness in the joint after rest; this improves when you start moving the joint
- A creaking sound on moving the affected joint
- A smaller range of movement in the joint or it may even give way suddenly.

See your doctor if symptoms persist or cause you distress.

AN ARTHRITIC MOBILE JOINT IN CROSS-SECTION

Osteoarthritis is more common in women than in men, especially in the knees and hands; plus we tend to suffer from more severe symptoms. Compare the normal knee with the arthritic one and you will see how the cartilage at the bones' ends has roughened and thinned, and the bones have developed the tiny spurs typical of osteoarthritis. The capsule around the joint also thickens and stretches.

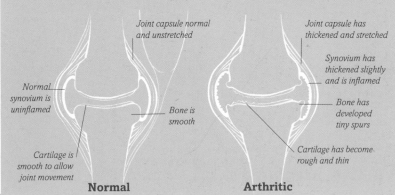

Joint capsule normal and unstretched

Joint capsule has thickened and stretched

Synovium has thickened slightly and is inflamed

Normal synovium is uninflamed

Bone is smooth

Bone has developed tiny spurs

Cartilage is smooth to allow joint movement

Cartilage has become rough and thin

Normal   **Arthritic**

normally carried out to exclude other types of arthritis (such as rheumatoid arthritis, see p266) as there are no specific tests that can detect osteoarthritis. You may also need an X-ray to see if there is any narrowing within a joint or if there are bony spurs. Do be aware that X-rays may be normal in the early stages of osteoarthritis.

MY TREATMENT OPTIONS

Unfortunately there is no cure for osteoarthritis – our joints just don't seem to be designed to work perfectly for a lifetime. But there are plenty of medicines to relieve any associated pain and stiffness. However, as with any drug, these can come with side effects.

Painkillers Paracetamol is the safest painkiller to take for short-term relief. It can also be used in combination with other analgesics, such as codeine-like drugs. Medicines known as non-steroidal anti-inflammatory drugs (NSAIDs), such as ibuprofen and diclofenac, can also reduce your pain, swelling, and stiffness. These may also be available as a gel for massaging into an affected joint.

Injections Steroids or hyaluronic acid (which is similar to the thick, viscous component of normal synovial fluid, see p258) can be given as injections into an affected joint. These injections may provide longer relief and can ease your pain for several weeks at a time.

Physiotherapy In sessions with a physiotherapist you can learn exercises that will help to stabilize and protect your joints. You may also have some hydrotherapy, which involves hot and cold water treatments, to increase your range of mobility in an affected joint, especially a knee.

Joint replacement If, despite taking medication, your pain continues to be severe and your joints become so badly swollen or damaged that they restrict your mobility, then your doctor may refer you to an orthopaedic surgeon. Depending on your particular problem, the surgeon may recommend that you have an operation to replace the affected joint with a prosthesis. As with any surgery there are risks that your doctor will discuss with you.

Replacing an osteoarthritic hip

This X-ray image shows a hip joint after joint replacement surgery. Osteoarthritis had damaged the cartilage around the ball-and-socket joint where the thigh bone meets the pelvis at the pelvic socket.

> ### AM I AT RISK?
>
> Osteoarthritis becomes more common as you get older; it is rare before the age of 40. It's not known why one woman and not another will develop osteoarthritis, but there are some known risk factors:
> - Being overweight or obese. The heavier you are the more weight your knees and hips have to bear; being overweight or obese also increases the chances of osteoarthritis worsening
> - Doing hard and repetitive exercise, such as seen in ballet dancers or gymnasts
> - Having a history of osteoarthritis in the family
> - Having a joint abnormality at birth
> - Having had an injury or operation on a joint.

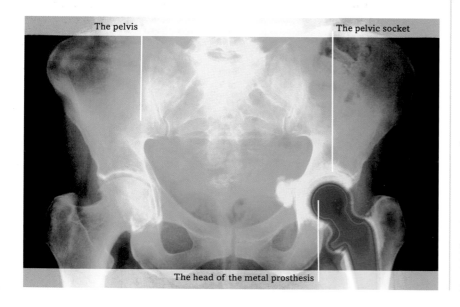

The pelvis

The pelvic socket

The head of the metal prosthesis

Advances in surgical techniques and materials technology mean that artificial joints may last 10–25 years. The implants can provide you with mobility that is both stable and pain-free.

Hips and knees are the most commonly replaced joints, and surgery for these is generally very successful. However, other joints, such as the shoulder, ankle, elbow, and knuckles, can also be replaced with varying amounts of success.

Depending on the procedure you have, you can expect to stay in hospital between two and five days. Afterwards, your recovery is likely to be slow and steady; many people feel much better three to six months after a joint replacement operation, but it can take up to a year to feel totally back to normal.

HOW CAN I HELP MYSELF?

There are several measures you can take to help you relieve the symptoms of osteoarthritis.

> "There are plenty of osteoarthritis treatments so that you can still enjoy life to the full."

Lose excess weight First and foremost, losing weight if you are overweight will be a great help; you'll be significantly reducing everyday stress on your hips, knees, and feet. Try to keep active, and pace your activities throughout the day with regular breaks. Turn to a healthy diet (see pp52–5), exercise (see pp56–7), and weight issues (see pp58–9).

Wear comfortable shoes You might find that certain footwear helps: shock absorbing trainers with thick soft soles or flat shoes may be much more comfortable and help lessen any aches and pains. If you suffer with bunions or the beginnings of one, then steer clear of pointed toes or high heels, or at least restrict your wearing of them to short periods.

You may take a supplement Many people take glucosamine and/or chondroitin supplements, which are available from health food stores, to "help with their joints". Such substances may have a modest effect on cartilage loss, and some people find that they provide pain relief. There is no evidence, however, that cod liver oil has any noticeable impact on osteoarthritis.

Use a walking aid If you find that a joint simply gives way from time to time, try using a walking stick (you can get collapsible ones that are easy to store and transport). Wearing a joint brace to support a knee, for example, can also help.

Modify your home and work Occupational therapists can give you advice on modifications to both your home and your work environment, as well as useful gadgets, such as jar and bottle openers, to help with daily life.

BUNIONS

Osteoarthritis at the base of the big toe may result in stiffness of the joint and a bony deformity – one of the causes of painful bunions. The big toe leans towards the other toes and the joint at the base sticks out (see right). The tissues overlying the bunion can become inflamed, causing pain and swelling. Bunions are more likely to cause symptoms when you wear shoes with a tight toe box or high heels. Standing for a long time may also aggravate symptoms. Your doctor may recommend that you wear pads over the bunion or wear a custom-made device inside your shoes. Alternatively, you may want to visit a podiatrist for exercise recommendations and orthoses (special devices inserted into shoes). In severe cases, surgical treatment may be necessary.

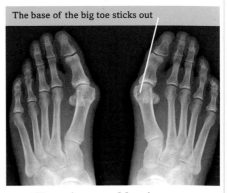

The base of the big toe sticks out

X-ray image of bunions

Autoimmune diseases

In this section, we look at rheumatoid arthritis, lupus, Raynaud's phenomenon, and Sjögren's syndrome. These diseases, in which your body attacks itself, are more common in women. As with so many conditions, it is not yet known what causes the body to prompt such an attack, or how this assault will affect the body.

Rheumatoid arthritis

This autoimmune disease can affect people of any age, although it most often occurs in people in their early 40s, and is three times more common in women than in men.

WHAT IS IT?

Arthritis means inflammation of joints, and rheumatoid arthritis is a common form of arthritis. In rheumatoid arthritis (RA), the body's own immune system attacks the lining (synovium) of joints, in particular those of the hands, wrists, and feet, or other joints in the body. This results in inflammation, swelling, stiffness, warm joints, and pain. The joint can become painful when the nerves are irritated by chemicals produced by the inflammation and the stretching of the outer part of the synovium by the swollen joint.

It is not known exactly what triggers this joint inflammation (see p259), which over time can also damage the cartilage, the ligaments, and the bone near to a joint. Rheumatoid arthritis may also affect tendons and sometimes other body parts, such as the lungs, eyes, and blood vessels, and lumps called rheumatoid nodules may occur in elbows, hands, and feet. Patients with rheumatoid arthritis are more at risk of cardiovascular disease (see Chapter 7, pp158–74). Treatment with steroids and NSAIDS may also play a role.

In most cases, RA symptoms develop gradually over several weeks or so. The disease is usually characterized by recurrent moderate attacks. The frequency of attacks, the number of affected joints, and the severity of symptoms are variable. Some people have a mild form of the disease, with very few symptoms. Most people have periods of flare-ups when their joints become more painful and inflamed. Such flare-ups may last for months or years, but are then often followed by better spells. For a few people, their rheumatoid arthritis becomes progressively worse quite quickly.

WHAT NEXT?

There is no single test to diagnose rheumatoid arthritis, and because there are many other possible conditions that may cause your joints to be painful, it can be quite difficult to diagnose RA. Your doctor will make a diagnosis based on a discussion with you about your symptoms, medical history, the findings of a physical examination, and the results of

HAVE I GOT THE SYMPTOMS?

There are several main and "extra-articular" ("outside of the joints") symptoms to look for:

- Pain and swelling in the fingers, wrists, or balls of feet
- Morning stiffness
- A general feeling of being unwell
- Tiredness
- Feeling hot and sweaty
- Feeling depressed or irritable
- Unexplained weight loss
- Dry, irritable eyes

See your doctor if you have one or more symptoms in addition to stiff, aching joints.

"You can reduce your risk of developing RA by adopting a healthy lifestyle."

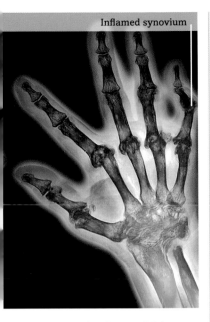

Inflamed synovium

Hand with advanced RA
This X-ray shows the swelling of the joint caused by the collection of fluid and cells in the synovium.

any blood tests and X-rays that he or she thinks might be appropriate. Blood tests can check for:

- Inflammation – erythrocyte sedimentation rate (ESR) and C-reactive protein (CRP)
- Rheumatoid factor (80 per cent of people with rheumatoid arthritis have this protein in their blood)
- Anti-cyclic citrullinated peptide (CCP) antibodies (these are specific to rheumatoid arthritis).

Any X-rays may show up damage caused by the disease process. There are also newer techniques, such as ultrasound scanning and magnetic resonance imaging (MRI), which may be pick up earlier changes due to the disease.

AM I AT RISK?

Rheumatoid arthritis exists all over the world, and approximately 1 person in every 100 of the population is affected by it. Rheumatoid arthritis can begin at any age, but it most commonly starts between the ages of 30 and 50 and symptoms typically appear when people are in their early 40s. As with many diseases, rheumatoid arthritis can run in families, but genes are only part of the picture.

Certain lifestyle factors may increase your risk of contracting rheumatoid arthritis, so the best way to help reduce this risk is by adopting a healthy lifestyle. Cigarette smoking is thought to increase the risk of rheumatoid

arthritis, so if you are still a smoker, turn to page 64 for tips on how to quit. It's also important to eat a balanced, varied diet, because a diet that is typically high in caffeine and red meat, and low in antioxidants, may increase the risk of this condition (see pp52–5 for advice on a healthy diet). Rheumatoid arthritis has also been found to be slightly less common in people who drink alcohol in moderation, or who have a high intake of vitamin C. If you are overweight or obese (see pp58–9), the excess weight that your body carries can put extra pressure on joints, so losing any excess weight can make a positive difference to your health.

JOINTS AFFECTED BY RHEUMATOID ARTHRITIS

Rheumatoid arthritis is likely to affect the joints highlighted *(below)*, and tends to affect the body symmetrically. The degree of joint damage, and the number of joints affected, will vary from person to person, since RA seems to affect everyone differently.

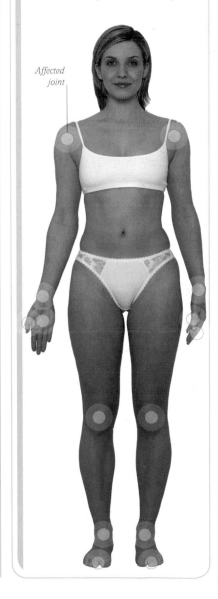

Affected joint

MY TREATMENT OPTIONS

The main aim of RA treatment is to suppress the inflammation in the joints as early as possible in order to prevent any more damage being done. (Once the joints have been damaged by inflammation, they do not heal very well.) Key treatments for rheumatoid arthritis include:

Painkillers, such as paracetamol, will help to reduce pain, and can be given in combination with stronger codeine-like drugs. However, painkillers alone are often not enough, and are usually prescribed together with NSAIDS.

Non-steroidal anti-inflammatory drugs (NSAIDS) reduce both the pain and the swelling of joints.

Disease-modifying antirheumatic drugs (DMARDs) can treat more than just the symptoms of rheumatoid arthritis – they also slow down the course of the disease itself. These drugs may take many weeks or months to become effective, and tend to be taken for many years. Since they can all potentially cause side effects, these drugs require regular monitoring by doctors and nurses. There are a number of drugs in this group:

- Methotrexate, sulphasalazine, leflunamide, gold, azathioprine, and penicillamine
- Newer biological therapies, such as antiTNF drugs and rituximab, are very effective and may work more quickly.

Steroids, which can cause a number of side effects if used in the long term.

HOW CAN I HELP MYSELF?

There are several ways to look after yourself to minimize the disability of rheumatoid arthritis as much as possible:

Take a fish oil supplement, which can have a modest beneficial effect on the symptoms of rheumatoid arthritis.

Keep your weight within healthy levels. Eating a good, healthy diet may also help, and lose weight if you are overweight.

RHEUMATOID ARTHRITIS AND PREGNANCY

Most women with rheumatoid arthritis feel better during pregnancy. Unfortunately, the disease can flare up again after the baby is born. Also, some of the drugs cannot be taken during pregnancy, so if you are thinking of becoming pregnant (or even if you are already pregnant), discuss this condition with your doctor.

Try to be as active as possible, because the muscles around the joints will become weak if they aren't used. Regular exercise to increase muscle strength may also help to reduce pain and improve joint function. However, you should work within your limits; you don't want to harm your muscles and joints.

Vary your level of activity from day to day, depending on how you feel. Swimming, cycling, and walking with supportive shoes, are all very beneficial. Physiotherapists and occupational therapists can also advise on particular exercises to keep the joints mobile and the muscles around the joints as strong as possible, and also on joint protection, adaptations to your home to make daily tasks easier, and useful aids.

Beneficial treatment
Swimming is a good way to exercise if you suffer from an autoimmune disease. Being in water reduces strain on the joints.

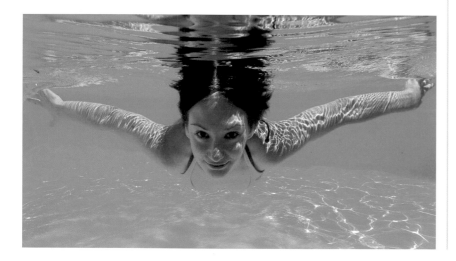

Lupus

Systemic lupus erythematosus (its full name) is usually called lupus for short. This autoimmune disease is nine times more common in women than in men, and it affects approximately 1 person in every 1,000 people.

WHAT IS IT?

Lupus causes inflammation in various parts of the body. It can be mild or severe; it can flare up and then simply subside; and it can present in many ways and mimic many diseases.

HAVE I GOT THE SYMPTOMS?

Lupus can cause a variety of symptoms, of which these are the most common:
- Joint pain
- Tiredness
- Skin rashes
- Increased sensitivity to light
- Fever
- Weight loss
- Swollen lymph glands
- Hair loss
- Mouth ulcers
- Poor circulation to the fingers and toes (Raynaud's phenomenon, see p270).

An individual suffering from lupus may have a different range of symptoms from another person with the condition.
See your doctor if you have any of these symptoms.

Lupus most typically develops in women of child-bearing age, though people at any age can be affected, and it has been found to be more prevalent among women of Afro-Caribbean and Asian origin.

It's not known why lupus and other autoimmune diseases occur. Some factors may trigger the immune system to make abnormal antibodies, which cause the inflammation and damage to various body tissues. Possible triggers may include viruses, environmental factors such as sunlight and infections, hormones, and genetic factors, although lupus is not a simple hereditary disease. Some women also have specific (antiphospholipid) antibodies that can result in a miscarriage during pregnancy, or in blood clots.

Lupus has wide-ranging effects on various body organs and systems, including:
- The kidneys (inflammation here leads to high blood pressure)
- The brain and nervous system (causing anything from a simple headache to anxiety and depression, epilepsy, and even mental health problems)
- The heart and lungs (resulting in breathlessness and chest pain)
- The digestive tract and liver (leading to loss of appetite, sickness, vomiting, as well as diarrhoea)
- The spleen (an enlarged spleen can be found when a patient is examined)
- The eyes (causing dry eyes and a dry mouth).

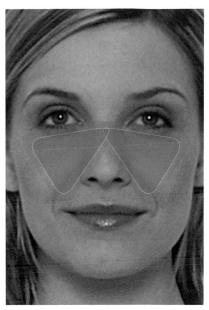

Butterfly rash
A red raised rash across the nose and cheeks in the shape of a butterfly is a common characteristic of lupus.

WHAT NEXT?

Your doctor will make a diagnosis based on your symptoms (see Have I Got the Symptoms?, left), medical history, a physical examination, as necessary, and the results of a range of specific blood tests. The tests can detect certain types of antibodies (ANA, antiDNA and other antibodies) or signs of disease activity in your blood. The blood tests may also show evidence of anaemia and abnormalities of other blood cells, and assess kidney and liver function.

MY TREATMENT OPTIONS

Although there is currently no cure, much progress has been made in the treatment and management of the disease, and the outlook for patients with lupus has improved dramatically. Most people with lupus are seen by a specialist who will advise on the right treatments. If you have very mild symptoms, you may not even need any treatment.

Medication can ease symptoms in most cases. Depending on how many of the symptoms you are suffering from, your doctor may prescribe one or more of the following effective medications:

- Painkillers and NSAIDs (for the relief of joint pain)
- Hydroxychloroquine tablets and steroid cream (both are used to treat skin rashes; hydroxychloroquine tablets also treat joint pains and tiredness)
- Steroid drugs (to treat inflammation in other parts of the body, such as the heart or the lungs)
- High-dose steroids and immunosuppressant drugs (for severe forms of the disease).

HOW CAN I HELP MYSELF?

There are some simple measures you can take:

Avoid the sun Strong sunlight can aggravate lupus symptoms (and not just the skin symptoms). Cover up as much as possible and apply sunscreen of SPF25 or above on exposed skin.

Stop smoking because smoking can increase the risk of lupus.

Try to avoid infections, since you are more prone to infection – particularly if you take steroids or immunosuppressant medication.

Avoid using certain drugs, such as blood-pressure drugs, which are known to cause drug-induced lupus or lupus flares.

Take a fish oil supplement, as this may be helpful.

Raynaud's phenomenon

This common disease affects the extremities (usually the fingers), which change colour and become painful. About 1 in 20 people develop the symptoms and it can affect all ages, but symptoms are usually mild. Fewer than 1 in 10 people affected by this condition have an underlying disease (such as an autoimmune disease), but it can also be a side effect of drugs, such as beta blockers.

WHAT IS IT?

Raynaud's phenomenon is due to constriction of the small blood vessels when exposed to the cold, or a change in temperature. The skin on your fingers, for example, changes colour: first becoming pale and cool, then blueish, and finally pink (muscle spasm in the arteries restricts the blood supply briefly). Along with colour change comes pain, numbness, and tingling. It can affect your feet and nose, earlobes, or tongue, but it's your hands that are usually the problem. Attacks are usually mild, with brief, infrequent bouts.

WHAT NEXT?

If you're unable to control the condition on your own, your doctor may prescribe medication to dilate the blood vessels.

MY TREATMENT OPTIONS

Discuss your symptoms with your doctor and see what kind of treatment is most suitable for you.

HOW CAN I HELP MYSELF?

There are several ways to self-treat:

Keep your hands warm with hand-warmers and heated gloves.

Avoid sudden exposure to cold.

Give up smoking, as it constricts the blood vessels in your hands.

Reduce stress in your everyday life and learn to relax as much as you can (see pp62–3).

HAVE I GOT THE SYMPTOMS?

Typically, these symptoms develop when you become cool, for instance in cold weather:

- Pain, numbness, throbbing, and tingling in fingers
- Skin on fingers changes colour when cold due to the constriction and dilation of blood vessels in the fingers
- Occasional problems with your feet.

See your doctor if these symptoms develop when you experience cold weather.

Sjögren's syndrome

Sjögren's (pronounced "show-grins"), syndrome is probably the second most common autoimmune disease after rheumatoid arthritis (see p266). Although this disease can strike at any age, women between the ages of 40 and 60 are the most likely group to get it.

WHAT IS IT?

In this autoimmune condition, your immune system attacks and damages the tissues of the salivary glands and the tear glands. The resulting symptoms (see Have I got the symptoms?, right), may prove to be uncomfortable, but can be treated. In addition to the attack on your salivary and tear glands, your body's immune system may also cause the inflammation of your joints, liver, kidneys, and lungs. If you have Sjögren's syndrome and become pregnant, there is a risk that some

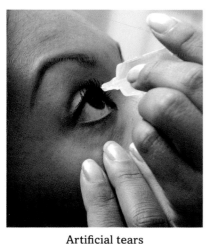

Artificial tears
Drops provide eye lubrication. Tilt your head back and pull the lower lid down to apply drops inside the lower lid.

of the autoantibodies your body has created may pass across the placenta to your growing baby and cause a disturbed heart rhythm. The babies of patients who carry these antibodies need to be monitored carefully during pregnancy, and may also need to have steroid treatment.

WHAT NEXT?

After taking your medical history and examining you, if necessary, your doctor will measure your tear and saliva production, arrange for blood tests to detect any autoantibodies, and perhaps ask for a lip biopsy (when tiny salivary glands are removed from the lower lip for close examination under a microscope). To determine your tear production, your doctor will gently insert a small piece of paper under your lower eyelid for several minutes and ask you to keep your eyes closed. How much saliva you can produce is measured simply by how much you can spit into a pot.

MY TREATMENT OPTIONS

Although there is as yet no cure for Sjögren's syndrome, doctors can prescribe a variety of treatments:
Artificial tears can help to lubricate dry eyes.
Special spectacles keep in moisture and reduce eye dryness.

HAVE I GOT THE SYMPTOMS?

The symptoms to look for are:
● Aching in the joints
● Dry eyes
● Dry mouth and dental problems
● Tiredness
● Swollen salivary glands and lymph nodes

Other organs of the body can also be affected by this condition.
See your doctor if you think that you have more than one of these symptoms.

Artificial saliva, given as a mouth spray or as lozenges.
Painkillers (including NSAIDs) can be helpful.
Hydroxychloroquine, the antimalarial drug, helps with joint pain and tiredness.
Steroid drugs can be used for arthritis and swollen glands or other organs, such as the lungs.
Minor surgery is offered for particular cases.

HOW CAN I HELP MYSELF?

There are several general measures to take to help your condition:
To treat dry eyes, avoid wind, air conditioning, dust, and smoke.
To treat a dry mouth, drink lots of water, chew sugarless gum, keep your teeth, gums, and mouth clean, and visit your dentist regularly.

"Some people may only notice mild symptoms, such as dry eyes and a dry mouth."

Back and neck pain

More working days are lost to back pain than any other condition – in the UK back pain accounts for 4.5 million days off work a year. Neck pain is also common and occurs more often in women. The good news is that most pain resolves itself within a few weeks. But do see your doctor if the pain persists.

HAVE I GOT THE SYMPTOMS?

Symptoms may come on over weeks or appear suddenly.
- Pain, which could be referred to arms or legs
- Stiffness, clicking, or cracking felt with movement (neck pain).

See your doctor urgently if you have weakness, numbness, or tingling in your arms or legs; numbness in your bottom; bowel problems or with passing urine; dizziness when looking up.

WHAT IS IT?

Pain due to bad posture or straining muscles or ligaments – so-called mechanical pain – is very common. Largely worse after movement and relieved by rest, the pain doesn't usually radiate (called "referred pain") to your arms or legs and tends to settle fairly quickly. However, the painful muscle spasm that's sometimes associated with it may last for several weeks.

"Referred" pain in your limbs may also be accompanied by numbness or tingling. Conversely, a painful shoulder (see p282) may result in pain felt in the neck.

Common causes of neck and back pain are:
- Bad posture
- Abnormal exertion
- Injury, such as whiplash
- A "slipped disc"
- Osteoarthritis of the spine
- Narrowing of the spinal canal (spinal stenosis)
- Abnormal curvature of the spine.

Bad posture whether hunching over a steering wheel or slumping at a desk can wreak havoc on your muscles, often triggering painful muscle strains.

Abnormal exertion can happen when over-reaching or lifting something too heavy or at an awkward angle. The resulting pain is a symptom of stress or damage to any of your spine's ligaments, muscles, tendons, or discs.

Whiplash injuries, where a person's head is thrown forwards and then backwards violently (as in a road traffic accident when a car is hit from behind) is a common cause of neck pain.

A "slipped disc" is more accurately described as a "prolapsed" (bulging) or "herniated" (ruptured) disc. The cause of this serious back pain is the jelly-like material held within the cushioning intervertebral discs. This prolapsed or ruptured disc can squash a nearby nerve root or the spinal cord. This pressure causes pain as well as symptoms in other parts of the body, such as numbness or tingling in your arms or legs, and can even affect bladder and bowel control.

Osteoarthritis of the spine is also referred to by doctors as spondylosis: cervical spondylosis if the osteoarthritis is in the neck or lumbar regions, spondylosis, if

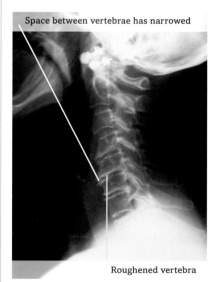

Space between vertebrae has narrowed

Roughened vertebra

Cervical spondylosis
This X-ray shows the vertebrae of the cervical spine. The osteoarthritic vertebrae are close together and have roughened edges.

in the lower back. Osteoarthritis (see p263) is a "wear and tear" arthritis. In the spine it affects both the facet joints and the intervertebral discs (see below). As we age, these discs become thinner and the spaces between the vertebrae become narrower. Bony outgrowths or spurs, called osteophytes, form at the edges of the vertebrae and the facet joints. These bony growths may cause localized pain or referred pain in an arm or leg, for example, if they squash a nerve.

Spinal stenosis Narrowing of the spinal canal by a disc or a bony growth is known as spinal stenosis. This narrowing puts pressure on the spinal cord and can be associated with numbness, weakness in the legs, or bladder or bowel problems.

Abnormal curvature of the spine If your spine curves in an abnormal way or if the curve is exaggerated, it may result in pain. Scoliosis, where the spine curves to the side, may also cause pain.

Rare causes of back and/or neck pain include: rheumatoid arthritis (see p266), ankylosing spondylitis, fibromyalgia (see p276), polymyalgia rheumatica, fractures associated with osteoporosis (see p260), infection (such as tuberculosis) or certain cancers that may have spread to the vertebrae.

WHAT NEXT?

Normally, your doctor will make a diagnosis based on your medical history and a physical examination.

Your doctor will want to find out where the pain is coming from,

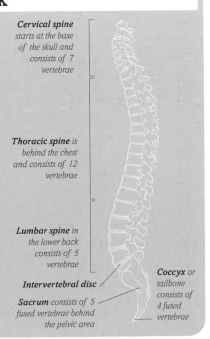

Prolapsed disc

Spinal cord

Lumbar disc prolapse
In this MRI scan, a prolapsed disc between the lumbar spine and the sacrum is putting pressure on the spinal cord

how much you can move before the pain kicks in, and whether any muscles are in spasm. To this end, he or she may want to examine your back and assess your ability to sit, stand, bend over, walk, and lift your legs.

If it's your neck that's painful, your doctor will want to see your range of movement and the exact location of the pain as well as determine the kinds of activities that bring it on. Your reflexes may also be tested.

Further tests, such as X-rays, CT, or MRI scans, are usually done only if there is suspicion of a trapped nerve, spinal stenosis, spinal fracture, inflammation, infection, or a tumour.

You may have to give a sample of blood for laboratory testing to help determine the diagnosis.

THE BONES OF YOUR BACK

Your back consists of stacked vertebrae forming the spinal column from skull to pelvis. It is divided into 3 main sections: the cervical spine (7 vertebrae); the thoracic spine (12 vertebrae); and the lumbar vertebrae (5 vertebrae). The sacrum is 5 fused vertebrae; the coccyx is 4. Cushioning discs sit between the vertebrae, while facet joints connect them at the back. The vertebrae are held together by ligaments, allowing flexibility. Your spinal cord lies within the spinal column. Nerves run from your brain through your spinal cord to the rest of your body.

Cervical spine starts at the base of the skull and consists of 7 vertebrae

Thoracic spine is behind the chest and consists of 12 vertebrae

Lumbar spine in the lower back consists of 5 vertebrae

Intervertebral disc

Sacrum consists of 5 fused vertebrae behind the pelvic area

Coccyx or tailbone consists of 4 fused vertebrae

LOWER-BACK PAIN

Because of the complex and interconnected nature of your lower back, any small amount of damage to a muscle, ligament, tendon, or disc can result in a lot of discomfort. The location of the pain – be it high up in the middle of the back or radiating down one leg, as shown below – will give your doctor clues as to the cause of your pain.

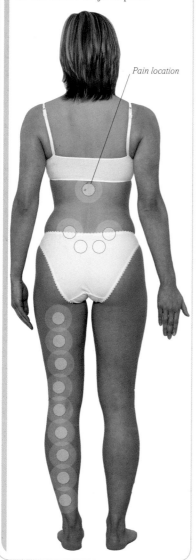

Pain location

MY TREATMENT OPTIONS

Most instances of back or neck pain settle within weeks and need little or no treatment, except for some pain relief. But if your pain is severe or your doctor has identified the cause of your pain, then other options, which may have potential side effects, are available.

Pain relief While your pain settles you may get enough relief from regular doses of paracetamol or ibuprofen. If these drugs are not quite enough, then your doctor can prescribe stronger non-steroidal anti-inflammatory drugs (NSAIDs), such as diclofenac or naproxen.

Steroid and local anaesthetic injections These can help with pain from a prolapsed or herniated disc or facet joint arthritis.

Other drugs Many people get relief from sciatic pain (pain in the buttocks and down the back of the thigh caused by pressure on the sciatic nerve) from the antidepressant drug amitriptyline and the anticonvulsant drugs gabapentin and pregabalin.

Manipulative therapies Your doctor may refer you to a physiotherapist, who can use various treatments to lessen the pain, such as heat, ice, ultrasound, TENS (transcutaneous electrical nerve stimulation), and muscle-release techniques. What's more, he or she will be able to teach you exercises and stretches to restore muscle function and strengthen your neck and/or back muscles.

Surgery If all forms of pain relief and/or manipulative therapies fail, then surgery may be necessary. In cases of spinal stenosis or a prolapsed or herniated disc, a surgeon can remove the cause of the pain. After such an operation, it's usual to spend a few days in hospital. It may take a few weeks afterwards for the pain to settle.

A pain-management programme If, despite all treatments, the pain persists then your doctor may refer you to a pain-management programme. Usually run as outpatient group sessions, these involve a multidisciplinary team (doctors, nurses, physiotherapists, and psychologists) to give advice and information about exercise, coping strategies, pacing of activities, and the use of medications.

HOW CAN I HELP MYSELF?

As well as following the advice of your doctor, there are some things you can try to help relieve the pain. Then, it's a good idea to learn how to prevent future occurrences by strengthening your muscles and keeping healthy (see opposite).

Rest It may help to spend a few days resting, but it's not a good idea to spend a long time in bed.

"Walking, swimming, and cycling are all excellent to strengthen your back muscles."

Try to get back to normal activities and work as soon as possible. Resting for too long may hinder your progress and weaken muscles, and a significant spell off work may also dent your confidence.

Gentle stretches For neck pain, gently move your head to one side and hold for 30 seconds. Then, repeat on the other side. Stretch your neck in as many directions as your pain allows. Stretching, strengthening, and stabilizing exercises can help relieve back pain. Such exercises are designed to restore the strength of your back muscles and the flexibility of your spinal column.

Sleep right You spend a third of your life sleeping and if you sleep in an awkward position – hugging a pillow, for instance, or even just lying on your front – you can be putting extra stress and strain on your back and neck muscles every single day. Try to train yourself to sleep lying on one side rather than on your front. Choose a supportive mattress and change it if you wake up first thing in the morning with backache; experts recommend that you change your mattress every 10 years.

Osteopathy, physiotherapy, and chiropractic Many women seek the services of an osteopath, physiotherapist, or a chiropractor. Each professional has a different approach to problems relating to the spine. Normally, a short course is all that's needed, along with paying attention to your posture in your day-to-day life.

KEEP YOUR BACK HEALTHY

By following these few simple guidelines you can build a strong, healthy back and lead a full and pain-free life.

- Exercise your back regularly – walking, swimming, and using exercise bikes are all excellent to strengthen your back muscles
- Always bend your knees and your hips, never your back, when lifting an object
- Exercises, such as pilates, that build "core strength" work your pelvic and abdominal muscles to support your back by working like a natural "corset"
- Never twist and bend at the same time
- Always lift and carry objects close to your body
- Try to carry loads in a rucksack, and avoid shoulder bags
- Always maintain a good posture – avoid slumping in your chair or walking around with your hands in your pockets
- When working at a desk, always use a chair with a back rest and sit with your feet flat on the floor or on a footrest under the table
- Choose a firm mattress and ensure you sleep in a comfortable position.

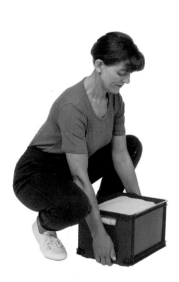

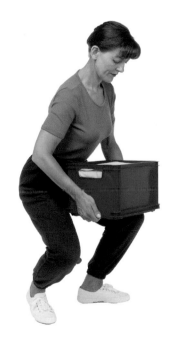

Good lifting technique
Step 1 To prevent back problems, learn how to lift correctly, using the power of your legs. Squat down in front of the object you need to lift.

Step 2 Then, while keeping your body straight and the object in front of you, straighten your legs and stand up.

Fibromyalgia

You may well know someone who has this common condition as it affects 1 person in 20, and 9 out of 10 sufferers are women. Fibromyalgia causes widespread and unremitting muscle pain, along with specific tender points. This discomfort is often accompanied by sleep disturbance and severe fatigue.

WHAT IS IT?

As with many conditions, the cause of fibromyalgia is unknown. It may be that chemical changes in the brain and nervous system lead to an increased sensitivity to pressure, so that what's normally felt as pressure becomes acutely painful. Recent research has suggested that fibromyalgia sufferers have lower than normal levels of a chemical called serotonin in the brain. Serotonin is involved in pain control and also in the regulation of sleep. Fibromyalgia may run in families; you're most likely to be affected if you have a relative who also suffers from it.

No one knows exactly what triggers fibromyalgia, but it often comes on after you've had a period of emotional stress or illness, or following surgery or an accident. Fibromyalgia often occurs together with other conditions, including irritable bladder, premenstrual syndrome (see pp92–3), painful periods (see p91), and irritable bowel syndrome (see pp304–5).

WHAT NEXT?

Your doctor may suspect you have fibromyalgia if you've had widespread pain for at least three months and you have tenderness in 11 out of the 18 characteristic locations (see opposite). If, after reviewing your medical history and carrying out a physical examination, your doctor thinks that fibromyalgia may be the cause of your symptoms, he or she will organize X-rays and blood tests to rule out other conditions that may cause similar symptoms, such as overactivity of the thyroid gland (see pp328–9). There's no specific test that will positively confirm the diagnosis of fibromyalgia.

MY TREATMENT OPTIONS

Fibromyalgia can be treated in a combination of ways and, in addition to appropriate medication (which may have side effects), includes learning about the condition and looking at how your behaviour could be contributing to your symptoms. A carefully planned programme of exercise is often integral to treatment.

Pain relief Paracetamol is recommended for the relief of pain. If this doesn't provide adequate relief, you might also be given opioid painkillers, such as tramodol. Low doses of antidepressants, including amitriptyline, fluoxetine, duloxetine, and milnacipran (sometimes used in combination), can be used for relieving pain and can also help with sleep problems. For some, the anticonvulsant drugs

HAVE I GOT THE SYMPTOMS?

Fibromyalgia is likely to cause a combination of any of the following symptoms:
- Pain at many sites
- Tender points (see opposite)
- Stiffness, which is often worse in the mornings
- Feeling exhausted, even when you've just woken up
- Frequently waking at night and having trouble getting back to sleep
- Joints that feel swollen, although they look normal
- Tingling
- Poor concentration
- Memory problems
- Headaches
- Light-headedness, anxiety, and/or depression.

See your doctor if you have been suffering from a number of these symptoms.

pregabalin and gabapentin are effective both for relieving pain and for helping to counteract any sleep disturbances.

Cognitive behavioural therapy This form of talking therapy aims to help you understand that your thoughts, beliefs, and expectations can all have an impact on your symptoms. Changing the way you think about your symptoms can sometimes lessen their severity.

Exercise plan By taking some exercise you'll be able to carry on with your everyday activities. Regular exercise also has a beneficial effect on sleep patterns. Your doctor may refer you to a physiotherapist, who'll be able to help design an exercise programme that will increase your strength, provide aerobic conditioning, and improve your flexibility and balance. Some of the best forms of exercise for fibromyalgia sufferers include low-impact aerobic exercise, such as swimming and walking, and activities such as yoga that involve stretching.

HOW CAN I HELP MYSELF?

Together with any medical treatment your doctor may prescribe, making a few simple changes to your lifestyle can reap big rewards in terms of a reduction in the severity of your symptoms and improving the frequency and length of your pain-free interludes.

Try to get a good night's sleep, training yourself to do so if necessary (see pp60–1).

Eat a healthy, balanced diet; though there are no special foods that will help the condition, it can make a difference (see pp52–5).

Learn how to relax and handle stress (see pp62–3).

Physical therapies such as massage can sometimes relieve pain and eliminate stiffness as well as help you relax.

Join a fibromyalgia support group. The opportunity to share your experiences with others who are going through the same thing can be a great source of comfort and self-help ideas.

CLASSIC TENDER SPOTS

Your doctor will test each of the highlighted areas for tenderness. If 11 out of 18 sites are tender, then it's likely you have fibromyalgia.

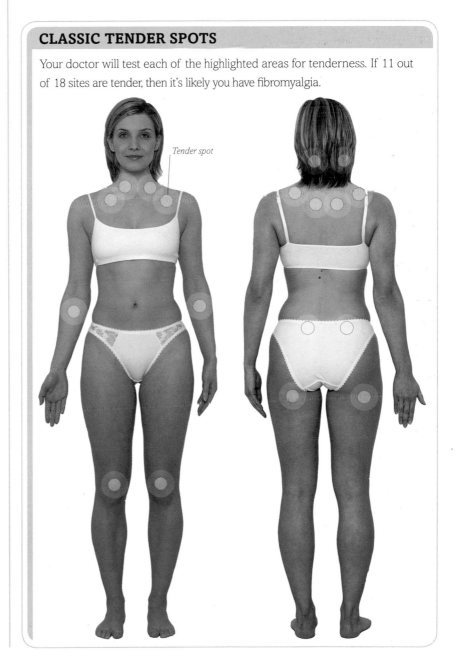

Tender spot

Chronic fatigue syndrome

Many of us in today's busy world complain of being "tired all the time", but if you have chronic fatigue syndrome (CFS), you literally are tired all the time. This long-term, often disabling, exhaustion persists even if you've had a good night's sleep. However, there are treatments to try, and ways to help yourself.

HAVE I GOT THE SYMPTOMS?

CFS causes persistent physical and mental tiredness for at least six months, and any four primary symptoms:

- Weakness and extreme exhaustion, lasting more than 24 hours, after any mental or physical activity
- Unrefreshing sleep, insomnia, or excessive daytime sleepiness
- Substantial impairment of short-term memory or concentration
- Unexplained muscle soreness
- Pain that moves from joint to joint without swelling or redness
- Headaches of a new type, pattern, or severity
- Tender lymph nodes in your armpit and/or neck
- Persistent or frequent sore throat.

In addition, there are some common secondary symptoms:

- Unexplained abdominal pain
- Hypersensitivity to light, noise, and to emotional overload
- Dizziness, fainting, lack of balance
- Palpitations, irregular heartbeat
- A need to urinate often
- Shortness of breath
- IBS (see pp304–5)
- Chills and inappropriate sweating, often at night
- A new allergy or sensitivity to a food, medication, or chemical.

See your doctor if you have any four primary symptoms and any secondary symptoms.

WHAT IS IT?

Also known as ME (myalgic encephalomyelitis or myalgic encephalopathy), CFS is recognized as a serious illness marked by prolonged exhaustion and wide-ranging symptoms (see box, above).

CFS is a complex, mysterious condition and research is still ongoing into the exact cause; it is discussed in this chapter because of its close relationship with fibromyalgia (see pp276–7). CFS tends to affect people from their early twenties to mid-forties, and can either develop suddenly or appear gradually over a period of years. Three to five times more women than men have CFS.

WHAT NEXT?

Currently, there's no diagnostic test for CFS, so your doctor will make a diagnosis based on your medical history and a physical examination, as well as tests to rule out all other possible causes of your symptoms. To be given a diagnosis of CFS, you have to meet some of the criteria set out in the Have I got the symptoms? box (see above). As tiredness can have other causes, your doctor may take a blood sample to exclude autoimmune

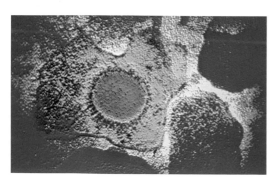

Cytomegalovirus
Although the cause of CFS is not yet known, one theory centres on a viral infection, such as might be caused by cytomegalovirus (left). It is also believed that a head trauma can trigger CFS.

diseases (see pp259, 266–71), iron-deficiency anaemia (see pp248–9), underactive thyroid gland (see p327), depression (see pp210–11), or viral infection.

Doctors generally find it hard to diagnose CFS because its signs and symptoms are similar to many other diseases. There are, however, a small number of self-designated CFS specialists in the UK, mostly in major teaching hospitals. If you want a referral to see one of these specialists, discuss this option with your doctor.

MY TREATMENT OPTIONS

Although a cycle of relapses and remissions – triggered by overexertion, infectious illnesses, or seasonal changes – is a common pattern of CFS, many people gradually improve over time after trying these treatments:

Medications to ease the various symptoms can be prescribed by your doctor. Although there are no specific medications to treat CFS, painkillers, such as paracetamol, or NSAIDs, such as ibuprofen or diclofenac, can relieve existing muscle or joint pain, or headaches. Some antidepressants can help regulate your sleep, promote appetite, and relieve pain; types commonly used are tricyclics (see p227) and selective serotonin reuptake inhibitors (SSRIs) (see p227). Blood pressure drugs, such as fludrocortisone, may help to stop you feeling dizzy and faint. Sleep-inducing drugs, such as amitriptyline, can help you get a

---

THE CFS SPECTRUM

Chronic fatigue syndrome is often organized into four categories: mild, moderate, severe, or very severe.

Mild CFS You can look after yourself, but you may need to take days off work to rest.

Moderate CFS You may only be able to do a little, though symptoms vary. You may have disturbed sleep patterns and doze in the afternoons.

Severe CFS You can carry out daily tasks like brushing your teeth, but may need a wheelchair for bigger chores. Concentrating may be hard.

Very severe CFS You can't carry out any daily tasks, and spend most of your day in bed. You may be highly sensitive to noise and bright lights.

---

good night's sleep. Antihistamines and decongestants, such as pseudoephedrine and fexofenadine, may help alleviate any allergy-related symptoms.

Pace yourself to strike the right balance: you need adequate rest, but too much rest can make you weaker. Your doctor may also encourage you to slow down and eliminate any unnecessary or excessively stressful activities. Ideally, you should follow a gentle, graduated exercise programme, such as walking, under your doctor's supervision, to increase your activity by no more than one minute a day.

Cognitive behavioural therapy helps to identify negative beliefs and behaviours that may be making your condition worse, or delaying recovery, and replaces them with healthy, positive ones.

Nutritional counselling and lifestyle counselling can be very beneficial. Many patients benefit from dietary supplements, such as daily multivitamins, omega-3 DHA, and probiotics for those with gastrointestinal symptoms.

HOW CAN I HELP MYSELF?

You can make simple changes to your lifestyle to help your recovery. **Complementary therapies,** such as acupuncture, massage, t'ai chi, and biofeedback therapies (see p225), may prove helpful.

Develop good sleep habits, such as going to bed and getting up at the same time, and skipping daytime naps (see pp60–1).

Avoid caffeine so it can't affect your sleep patterns.

Don't smoke For advice, see p64.

Learn to relax by avoiding stressful situations and knowing when to take "time out". If you feel like doing certain activities, that's fine, just make sure that you relax regularly. Even people who feel they've recovered from CFS find they need more rest than their peers.

Localized problems

All of us have had niggling aches and pains in joints at one time or another. It's when a niggle in a knee or a wrist, for example, turns into a persistent ache or sudden intense pain that you know there's a problem. With the appropriate treatment and then some preventive measures, you'll soon be as good as new.

Repetitive strain injury

WHAT IS IT?

Better known as RSI, repetitive strain injury is not one condition but a term used for various disorders that develop as a result of repetitive movements, awkward postures, and sustained force. RSI is common in adults of working age and is more common in women. It mainly affects soft tissues in the upper parts of the body: the shoulder, forearm, elbow, wrist, hands, and neck.

Initially, symptoms may be felt when carrying out a particular activity and subside when you finish that work and rest. If such symptoms remain untreated, however, they can worsen so that you feel pain all the time.

Certain occupations put you at risk of developing RSI, including:
- Working in any manufacturing industry
- Typists and those working in computer data entry
- Dressmakers and tailors
- Musicians
- Hairdressers
- Professional sports people.

Even activities carried out as part of your favourite hobby or sport can put you at risk of strain, so you must always take care.

WHAT NEXT?

Your doctor will be able to make a diagnosis based on your medical history and a thorough physical examination. If your pain is in your wrist and forearm, he or she may tap gently in different areas to elicit a response that will indicate one condition over another.

MY TREATMENT OPTIONS

Some people get better without any treatment but many need a

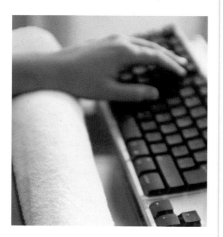

Wrist support
An occupational therapist may advise that a wrist support could alleviate your RSI when you are working at the computer.

HAVE I GOT THE SYMPTOMS?

Symptoms of RSI can vary with the person and most commonly affect the neck, shoulder, elbow, hand and wrist, or carpal tunnel (see p283). They include:
- Pain
- Stiffness
- Tenderness
- Swelling or tingling (pins and needles)
- Loss of strength or sensation.

See your doctor if you experience any of the symptoms listed above.

combination of the following. When discussing potential treatments with your doctor, ask about any side effects.

Rest If you can, you should stop doing the activity that has caused your RSI. If this is impossible since it involves your job, then talk to them so that they can make adjustments to your work.

Firm splints can be used to support the injured soft tissues during the healing process. Your doctor may be able to prescribe you one but you can buy them too.

A course of non-steroidal anti-inflammatory drugs, such as ibuprofen and diclofenac, may be prescribed by your doctor for effective pain relief and to address any inflammation or swelling.

Physiotherapy can help to improve strength in targeted muscles to speed recovery and prevent future episodes.

Occupational therapy can address any ergonomic issues in your work place.

HOW CAN I HELP MYSELF?

To relieve your symptoms and to prevent any more episodes in the future, you make need to take a long, hard look at your lifestyle. If you're a sporty person, you need to be conscientious about warming up and cooling down before and after your chosen activity.

A lot of cases of RSI result from our highly computerized world. But a few simple steps can limit the impact of keyboarding.

Adjust your screen, seat, keyboard, and mouse if you sit at a desk all or most of the day so that they cause the least amount of strain on your back, wrists, hands, and fingers.

Try to be aware of your posture (see p67). Sit tall and ensure your eyes are level with the top of your screen.

Take frequent breaks.

Stop and stretch out your neck, hands, and fingers regularly.

Golfer's elbow and tennis elbow

WHAT ARE THEY?

Such soft-tissue problems occur when the tendons attaching the muscles that straighten or bend your fingers and wrist to the upper arm bone (humerus) become inflamed where they attach to the elbow. It's normally a short-lived complaint, although some people suffer repeat episodes. Any strain on the tendons can cause golfer's elbow and tennis elbow, as can any repetitive activity that involves gripping and twisting, such as using a screwdriver. Pain normally lasts for six to 12 weeks, or longer.

WHAT NEXT?

Consult your doctor or physiotherapist on the best course of action for you.

MY TREATMENT OPTIONS

Rest your arm. Ask your doctor about potential side effects of drugs prescribed.

A course of non-steroidal anti-inflammatory drugs (NSAIDs), such as ibuprofen, can help to relieve pain as well as reduce inflammation.

Cold treatment Ice packs can help counter any pain.

Steroid injections can reduce inflammation around the tendon if the pain doesn't settle with a course of NSAIDs.

HOW CAN I HELP MYSELF?

Physiotherapy can be helpful in restoring the strength and the tone of the muscles.

Rest from the sport or repetitive action that caused the injury in the first place.

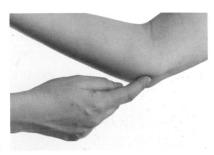

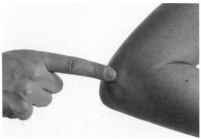

Location of the pain
In golfer's elbow (top), it's the tendons on the inner side of your elbow that are painful. In tennis elbow (below), it's those on the outer side of your elbow.

> **HAVE I GOT THE SYMPTOMS?**
>
> Symptoms are worse when you use or twist your elbow.
> - Pain on the inside, just by the bony lump of your elbow
> - Pain on the outside, just by the bony lump of your elbow
> - Pain that radiates down the arm towards the wrist.
>
> **See your doctor** if you have any of these symptoms.

Painful shoulder

WHAT IS IT?
Your painful shoulder may be caused by a process within the shoulder joint itself; the pain can be over the front of your shoulder, in your upper arm, or at the tip of your shoulder. Often shoulder pain produces secondary pain in the neck muscles. Conversely, neck problems (see pp272) can also result in shoulder pain. Osteoarthritis (see pp263–5) and rheumatoid arthritis (see pp266–8) can also cause shoulder pain, as can calcific tendinitis (calcium deposits in the rotator cuff tendons) or tears in the rotator cuff tendons, and subacromial bursitis (inflammation of the subacromial bursa).

WHAT NEXT?
Your doctor will be able to make a diagnosis based on your medical history and a physical examination. A diagnosis can be made in most cases without an X-ray. In complicated cases an MRI scan may be needed.

MY TREATMENT OPTIONS
Ask your doctor whether your treatment has any potential side effects.

Non-steroidal anti-inflammatory drugs can relieve pain and reduce inflammation.

Physiotherapy can help alleviate any stiffness and improve your range of movement.

Steroid injections can reduce inflammation within the joint itself if the pain is severe.

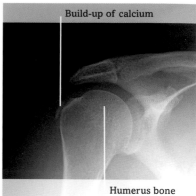

Build-up of calcium

Humerus bone

Calcific tendinitis
This X-ray of a shoulder joint shows a crescent-shaped build-up of calcium in the rotator cuff, causing pain and stiffness.

HOW CAN I HELP MYSELF?
Follow the treatment plan recommended by your doctor.

HAVE I GOT THE SYMPTOMS?

- Pain and tenderness in your shoulder, especially when reaching, lifting, pulling, or sleeping on the painful side
- Shoulder weakness, especially when trying to lift your arm straight out to the side
- Any loss in the range of motion of your shoulder.

See your doctor if you have any of these symptoms.

WHAT'S GOING ON INSIDE YOUR SHOULDER JOINT?

Inflammation of the tendons within the shoulder joint, known as the rotator cuff, often causes shoulder joint pain. The rotator cuff actually comprises four tendons: supraspinatus, subscapularis, teres minor, and infraspinatus. If you injure one of these, your doctor will probably refer you for some physiotherapy.

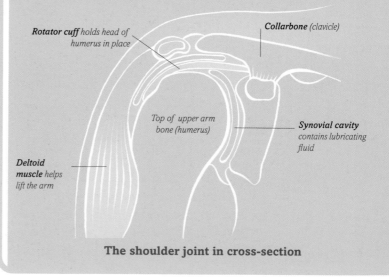

Rotator cuff holds head of humerus in place

Collarbone (clavicle)

Top of upper arm bone (humerus)

Synovial cavity contains lubricating fluid

Deltoid muscle helps lift the arm

The shoulder joint in cross-section

Carpal tunnel syndrome

WHAT IS IT?

Women are far more likely to have carpal tunnel syndrome than men and it's a condition that can strike at any age. It is due to entrapment of the median nerve at the carpal tunnel, which lies in the wrist. Tendons in the forearm that help move the fingers and the median nerve all pass through it. The main nerve to your hand is called the median nerve. Before it branches into smaller nerve bundles in the palm of your hand, it passes through the carpal tunnel at your wrist. Space in the carpal tunnel is tight. So if a tendon is injured and inflamed, there is no room for it to expand. Swelling puts pressure on the median nerve, resulting in pain, tingling or pins-and-needles sensation.

In addition to tendon injuries from repetitive movements, for example, the nerve may be squeezed if there is arthritis of the wrist joint or a wrist fracture. Furthermore, any fluid retention, for example during pregnancy (see p128), or accumulation of fat, for instance in weight gain or in an underactive thyroid gland (see p327), may also result in carpal tunnel syndrome.

WHAT NEXT?

After carrying out a thorough examination, your doctor may refer you for a nerve conduction test. Such tests will indicate to the doctor if the problem is related to the median nerve or the nerves originating from the neck.

MY TREATMENT OPTIONS

Your doctor will advise you as to which of the following treatment options is best suited to your case. He or she should also let you know about the potential side effects of any medication you're prescribed.
Rest your wrist when you can.
Non-steroidal anti-inflammatory drugs can relieve pain and reduce inflammation.
Support your wrist by wearing a splint (your doctor will prescribe one) in the short term.
Steroid injections can cure it.
Surgery may be necessary in severe cases and can be done as a day case in hospital.

HOW CAN I HELP MYSELF?

Follow the treatment plan recommended by your doctor.

HAVE I GOT THE SYMPTOMS?

Symptoms are usually worse in the thumb, index, and middle fingers (and in one half of your ring finger). They are also often worse at night-time.
- Pain or aching in your hand; sometimes this pain radiates into your forearm
- Numbness
- Tingling and weakness in one or both hands.

See your doctor if you have any of these symptoms.

WHERE IS THE CARPAL TUNNEL?

The carpal tunnel is formed by the bones of the wrist (the carpal bones) and a strong ligament that lies over them. The median nerve, which both controls movement in the thumb, index, middle, and half of the ring fingers and relays sensations from them, runs through this tunnel, alongside the tendons. Everything fits just so within the carpal tunnel, so any injury that results in inflammation will impact on the function of the median nerve, and cause pain.

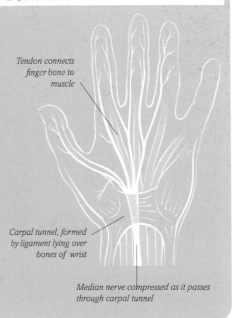

Tendon connects finger bone to muscle

Carpal tunnel, formed by ligament lying over bones of wrist

Median nerve compressed as it passes through carpal tunnel

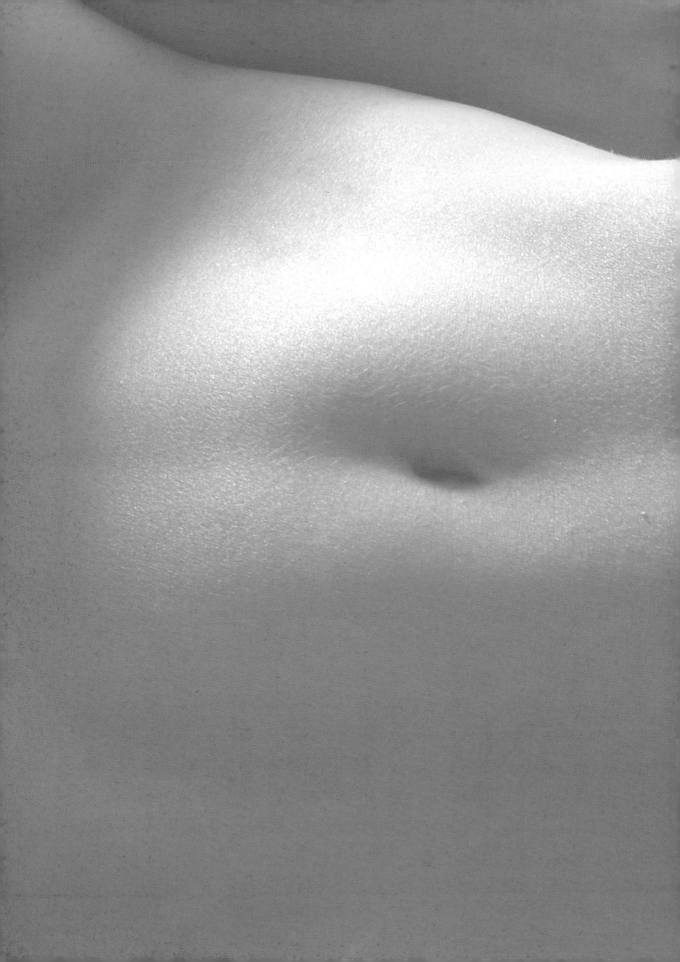

Digestive system

Dr Anne Ballinger MD FRCP

Your digestive system

The gastrointestinal system is a remarkable piece of machinery, most of which is contained within the chest and abdomen. One of the most important of the body systems, its main function is to process the food we eat so that the body can absorb and use nutrients in the diet for energy and as building blocks for the growth and repair of muscles, bones, and other tissues in the body. The various parts of digestive system are subject to a variety of disorders, the most common of which are minor and easily treated by simple measures.

THE DIGESTIVE SYSTEM

The entrance to the digestive tract is the mouth (below), which is connected to the oesophagus. The organs of the digestive system are shown in cross section (right). The tract itself is a long tube to which a number of organs are connected. These send digestive juices into the tract to help break down the food you eat. One of those organs is the liver, which produces bile, a digestive juice that helps the breakdown of fats. Bile drains from the liver into the gallbladder, where it is stored, to be released next time you eat.

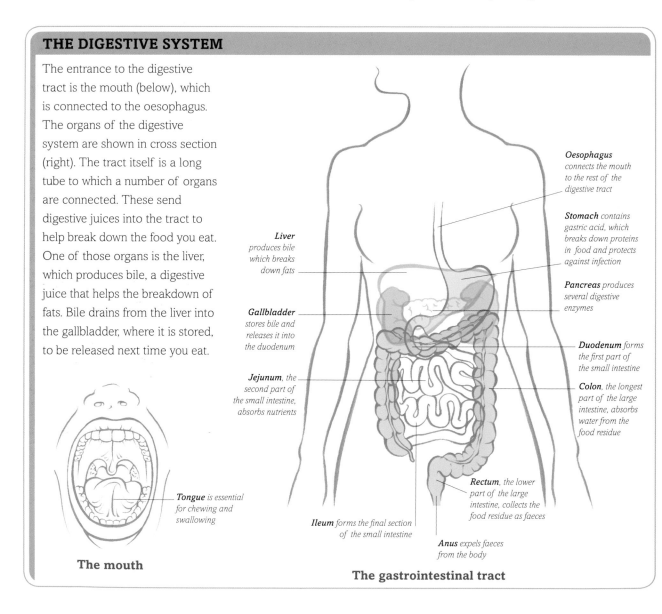

Liver *produces bile which breaks down fats*

Gallbladder *stores bile and releases it into the duodenum*

Jejunum, *the second part of the small intestine, absorbs nutrients*

Tongue *is essential for chewing and swallowing*

The mouth

Oesophagus *connects the mouth to the rest of the digestive tract*

Stomach *contains gastric acid, which breaks down proteins in food and protects against infection*

Pancreas *produces several digestive enzymes*

Duodenum *forms the first part of the small intestine*

Colon, *the longest part of the large intestine, absorbs water from the food residue*

Rectum, *the lower part of the large intestine, collects the food residue as faeces*

Ileum *forms the final section of the small intestine*

Anus *expels faeces from the body*

The gastrointestinal tract

The gastrointestinal system is essential for life, but we are able to survive and function quite well even if large parts are damaged or removed. Gastrointestinal diseases are common and, not surprisingly, diet plays a part in the cause or treatment of many of them. For instance, heavy alcohol drinking not only damages the liver but also causes pancreatic disease and is a risk factor in the development of mouth and oesophageal cancers and polyps in the colon, while a low-fibre, high-fat diet increases the risk of colon cancer. Although the structure of the digestive system is the same in both sexes, the effects of female sex hormones, particularly in pregnancy, on muscle contraction means that women may be more likely to suffer from certain digestive-tract problems, such as constipation. Moreover, women are more likely to suffer liver damage as a result of drinking alcohol.

THE PROCESS OF DIGESTION

During the digestive process, the proteins, fats, and carbohydrates in the food you eat are broken down into amino acids (from dietary proteins), fatty acids (from dietary fats), and simple sugars (from dietary carbohydrates). These small molecules are all produced by a combination of mechanical churning of your food and the work of the digestive juices on it. These juices contain acid and digestive enzymes produced by the pancreas gland and bile from the gallbladder.

The small molecules that are the result of these actions are then absorbed via the wall of your small intestine and are carried in the lymph ducts and in the bloodstream, via the liver, to all parts of your body ready for use as needed.

The starting point of the whole digestive process is your mouth, which is the entry point for the food that you eat and the liquids that you drink. The first part of the process takes place here – the initial breakdown of food by chewing and by the action of the digestive enzymes found in your saliva.

From your mouth, the chewed-up food moves into the oesophagus. This is a long muscular tube that pushes food and liquid on and into your stomach. The stomach behaves like a mixer; it churns the food

HOW WE ABSORB NUTRIENTS

Semi-liquid food passes from the stomach into the small intestine. Here the nutrients are absorbed through the inner lining of the small intestine. In order for them to be absorbed as quickly as possible, this inner lining is covered in millions of tiny finger-like projections called villi, which in turn are covered in brush like structures called microvilli. These give the small intestine a huge surface area – the equivalent in size to a tennis court – through which the nutrients can rapidly be absorbed.

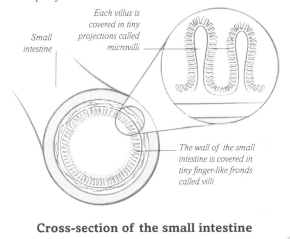

Small intestine

Each villus is covered in tiny projections called microvilli

The wall of the small intestine is covered in tiny finger-like fronds called villi

Cross-section of the small intestine

around and mixes it with acid that it secretes. This acid helps continue the process of digestion.

The semi-liquid food then leaves the stomach and enters the small intestine. This can be anything from four to seven metres (13–23ft) long and is made up of three parts – the duodenum, jejunum, and ileum. It is where the food is broken down even further and the small molecules are produced, ready to be absorbed.

The mainly digested food residue then passes into your large intestine (colon). Here, excess fluids are absorbed and any food residues that cannot be absorbed (mostly indigestible cellulose or fibre) are formed into faeces (stools) and eliminated via the rectum and then the anus. There is enormous variation between different people in gut transit time (that is, the length of time food takes to travel from the mouth to the anus), but the usual range is from one to three days.

Mouth and tongue disorders

Disorders of the mouth and tongue are common, and rarely serious. However, because you use your mouth for speaking, eating, swallowing, and for making facial expressions, these disorders can cause a great deal of discomfort and, in some cases, embarrassment.

Tongue conditions

Problems with your tongue may involve changes in its appearance and/or discomfort.

WHAT IS IT?

Your tongue may be affected by nutritional deficiencies, mouth ulcers, oral thrush (see below), and, rarely, cancer (see opposite). Other conditions that may cause your tongue to appear abnormal include:

Glossitis This is inflammation of the tongue due to injury (for example, scalding) or infection.
Geographical tongue This is a harmless condition in which irregular red, smooth patches appear on the tongue It is not known what causes it.
Black hairy tongue In this condition dark, "hairy" areas appear on the tongue caused by bacterial growth on its surface.

WHAT NEXT?

Your doctor is likely to be able to diagnose your tongue problem by a simple visual examination.

MY TREATMENT OPTIONS

Treatment depends on the cause. Minor tongue conditions, such as glossitis and geographical tongue, usually get better without specific treatment. If your doctor suspects an infection, you may need to take antibiotics or antifungal medication, perhaps in the form of lozenges.

> ### HAVE I GOT THE SYMPTOMS?
>
> Tongue disorders can appear as any of the following:
> - Painless bald, smooth areas on the tongue
> - Brown or black discoloration on the tongue
> - White patches on the tongue
> - Soreness.
>
> **See your doctor** if you notice any of these symptoms.

Ask your doctor about any possible side effects of the medication.

HOW CAN I HELP MYSELF?

To keep your tongue healthy, pay attention to oral hygiene (see p68).

Oral thrush

Thrush infection of the mouth usually occurs only if you're run down and the natural defences of your body are disrupted.

WHAT IS IT?

This condition, in which you get white patches in your mouth, is more common if you suffer from

> ### HAVE I GOT THE SYMPTOMS?
>
> Oral thrush causes the following symptoms:
> - White patches inside the mouth or on the tongue under which the area is red and sore.
>
> **See your doctor** if you notice these symptoms.

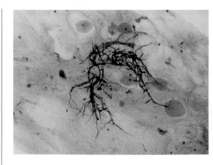

Candida albicans
Light micrograph of human saliva, showing the fungus that causes thrush.

diabetes, if you are malnourished, or if you have an immune deficiency, which can occur as you age, or if you have AIDS (pp120–1). You may also get it if you have poorly fitting dentures, have been taking antibiotics, or have been treated with drugs such as chemotherapy.

WHAT NEXT?

Your doctor will confirm the diagnosis by carrying out a simple visual examination. If the cause of the thrush is not obvious, he or she will probably advise tests to help identify the underlying cause of your infection.

MY TREATMENT OPTIONS

You will be prescribed an antifungal lozenges or paste.

HOW CAN I HELP MYSELF?

Use a soft toothbrush (change often), and avoid acidic or spicy food that may cause discomfort.

Leukoplakia and oral cancer

Both these conditions are characterized by abnormal-looking but painless areas in the mouth or on the tongue.

WHAT IS IT?

Leukoplakia is a condition in which painless white patches occur, often as a result of repeated damage to the mouth of tongue – for example, from a jagged tooth –

AM I AT RISK?

Both leukoplakia and oral cancer are more common in smokers and those who chew tobacco, and are more likely over the age of 40. Those who have an excessive intake of alcohol are also more susceptible.

but for which often no cause can be easily found.

Leukoplakia patches may clear up after the source of the irritation has been taken away. Very rarely, the patches may develop into oral cancer so you should be sure to see your dentist for a follow up. Oral cancer, a rare condition that often first appears as a slowly growing sore or ulcer in the mouth that doesn't heal, may also develop without being preceded by leukoplakia.

WHAT NEXT?

Your doctor may arrange for a biopsy of the tissue to be taken from the affected area. The laboratory results from the sample will help your doctor to make a firm diagnosis of the cause.

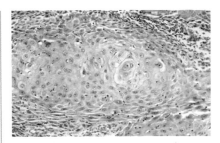

Oral cancer
Light micrograph of cancer cells (areas in pink) in the mouth.

MY TREATMENT OPTIONS

Leukoplakia patches often require no treatment, but your doctor may suggest that you have them regularly monitored. In some cases of leukoplakia, and often in the case of small oral cancers, the abnormal tissue may be removed surgically or by laser treatment. Follow-up treatment with X-rays may be advised in the case of oral cancer. Ask your doctor about any side effects of the treatment.

HOW CAN I HELP MYSELF?

To reduce your risk of developing these conditions, don't smoke and keep your alcohol intake to a minimum. In addition, going for regular check-ups at the dentist will help you to avoid leukoplakia caused by dental problems.

HAVE I GOT THE SYMPTOMS?

The symptoms of these conditions are usually painless and may include the following.
- White patches in the mouth or on the tongue, which may have a hard surface, and that cannot easily be scraped away
- An isolated nodule inside the mouth that is perhaps slowly growing
- A persistent mouth ulcer that fails to heal.

See your doctor if you notice any of these symptoms.

Gastro-oesophageal reflux disease

Heartburn caused by acid reflux is very common, especially when we have over-indulged in food or have eaten too close to bedtime. Although not usually life-threatening, frequent episodes of acid reflux can damage your oesophagus.

WHAT IS IT?

Food travels from your mouth through the oesophagus into your stomach via a valve-like muscle (the lower oesophageal sphincter). The food starts to be broken down by the acid in your stomach, while the sphincter helps to prevent food and acid flowing back into the oesophagus. Unfortunately, the sphincter sometimes allows acid to flow back into the oesophagus (acid reflux). Although your stomach is designed to withstand the acid, the lining of the oesophagus is very sensitive to it and when you have acid reflux, you'll be aware of heartburn – a burning sensation in your chest.

Heartburn affects many pregnant women. The increased pressure in the abdomen from the growing baby has a tendency to force the acidic stomach contents back into the oesophagus.

Frequent and recurrent attacks of acid reflux (gastro-oesophageal reflux disease, or GORD) may damage the oesophagus, causing inflammation and ulceration.

Although it causes discomfort, GORD rarely leads to any life-threatening complications. However, in Barrett's oesophagus, the cells of the lower part of the oesophagus change in response to repeated exposure to stomach acid. These cells are associated with an increased cancer risk and if your doctor suspects this, he or she will monitor you by regular endoscopy. An endoscope is a small flexible tube that contains a tiny light and video camera that is used to examine various parts of the body. Here, it is passed down into oesophagus so that the doctor can inspect the lining of the oesophagus. Persistent and untreated reflux can lead to scarring and narrowing of the oesophagus, in which case the oesophagus may need to be stretched using an endoscope.

AM I AT RISK?

Risk factors for the development of acid reflux include:

- Being pregnant
- Being overweight
- Eating a high-fat diet
- Consuming excessive amounts of alcohol or coffee
- Being a smoker
- Having a hiatus hernia.

HAVE I GOT THE SYMPTOMS?

Symptoms vary between people and between episodes. They are most noticeable after eating and may include:

- Heartburn (often worse on lying down)
- Acid taste in mouth
- Persistent sore throat
- Difficulty or pain during swallowing
- Persistent cough.

See your doctor if your symptoms are persistent, do not respond to self-help remedies (see opposite), or if heartburn often interrupts your sleep.

WHAT NEXT?

You rarely need tests and examinations to diagnose GORD and your doctor will be able to diagnose it from your description of your symptoms. If lifestyle changes and standard drug treatments do not help, or if you have additional symptoms, such as

HIATUS HERNIA

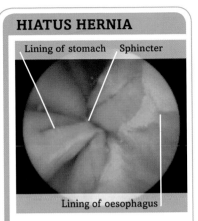

Lining of stomach   Sphincter

Lining of oesophagus

Junction of the oesophagus and stomach

A hiatus hernia occurs when the upper part of the stomach (dark pink) pushes upwards through the lower oesophageal sphincter into the oesophagus (light pink). Having a simple hiatus hernia makes it more likely that you will have GORD, but it does not cause the symptoms. If you need surgery for GORD (see right), your hernia will be repaired at the same time.

weight loss or vomiting blood, your doctor will probably arrange for you to have a gastroscopy, in which an endoscope is passed down your oesophagus and into your stomach so that your doctor can inspect the stomach lining.

MY TREATMENT OPTIONS

There are three types of medication that are commonly prescribed in the treatment of GORD. Ask your doctor about any possible side effects when discussing your treatment options.

Antacids These medications neutralize the acid from the stomach and prevent the oesophagus from being damaged.
Histamine receptor blockers (H2 blockers) and proton pump inhibitors (PPIs) These reduce acid output. PPIs are the most effective.
Pro-motility drugs These help the oesophagus to empty itself of any stomach contents.

Medication for GORD rarely has side effects. Although not licensed to be taken during pregnancy, most of these drugs have not caused any adverse effects to a developing baby. Nevertheless, always discuss any drug treatment with your doctor if you are pregnant.
Surgery Occasionally, surgery is necessary to tighten the lower oesophageal sphincter.

HOW CAN I HELP MYSELF?

Lifestyle changes are the first course of action to improve your symptoms, particularly if they are mild and infrequent:

Watch your weight There is a close relationship between body weight and reflux symptoms and losing weight by diet and exercise (see pp52–7) may help. You should try to maintain your weight within a healthy range (see your body mass index, pp58–9).
Give up smoking (see p64) as smoking relaxes the sphincter between the stomach and the oesophagus and encourages reflux.
Don't eat late at night Allow at least four hours between eating and going to bed, to allow your stomach to empty. It may help to have a light meal at night. Coffee, chocolate, and fatty foods may trigger symptoms, and should therefore be avoided by anyone with a tendency to acid reflux. Avoid tight-fitting clothing that increases pressure in the abdomen and promotes reflux.
Prop up your bed to raise the level of your head to help prevent night-time acid reflux through the simple action of gravity.

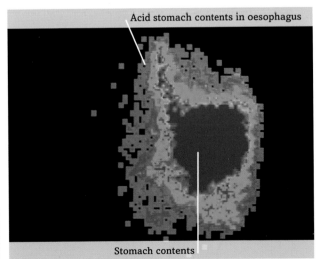

Acid stomach contents in oesophagus

Stomach contents

Acid reflux on camera
Here, acid stomach contents can clearly be seen in the oesophagus as a result of a hiatus hernia. The stomach contents are the red mass at the centre; the area of reflux is the red "horn" in the upper left of the picture.

Indigestion and ulcers

Most of us have indigestion at some time and we can usually treat it with over-the-counter remedies. Having indigestion doesn't usually mean there is anything seriously wrong with you, but if you suffer from it frequently, you should ask your doctor to investigate it further.

WHAT IS IT?

Some people have indigestion because their stomach does not empty itself of its contents as fast as it should. Specific problems that may cause the symptoms of indigestion are gastro-oesophageal reflux disease (see pp290–1), ulcers in the upper intestine (peptic ulcers), or – in rare cases – cancer of the stomach or oesophagus.

WHAT NEXT?

Your doctor may treat your indigestion without any further investigations. However, if you are over the age of 55 or have any of the symptoms in the right-hand column of the box below, you will usually need an endoscopy of your upper intestinal tract (see p290) before treatment to make sure nothing serious is causing your symptoms. Otherwise, your doctor may do a simple test to look for the bacteria *Helicobacter pylori*, which is the main cause of peptic ulcers. He or she may suggest lifestyle modification (see Am I at risk? right) and may prescribe acid-suppressing medication.

MY TREATMENT OPTIONS

Treatment depends on what seems to be the cause of the problem. Ask your doctor about any possible side effects.

A combination of antibiotics and acid blockers These are recommended if your bacteria test is positive; they kill the bacteria and heal any ulcers.

AM I AT RISK?

There are several lifestyle habits that often contribute to, or cause, indigestion. These include:
- Eating heavy meals, especially late in the evening (leave a four-hour interval between eating and going to bed)
- Irregular meal times
- Smoking
- Drinking excess alcohol
- Stress and anxiety
- Regular use of a painkiller such as aspirin or a non-steroidal anti-inflammatory drug (often used to treat arthritis).

Acid blockers These treat peptic ulcers caused by aspirin and non-steroidal anti-inflammatory drugs (NSAIDs). They also work when sensitivity to acid is the cause.

Promotility agents These help your stomach to empty faster.

Lifestyle modification See Am I at risk? above.

HOW CAN I HELP MYSELF?

Check the risk factors identified in the panel (above) and if any of these apply to you, try to eliminate them from your lifestyle.

HAVE I GOT THE SYMPTOMS?

If you have indigestion, you may feel the following:
- Pain or discomfort in the upper abdomen or chest often associated with eating
- Nausea
- Bloating
- Heartburn (see pp290–1)
- Belching.

See your doctor if you have indigestion regularly and especially if attacks of indigestion are a recent development for you, are over 55 years of age, or have any of the following symptoms:
- Unintended weight loss
- Vomiting,
- Difficulty in swallowing.

Oesophageal disorders

If you have trouble swallowing, together with chest pain, it could be that the problem lies in the muscles of your oesophagus. Although these often distressing disorders are not particularly common, they are more likely to occur in young and middle-aged women.

WHAT ARE THEY?

There are three main types of disorders that can prevent your food from passing normally from the oesophagus into your stomach. They give you discomfort when you swallow.

Achalasia See the panel (right).

Diffuse oesophageal spasm In this disorder, the muscles of the oesophagus contract irregularly.

Hypertensive ("nutcracker") oesophagus In this disorder, the contractions of the oesophageal muscles are too strong.

HAVE I GOT THE SYMPTOMS?

If you are suffering from an oesophageal disorder, you may notice the following symptoms:

- Difficulty swallowing, as though food, and sometimes liquid, is stuck behind your breastbone within seconds of swallowing
- Chest pain (often burning) that feels as though it is coming from the heart area – more common in younger people.

See your doctor if you experience either symptom.

WHAT HAPPENS IN ACHALASIA

If you have achalasia, the muscles of your lower oesophagus do not contract properly and the valve between the oesophagus and the stomach (the lower oesophageal sphincter) does not relax. This prevents food from passing through into your stomach.

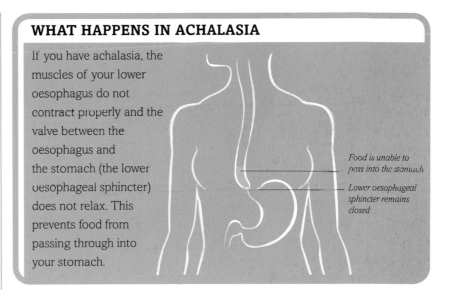

Food is unable to pass into the stomach

Lower oesophageal sphincter remains closed

WHAT NEXT?

Most muscular disorders are diagnosed by barium swallow (you swallow a white chalky mixture, after which X-rays are taken) or by oesophageal manometry (measuring the pressure in the oesophagus using a probe passed through the nose and guided into the oesophagus). Your doctor may recommend an endoscopy of your upper intestinal tract (see p290). This test will also reveal if there is any narrowing of the oesophagus or evidence of GORD (see pp290–1). It will also help the doctor to exclude oesophageal cancer as a cause of your symptoms.

MY TREATMENT OPTIONS

Treatment depends on the diagnosis.

Botulinum toxin injection to relax the muscle fibres.

Balloon dilation uses a small balloon at the end of an endoscope to stretch the muscle.

Myotomy disrupts the muscle fibres by surgically cutting the muscle.

Medication to relax the muscles.

HOW CAN I HELP MYSELF?

The following can often help:

Eat slowly and chew well.

Drink plenty when you eat.

Have a fizzy drink This can help shift food that gets stuck.

Gallstones

It a common saying that the typical gallstone patient is female, fertile, fat and forty and there is some truth in this. It is a fact that women are twice as likely as men to develop gallstones, and the condition is more common in those who are overweight and middle-aged.

WHAT IS IT?

Gallstones are small, solid lumps – the commonest type are made from cholesterol – that form in the bile (see pp286–7). They begin as tiny crystals, but then grow and may get as large as a few centimetres across. You may get one or several gallstones. Women are more often affected by this problem than men because the female hormones progesterone and oestrogen tend to relax the gallbladder. This slows the flow of bile, and makes it more likely that stones will form.

If a stone blocks one of the ducts that carry bile from your

HAVE I GOT THE SYMPTOMS?

Where gallstones cause symptoms, these may include:
- Fatty food intolerance
- Bouts of upper abdominal pain, often on the right
- Nausea and vomiting
- Yellowing of the skin or whites of the eyes
- Pale stools.

See your doctor if you have any of these symptoms.

AM I AT RISK?

The following are risk factors for developing gallstones:
- Being overweight and eating a high-fat diet: these two factors result in high levels of cholesterol being secreted in the bile, which increases the tendency of stones to form
- Being on a very low-calorie diet: surprisingly, gallstones often develop during the first few weeks of a very low-calorie diet, perhaps because the gallbladder cannot contract and empty normally
- Taking certain prescribed medications, including oral contraceptives, affect gallbladder functioning and may increase the risk of gallstones
- Having a family tendency to develop gallstones
- Being a woman: you're more likely to develop gallstones than a man with a similar lifestyle and genetic inheritance.

gallbladder to the intestines you may get symptoms (see box, left), including mild to severe abdominal pain, nausea, and vomiting. These symptoms are known as biliary colic. You will feel the pain in your upper abdomen, more often on the right, and it may extend to your back. It may last from between several minutes to several hours, and it can occur repeatedly. You may not feel any pain between "attacks". Some sufferers from this condition also develop jaundice (yellowing of the skin and whites of the eyes) and you may also notice that you pass pale faeces. This is

due to the lack of bile pigment in the gut. Gallstones can also cause inflammation of the gallbladder (cholecystitis) or pancreas (acute pancreatitis). If you have either of these complications, you are likely to have pain in your upper abdomen and you may also have a raised temperature. Each of these conditions needs urgent hospital assessment and treatment.

WHAT NEXT?

Gallstones don't always cause symptoms and they're often found while something else is being investigated. If you've been

WHERE GALLSTONES LODGE

Gallstones form within the gallbladder and may remain there. However, they may also pass into the bile duct, where they cause problems if they become stuck. Small stones may simply pass into the intestine.

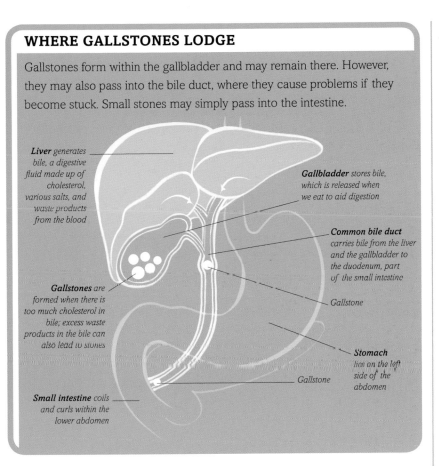

Liver *generates bile, a digestive fluid made up of cholesterol, various salts, and waste products from the blood*

Gallbladder *stores bile, which is released when we eat to aid digestion*

Common bile duct *carries bile from the liver and the gallbladder to the duodenum, part of the small intestine*

Gallstone

Gallstones *are formed when there is too much cholesterol in bile; excess waste products in the bile can also lead to stones*

Stomach *lies on the left side of the abdomen*

Gallstone

Small intestine *coils and curls within the lower abdomen*

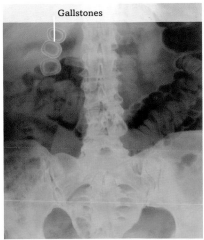

Gallstones

Gallstones

This coloured X-ray of the abdomen shows three large gallstones (coloured blue) in the gallbladder.

experiencing symptoms that may be caused by gallstones, your doctor will want to be sure of the cause before recommending treatment. An ultrasound examination of your gallbladder is usually the first test. You may also need blood tests and further special X-rays or an endoscopy (see p290), to see if gallstones have become lodged in your bile ducts.

MY TREATMENT OPTIONS

If you don't have any symptoms, you usually don't need treatment, otherwise your doctor will find the best treatment for you. Ask your doctor about any side effects when discussing treatment options.

More frequent meals If you don't have symptoms and the stones are small, your doctor may recommend you simply eat more frequent small meals. This will encourage the gallbladder to expel any stones that may have formed.

Surgery If you have symptoms from gallstones, your doctor will usually recommend removal of the gallbladder, which can usually be done by laparoscopic ("keyhole") surgery, leaving only three tiny scars. Most people who have had this treatment can leave hospital the next

day and return to normal activities within two weeks. Removing the gallbladder doesn't create problems, as the bile simply drains directly into the digestive tract.

Dissolving the gallstones Medication or mechanical methods to dissolve or fragment the gallstones while leaving the gallbladder in place are also occasionally used for the treatment of gallstones, but there is a risk that gallstones will form again.

HOW CAN I HELP MYSELF?

Most risk factors for gallstones are unavoidable, but you can reduce the chances of developing the problem by keeping to a healthy weight (see pp58–9) and sticking to a low-cholesterol diet (see p173).

"Because of our female hormones, women are twice as likely as men to develop gallstones."

Liver disorders

Your liver is your largest internal organ, and plays an essential role in regulating many aspects of your digestion and the way your body uses the nutrients in your food. Liver problems – many of them caused by drinking too much alcohol – are becoming more common, and many women are affected.

Hepatitis

The term hepatitis covers a group of conditions characterized by inflammation of the liver, which damages the liver cells.

WHAT IS IT?

Often caused by infection, hepatitis can be acute (starts suddenly and lasts less than six months) or chronic (long-lasting). Common causes are:

- The hepatitis viruses A, B, C, D, and E
- Other viral diseases such as glandular fever
- Overdose of drugs, such as paracetamol
- Drinking excessive amounts of alcohol (see opposite)
- Cirrhosis (see p298).

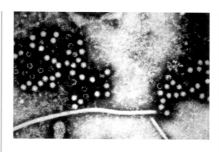

Hepatitis E virus
This virus, shown here as round particles (in purple), like Hepatitis A, is often spread via contaminated water.

The hepatitis A and E viruses only cause acute hepatitis, while the other hepatitis viruses can cause both acute and chronic hepatitis. If you have an attack of acute hepatitis, your liver will heal completely, whereas chronic hepatitis may eventually lead to permanent damage to the liver (see Cirrhosis, p298).

AM I AT RISK?

Hepatitis A is easily transmitted in contaminated water or food (often shellfish). If you travel to areas of high risk (Africa, Asia, South America), it is very important to be vaccinated against it before you go.

Hepatitis B and C are transmitted through infected blood and blood products and, especially in the case of hepatitis B, through sexual intercourse. Intravenous drug-users who share needles and people who have sex with an infected person are among those most at risk.

Hepatitis D only occurs in people who already have hepatitis B, and then usually only in drug addicts, while hepatitis E mainly occurs in South East Asia. It can be severe in pregnant women.

HAVE I GOT THE SYMPTOMS?

Often the condition is symptomless. In the early stages of acute hepatitis, you may experience the following symptoms:

- Tiredness and aching muscles
- Jaundice (yellowish skin and whites of the eyes)
- Pale stools and dark urine
- Pain in the right of your upper abdomen.

Symptoms are similar in chronic hepatitis, but jaundice usually only develops in the late stages.

See your doctor if you have any of the symptoms described.

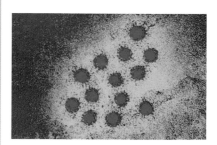

Hepatitis A virus
The hepatitis A virus (shown here as red dots) is a common cause of hepatitis infection for which you can be immunized.

WHAT NEXT?

Your doctor will diagnose hepatitis on the basis of your symptoms and the results of your blood tests. If you have chronic hepatitis, you will usually be recommended a liver biopsy to check for liver damage.

MY TREATMENT OPTIONS

Your doctor will work with you to find the best treatment.
Acute hepatitis There is no specific treatment.
Chronic hepatitis You may be prescribed antiviral drugs, and/or steroids or other drugs that suppress your immune system.

HOW CAN I HELP MYSELF?

For all forms of hepatitis, the best treatment is to rest, avoid alcohol, and eat well (see pp52–5).

Alcoholic liver disease

Alcohol-related liver disease is progressive liver damage caused by the excessive consumption of alcohol (see p299).

WHAT IS IT?

Alcohol affects the liver in the following ways:
Fatty changes in the liver This is the first stage of the disease and is reversible if you stop drinking. These changes do not cause symptoms and are often only revealed by blood tests that check your liver function (see also p298).
Alcoholic hepatitis If you continue to drink heavily, you can develop alcoholic hepatitis. In this condition your liver becomes enlarged and you get jaundiced. Alcoholic hepatitis can lead to the potentially life-threatening condition cirrhosis (see p298). Women are more sensitive than men to the effects of alcohol (see p65 and p299) and some people have an inherited susceptibility to alcohol-related liver damage. However, in simple terms, the more you drink, the more likely you are to experience liver problems.

WHAT NEXT?

If you have a history of excessive alcohol consumption and abnormal results of blood tests for liver function, the diagnosis of alcoholic liver disease can usually be made from your symptoms Your doctor may also arrange for you to have an ultrasound examination of the liver and perhaps a liver biopsy, too.

HAVE I GOT THE SYMPTOMS?

Symptoms of alcoholic liver disease may not appear for several years, but after less than 10 years of heavy drinking, you may experience:
- Nausea and occasional vomiting
- Discomfort in the upper right side of your abdomen
- Weight loss
- Fever
- Yellowing of the skin and the whites of the eyes
- Swollen abdomen.

See your doctor if you regularly consume alcohol and have noticed any of these symptoms.

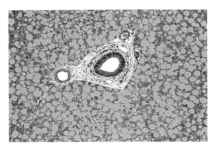

Liver changes in alcoholic hepatitis
This micrograph of a section through the liver shows how the normally regular cell structure of the liver is disrupted by fatty deposits (yellow areas).

MY TREATMENT OPTIONS

Once a diagnosis has been made, you may need to go into hospital.
Medication This may be given to help you cope with alcohol withdrawal and prevent cravings.

HOW CAN I HELP MYSELF?

There are important lifestyle changes you can make:
Stop drinking alcohol This is key to halting the disease. Abstaining from alcohol gives your liver a chance to return to normal, otherwise you run the risk of developing cirrhosis (see p298). Consider joining a support group.
Eat a healthy diet A balanced healthy diet and vitamin supplements are also important (see pp52–5 for advice).

Fatty liver

This is yet another of those common conditions that you can have without realizing it. In fact, it's so common that, in developed countries, about one-fifth of the population has it.

WHAT IS IT?

Fatty liver occurs when there's an excessive build up of fat in your liver cells. It's usually the result of too much fat being delivered to your liver, and your liver then being unable to process it normally. You're more likely to get it if you're obese or have diabetes, and a rare form can affect women during pregnancy.

HAVE I GOT THE SYMPTOMS?

Usually there are no symptoms and the condition is usually detected during tests for other reasons or because your lifestyle leads your doctor to suspect that fatty liver is a possibility.

WHAT NEXT?

If blood tests reveal abnormal liver function and if a scan of your liver supports this, then your doctor will suspect your liver is fatty. The only way definitely to prove the diagnosis of fatty liver is to perform a liver biopsy. However, this is not usually necessary if the blood tests reveal only a mild problem and the results of tests for other causes of liver disease are negative. Fatty liver caused by pregnancy corrects itself following the birth of the baby.

MY TREATMENT OPTIONS

There is much ongoing research into drug treatment for fatty liver, but the main treatment at present consists of measures you can take yourself (see below).

HOW CAN I HELP MYSELF?

Certain lifestyle changes will help to reduce the risk of fatty liver.
Lose weight If you're overweight, it's vital to reduce your weight by lowering your calorie intake and increasing your physical activity

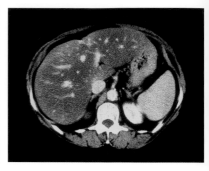

Fatty liver in cross section
This CT scan shows a cross section through the abdomen of a woman suffering from fatty liver. The liver is the large purple-coloured organ. Fatty deposits show up as blue patches.

(see pp56–7). This will help to improve the condition and may even reverse it in some cases.
Watch your diet A diet that's high in fibre and polyunsaturated fats, but low in other types of fat (you should have less than 30 per cent of your total calories as fat) will almost certainly help (see p173).
Avoid alcohol to stop damaging the liver further (see p65).
Watch your blood sugar Be sure to take measures to control your blood sugar levels if you have diabetes (see pp320–5).

Cirrhosis

This serious condition affecting the liver develops as a result of long-term damage.

WHAT IS IT?

The damaged liver cells are replaced by scar tissue and the remaining cells try to replace the dying ones, resulting in clusters (nodules). The liver's abnormal structure then affects its blood flow and the loss of healthy liver cells stops it from functioning normally.

Drinking excessive amounts of alcohol over many years is the most common cause of cirrhosis in the developed world, while long-standing hepatitis B or C infection is the most common cause worldwide. Haemochromatosis, a much rarer cause, is an inherited disease. In this, your intestine absorbs too much iron from what you eat and you get deposits of iron in your liver, heart, pancreas, and pituitary gland. In the long term, the excess iron in your liver causes cirrhosis. Severely fatty liver (above) may also cause cirrhosis and there are other rarer causes, too. If you have cirrhosis, it can lead to liver cancer.

You may experience very few symptoms until the late stages of the disease. The damaged liver is unable to function normally, leading to:

- Easy bruising
- Mild confusion
- Altered sleep patterns
- Jaundice (yellowing of the skin and whites of the eyes)
- Swollen abdomen
- Bleeding from the gullet.

See your doctor if you have any of these symptoms

WHAT NEXT?

The only way to confirm that you have cirrhosis is by having a liver biopsy. However, blood tests and ultrasound or CT scans can often give your doctor all the information needed to make a diagnosis.

MY TREATMENT OPTIONS

The most important part of your treatment is to remove the underlying cause (see How can I help myself?, right). Other aspects of the treatment of cirrhosis include managing the symptoms and detecting complications early.

Diuretic tablets Your liver helps the kidneys to get rid of unwanted fluids, but cirrhosis impairs this function. Fluid can build up in the abdomen, and diuretic tablets are often given to reduce excess fluids.

Checks on the oesophagus You may need an endoscopic

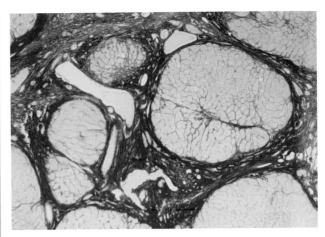

Cirrhotic liver tissue This micrograph shows a section through liver tissue with alcohol-induced cirrhosis. The pink areas are scar tissue. A cirrhotic liver has a knobbly appearance.

examination (see p290) of the lining of the oseophagus and, if necessary, you'll be given medication to reduce the pressure in the blood vessels and to prevent bleeding from the oseophagus.

Ultrasound Regular ultrasound scans are likely to be advised to check for any signs of liver cancer.

Vaccinations If you have cirrhosis, you'll be more susceptible to infection so your doctor may offer vaccinations against hepatitis A and B, pneumococcus, and influenza.

Liver transplant In advanced cases when liver function is dangerously reduced, a liver transplant may be offered.

HOW CAN I HELP MYSELF?

Whatever the cause of your cirrhosis, you must abstain from alcohol for the rest of your life.

HOW ALCOHOL AFFECTS THE LIVER

Once alcohol has been absorbed from the stomach and intestines (see p287), it goes straight to the liver via the blood stream. Here it is broken down, in the same way as your other food and drink. If you consume more alcohol than your liver can process, the imbalance means that your liver cannot break down the protein, fats, and sugars in your food as it should.

The first and commonest problem you get when you have drunk too much alcohol is that your liver is infiltrated by the excess fat that it cannot break down fast enough. This can develop in as few as eight days after the start of heavy drinking. It is reversible, but if you carry on drinking, you will get more serious and irreversible liver damage.

Women are more susceptible than men to the effects of alcohol on the liver because they absorb alcohol more quickly, have a smaller volume of blood, and have a higher ratio of fat to lean tissue – and alcohol is relatively insoluble in lean tissue.

Gastroenteritis

If you've ever had a holiday tummy bug with diarrhoea and vomiting, then you've had gastroenteritis, which is most commonly caused by an infection you've picked up. The condition, which affects women and men equally, usually subsides without you needing any specific treatment.

This common condition usually clears up without the need for medical treatment.

WHAT IS IT?

Gastroenteritis is inflammation of the lining of the stomach and intestines. It's usually caused by infection transmitted either from person to person or by eating contaminated food or drink. A variety of bacteria or viruses, among them staphylococcus and clostridium, may be responsible. Most people in previously good health recover quickly, but it

HAVE I GOT THE SYMPTOMS?

The symptoms of gastroenteritis include:
● Diarrhoea
● Vomiting
● Abdominal pain
● Fever.

See your doctor as a matter of urgency if you pass bloodstained diarrhoea, are unable to keep fluids down, have not passed urine for over 6 hours, become drowsy, listless or confused, or are in poor health.

PREVENTING GASTROENTERITIS

These measures help combat the spread of gastroenteritis from person to person or via contaminated food and water.
● Wash your hands thoroughly with soap and water before cooking and preparing food.
● Wash hands with soap and water after going to the toilet.

● Thaw frozen meat and poultry completely before cooking.
● Store cooked and raw foods in separate areas of the refrigerator.
● Cook meat and poultry thoroughly.
If you have gastroenteritis:
● Don't share towels or cutlery with other people.
● Disinfect the toilet after use.

creates a potentially serious risk of dehydration for babies, pregnant women, and those in poor health.

WHAT NEXT?

Your doctor is likely to diagnose gastroenteritis on hearing about your symptoms.

MY TREATMENT OPTIONS

You can usually manage the condition at home (see How can I help myself?, below). If you show serious signs of dehydration, you may need intravenous fluids.

HOW CAN I HELP MYSELF?

Follow the advice above to avoid spreading infection. Stay away from work until the symptoms have stopped completely. If your job

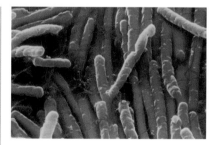

Clostridium difficile
These bacteria are sometimes the cause of gastroenteritis. There are normally small numbers of them in the human gut.

involves handling food, ask your doctor's advice before returning to work.

Drink plenty Aim to drink 2–3 litres (4–6 pints) of fluids a day in frequent small amounts.

Use rehydration salts These help maintain the correct fluid and salt balance in the body (see p302).

Coeliac disease

A condition that can only be controlled by diet, coeliac disease often means that sufferers must make significant changes to their lifestyle. This uncommon disorder occurs in between 0.5 and 1 per cent of the population. Women are, however, more often affected than men.

Coeliac disease is the result of an abnormal reaction of the immune system that damages the lining of the small intestine.

WHAT IS IT?

In coeliac disease, your immune system reacts against gluten – a protein contained in wheat, rye, and barley, and any foods that are made from these cereals. This reaction damages the villi of your small intestine and means that you can't absorb nutrients properly.

HAVE I GOT THE SYMPTOMS?

The disease often reveals itself in infancy, but can also appear later in life. Symptoms may include:

- Mouth ulcers
- Loose, bulky, greasy looking faeces
- Abdominal pains
- Bloating and flatulence
- Tiredness and weakness
- Persistent itchy rash on the knees, buttocks, elbows, and/ or shoulders
- Weight loss.

See your doctor if you have any of these symptoms.

WHAT NEXT?

Your doctor will carry out a blood test to look for increased levels of a certain antibody (protein) as a first step. A biopsy of the lining of the small intestine is the only way to confirm the diagnosis. Your doctor will also take a blood sample to check for anaemia (see p248). A DEXA scan (see p260) may be ordered to check for osteoporosis, which can occur because of reduced absorption of calcium and vitamin D. Your doctor may advise that your close relatives be tested for the disease.

MY TREATMENT OPTIONS

There is no medication that can help with coeliac disease, but your doctor will refer you to a dietician. Follow the advice given under How can I help myself? (below).

HOW CAN I HELP MYSELF?

Self-management is the only option for treating the symptoms of coeliac disease.

Avoid gluten You must avoid this in your diet for the rest of your life, which will involve quite major adjustments. There are now plenty of gluten-free foods on the market, so you'll have a wide choice and

AM I AT RISK?

The disease seems to run in families, and many sufferers have a least one close relative with the condition. In the long term, you have a slightly increased risk of certain types of cancers if you have untreated coeliac disease.

won't necessarily feel very deprived, but you'll need to watch what you eat carefully when you're eating out. Following a gluten-free diet is particularly important for the health of your baby if you're pregnant or are planning a pregnancy. There are a number of support groups that can offer information and advice.

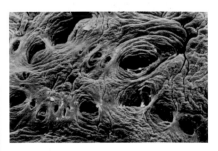

Coeliac disease close up
Coeliac disease leads to an unusually smooth wall of the small intestine caused by the loss of villi (see p287), as shown by this scanning electron micrograph (SEM).

Altered bowel habits

The majority of people move their bowels between three times a day and three times a week, but many have bowel movements more or less frequently than this and still have completely normal bowels. You only need to worry if there's a change in your normal habits.

Diarrhoea

If you pass loose stools unusually frequently, either suddenly or over a long period of time, it's a sign that you may have an underlying problem that should be checked out.

WHAT IS IT?

Diarrhoea is usually defined as passing loose or watery stools more than three times a day, or a large volume of stool. You might sometimes have it together with stomach pains, nausea, or an urgent need to go to the bathroom. Acute diarrhoea, which often starts suddenly, may be short-lived, lasting only a few days or up to three weeks. It's often due to an infection (see p300). If you have chronic diarrhoea, it's persistent and often lasts longer than a few weeks. Many people with this condition are diagnosed with irritable bowel syndrome (IBS) (see pp304–5), but there are many possible causes of diarrhoea other than IBS. For example, it can be a side effect of some medications.

WHAT NEXT?

If you have chronic diarrhoea, you should see your doctor so he or she can investigate the cause. This is especially important if you have a family history of inflammatory bowel disease (see pp310–11); colon cancer (see pp307–9); or coeliac disease (see p301); if you're aged 45 years or older; or if you've recently had abdominal surgery.

Often you'll need nothing more than simple blood tests. Your doctor may want to test a stool sample for infection, particularly if you've been treated with antibiotics or have recently returned from abroad. Your doctor may also want you to have a colonoscopy to check your colon (see p308). You'll usually only need other tests if your blood tests are abnormal or your symptoms are particularly troublesome.

REHYDRATION SALTS

Diarrhoea can deplete fluids and salts in your body, leading to dehydration. The signs of dehydration are passing small amounts of dark-coloured urine, a dry mouth, thirst, and feeling weak. Rehydration salts help to restore the natural balance. It's easy to make your own, and often cheaper than buying ready-made salts. You can buy the ingredients from any chemist and most supermarkets.

Ingredients

Glucose 20g
Sodium chloride (table salt) 3½g
Sodium bicarbonate
  (bicarbonate of soda) 2½g

Method

Add the powders to 1 litre (1¾ pints) of tap water and stir. Drink small amounts regularly throughout the day. You will need to make a fresh solution each day.

HAVE I GOT THE SYMPTOMS?

Along with chronic diarrhoea you may notice any of the following symptoms:

● Blood in the faeces
● Weight loss
● The need to get up at night to open your bowels

See your doctor if you have any of these symptoms.

MY TREATMENT OPTIONS

The treatment of chronic diarrhoea depends on the cause. If the problem is serious enough to bring to your doctor's attention, treatment options will be discussed once a firm diagnosis is made.

HOW CAN I HELP MYSELF?

If you have acute diarrhoea, follow the self-help measures advised for gastroenteritis (see p300), in particular, be sure to drink plenty of clear fluids such as water or dilute fruit juice. Be alert for any signs that you may be suffering from dehydration (see box, left).

Constipation

Not being able to pass a stool is one of the most common gastrointestinal complaints and, like diarrhoea, is usually a symptom of something else. It's more common in women than in men, and is often a particular problem when you're pregnant.

WHAT IS IT?

Constipation is the infrequent passage of stools, or difficulty passing a stool because it's hard and dry. You may also feel bloated. The more constipated you are, the harder it is to pass a stool, which may put you at risk of haemorrhoids (see pp314–15) and a weakened pelvic floor (pp341–2).

It's usually caused by having a diet that doesn't contain enough fibre (roughage) and/or fluids.

Leading a sedentary lifestyle can be a contributory factor, too, and if you regularly resist the urge to defecate, you may lose your normal bowel reflexes. Constipation is much more of a problem for women than for men. Some women notice that their constipation is worse at particular times of the menstrual cycle and during pregnancy. This may be due to the effect of female hormones on the intestine.

WHAT NEXT?

Although there's rarely any serious underlying cause for constipation, if your bowel habits suddenly change, it's important to seek your doctor's advice, especially if you've noticed blood in your faeces, severe abdominal pain, weight loss, or you're over 45 years old.

MY TREATMENT OPTIONS

Constipation often improves with a few simple lifestyle changes, involving adding fibre to your diet and taking more exercise (see How can I help myself?, right).

Laxatives If your constipation is severe, your doctor may decide to prescribe a laxative. Ask about any possible side effects.

Specialized investigations If your constipation doesn't respond to these measures, you may need more tests to investigate in detail the way your bowel muscles are working and if the sphincter muscle in your anus relaxes as it should to allow normal passage of a motion.

HAVE I GOT THE SYMPTOMS?

Constipation can be defined as any of the following:

- Passing fewer bowel motions than is normal for you
- Straining to pass a stool
- Passing faeces that are hard and pellet-like
- A feeling of incomplete bowel emptying.

See your doctor as a matter of urgency if you also have blood in the faeces or experience severe abdominal pain.

HOW CAN I HELP MYSELF?

Constipation can usually be alleviated by the following:

Eat plenty of fibre High-fibre foods include fruit (soaked prunes are helpful), vegetables, and pulses.

Try over-the-counter laxatives, but only for a short time; focus on adding more fibre to your diet.

Drink plenty of water Liquids add fluid to the colon and bulk to the stools, making bowel movements softer to pass. Drink 1.5–2 litres (2½ –3½ pints) of fluid per day. Avoid too many caffeine-containing drinks and alcohol, which can cause dehydration.

Exercise regularly Even gentle exercise, such as walking, helps to keep your digestive system active.

Don't ignore the need to go to the toilet Always respond promptly to your body's natural signals. This helps your reflexes return to normal.

Irritable bowel syndrome

The pain and discomfort of this unpleasant condition can come and go and you may feel perfectly normal in between episodes. It can start at any age, but mostly begins when you're a young adult. For reasons that aren't fully understood, irritable bowel syndrome (IBS) is more common in women.

IBS is a common condition of the intestines – it affects about 15 per cent of people at some time in their lives. It comes under the umbrella term of "functional bowel disorders". In these disorders, although the intestine appears normal when examined by X-ray and endoscopy (see p290), there is actually something wrong with its normal activity and sensitivity.

WHAT IS IT?

If you have IBS, you may have a variety of symptoms (see Have I got the symptoms?, below). These are the result of increased strength or frequency of the contractions of the muscles of your intestine, heightened sensitivity of the nerves of your intestine (intestinal hypersensitivity), or a change in the way in which your brain controls some of these functions. There is no single cause of IBS, but it's believed that stress or emotional upset may play a role. Some people get the symptoms after they've been having a particularly stressful time or have experienced a major life event.

Sometimes symptoms start after an intestinal infection, in which case it's called post-infectious IBS. About 10 to 20 per cent of people develop IBS after they've had gastroenteritis (see p300), even though the bacteria or virus that caused the gastroenteritis is no longer present.

WHAT NEXT?

Your doctor will probably diagnose IBS based on your symptoms. He or she may have some simple blood tests done, for instance, to check for coeliac disease (see p301) if you're mainly suffering from diarrhoea.

You may need further investigations if your symptoms aren't typical of IBS, if you develop symptoms for the first time when you're over 45 years old, or if a close relative has a bowel problem, such as Crohn's disease (see pp310–11).

MY TREATMENT OPTIONS

There is no single treatment that is suitable for everyone and you may have to try one or two before you find the one that helps you. The treatment will also depend on the particular type of symptoms you are having. If your symptoms aren't too troublesome, it's perfectly acceptable not to have any treatment, but if you are prescribed medication, be sure to

---

HAVE I GOT THE SYMPTOMS?

IBS may cause one or more of the following symptoms, which may be present every day, or may come and go and be interspersed with periods of feeling completely well:

- Abdominal pain that may be mild or severe, often in the lower abdomen. The pain may be eased by passing wind or a motion.
- Altered bowel habit, either loose, frequent stools, or hard, pellety stools. The stools may also vary, with alternating diarrhoea and constipation, and perhaps containing mucus. There may be urgency to defecate, and a feeling of incomplete evacuation.
- Bloating of the abdomen
- Other symptoms may include feeling sick, belching, tiredness, and feeling full soon after eating.

See your doctor if you have any of the symptoms of IBS described.

ask your doctor if there might be any side effects.

Medication Many IBS sufferers manage their condition without the need for medication (see How can I help myself?, right). Others benefit from one or more of the following drug treatments:

Antispasmodic drugs These can be useful for pain and are taken as needed. They may also be helpful if you take them about 30 minutes before you eat, if urgency to go to the toilet after mealtimes is a problem.

Antidiarrhoeal drugs If you suffer mainly from diarrhoea, you may find an antidiarrhoea medication, such as loperamide helpful. You can take this as needed.

Laxatives There are a variety of laxatives available if you suffer mainly from constipation; your doctor will recommend a product that is right for you.

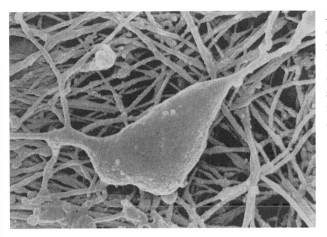

A nerve cell (neuron) in the intestine
In IBS, these nerve cells may be over-sensitive, causing irregular muscle contractions.

Antidepressants These are used in low doses if you are suffering from intestinal hypersensitivity, as they slow down the movement of the bowel, and may also alter the way the nerve impulses between the intestine and the brain are processed. They can be very effective if abdominal pain or diarrhoea are your main symptoms.

HOW CAN I HELP MYSELF?
Many IBS sufferers manage their symptoms effectively without the need for medication.

Watch your diet There is no single food that has been shown to worsen or relieve symptoms, but a few people find that certain foods do make them worse, so it may be worth keeping a food diary for a few weeks to try and identify any culprits. Adjusting your diet is more likely to be helpful if your main symptom is diarrhoea. Foods that commonly seem to trigger

symptoms are wheat and dairy products. A high-fibre diet may help if constipation is a particular problem for you, but this can make bloating and flatulence worse.

Keep hydrated Make sure that you drink enough fluids throughout the day but avoid caffeine-containing drinks as these may trigger the problem.

Make lifestyle changes Have regular mealtimes and avoid eating "meals on the go". Try relaxation techniques (see pp62–3) and regular exercise (see pp56–7) to help you to reduce and manage stress.

Try probiotics ("good bacteria") These are sold over-the-counter and may help to ease bloating and flatulence. You may need to try a number of different products before you find one that suits you.

Try hypnotherapy This can help some types of IBS. You need to commit to it to complete the course.

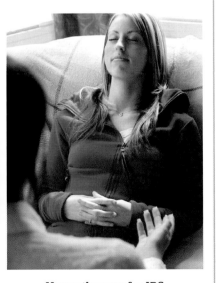

Hypnotherapy for IBS
Relaxation and visualisation techniques can help you cope with your symptoms.

"Many IBS sufferers manage their symptoms effectively without medication."

Gastrointestinal cancer

Any part of the gastrointestinal tract may be affected by cancer. Some of these cancers are relatively common, others are quite rare. Fortunately, it is also the case that many of these cancers can be successfully treated if diagnosed early.

Cancers of the upper gastro-intestinal tract

Cancerous tumours may occur in almost any part of the digestive tract. Those affecting the oesophagus, stomach, pancreas, bile ducts, liver, and small intestine are known collectively as upper gastrointestinal (GI) cancers.

HAVE I GOT THE SYMPTOMS?

Symptoms vary according to the specific cancer, and are often mild and therefore overlooked. The most common symptoms of upper GI cancers include:
- Upper abdominal pain
- Weight loss.

A symptom specific to oesophageal cancer is increasing difficulty in swallowing over a short period of time.
Jaundice (yellowing of the skin and whites of the eyes) may occur in cases of cancer of the liver, bile ducts, and pancreas.
See your doctor if you notice any of the symptoms described.

WHAT ARE THEY?

Like other forms of cancer, these cancers occur when normal cell division and renewal are disrupted and abnormal cells multiply uncontrollably, forming a tumour that prevents the affected organ from functioning normally. In some cases of liver cancer, the disease occurs as a result of the spread of abnormal cells from a tumour elsewhere in the body.

Luckily, most of these cancers are relatively rare. The exception is stomach cancer, which worldwide is the second most common cause of cancer death. However, the numbers affected by this cancer are diminishing, possibly due to changes in diet. In general, upper GI cancers tend to affect mainly people over the age of 50.

WHAT NEXT?

The initial tests your doctor suggests will depend on your symptoms, but usually include an endoscopy (see p290) of your upper gastrointestinal tract, or an ultrasound or CT scan of your abdomen. You may need a biopsy to confirm the diagnosis. If cancer is diagnosed, you will be referred to a specialist team of doctors.

AM I AT RISK?

You're more at risk from upper GI cancers if:
- You're over 50
- You smoke
- You're overweight
- You've a high alcohol intake.

Further tests may be needed to find out how far the cancer has developed and whether the tumour is confined to its original site or has spread beyond it to affect other organs.

MY TREATMENT OPTIONS

Your treatment will depend on the stage of the disease and your general health. In the case of medication, ask your doctor about any possible side effects.
Surgery Tumours that are confined to the original site can usually be removed by surgery. If you have a primary liver tumour, then, in a few selected cases, you may be given a liver transplant.
Chemotherapy and/or radiotherapy are often given before or after the operation to improve your overall outcome. Tumours that have spread beyond

the original site cannot be removed surgically and are usually treated with chemotherapy.

Other treatments may be used to improve your symptoms. For instance, depending on the part of the body affected, stents (see pp170–1) may be inserted in your oesophagus during an endoscopy to help with swallowing, or into in the bile ducts to relieve jaundice.

HOW CAN I HELP MYSELF?

A few simple lifestyle changes may reduce your risk of developing this type of cancer:

Stop smoking GI cancers are more common in smokers.

Maintain a healthy weight within the recommended range for your height (see pp58–9). Many forms of GI cancer are more prevalent in those who are seriously overweight.

Reduce your alcohol intake to within recommended limits (14 units a week for a woman).

Colorectal cancer and polyps

Cancer of the large intestine is one of the most common of the gastrointestinal cancers. The good news is that a recently introduced screening programme is detecting and treating the disease at an early stage when treatment is most likely to be successful.

WHAT IS IT?

The colon is the section of the gastrointestinal tract that connects the small intestine to the final section of the large intestine – the rectum. Cancer in any part of the body develops when the process of cell division, repair, renewal, and development of new cells becomes uncontrolled for some reason. In some cases these abnormal cells form a tumour (a growth or lump).

In the early stages of colorectal cancer, the tumour is confined to the colon or rectum, while more advanced cancers are likely to spread into the lymph nodes, or at an even later stage into the liver and/or lungs. In some people, cancer may start within an intestinal polyp (see p309).

Colon cancer is equally common in men and women, but is commoner among older people. In fact, it is extremely uncommon in anyone under the age of 40, unless there is a family history of the disease at a young age.

Rectal cancer is slightly more common in men and in a small percentage of sufferers, there is a genetic tendency to develop this form of cancer. Brothers, sisters, and children of people with colorectal cancer are thought to be more likely to get the disease in later life. They may be advised

HAVE I GOT THE SYMPTOMS?

Colorectal cancer is likely to cause one or more of the following common symptoms:
- Bleeding from the rectum
- Abdominal pain
- A change in bowel habit.

See your doctor if you develop any of these symptoms.

AM I AT RISK?

Although the exact cause, or causes, of colorectal cancer is not yet understood, there are certain lifestyle factors that are thought to contribute to this condition. These include:
- A high-fat, low-fibre diet
- Smoking
- Not getting enough exercise
- Obesity.

In addition, you are at increased risk of developing colorectal cancer if you have intestinal polyps or if a close family member has had the disease.

to go for regular screening (perhaps including a colonoscopy) to detect polyps or an early cancer – particularly if they had a relative who developed cancer before the age of 45.

WHAT NEXT?

After assessing your symptoms in the context of your age and your medical and family history, your doctor will decide whether you need further investigations.

WHAT HAPPENS DURING A COLONOSCOPY

Colonoscopy is the most commonly used technique for examining the colon and rectum to detect early colorectal cancer and polyps, for taking biopsies (tiny tissue specimens), and for removing polyps if they are present. The day before you have the colonoscopy, you will be given strong laxatives to empty your colon so the lining can be clearly seen. On the day, you will normally be admitted to hospital as a day case and given a mild intravenous sedative. Once you are sedated, a small flexible tube (colonoscope) with a light source and a camera is passed via the anus into the rectum and colon, and then to the junction of the colon and the small intestine. The specialist can see on a monitor what is going on in your colon and rectum and can remove any polyps. If these are attached to blood vessels, the blood vessels will be cauterized to prevent bleeding. The whole procedure usually only takes about 30 minutes.

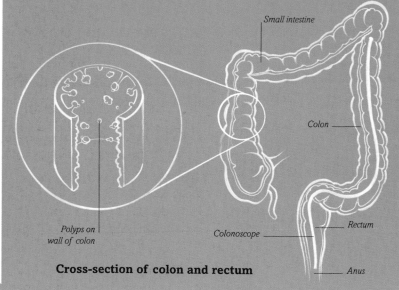

Small intestine

Colon

Polyps on wall of colon

Colonoscope

Rectum

Anus

Cross-section of colon and rectum

The symptoms of colorectal cancer (see Have I got the symptoms?, p307) are not specific to the condition, but may be caused by many less serious diseases, such as ulcerative colitis and Crohn's disease (see pp310–11).

Further investigations will involve taking a look at what is going on in the colon. This can be done by one of the following three methods: colonoscopy (see box, above), barium enema (when a white chalky barium-containing mixture is placed in the colon, which is then X-rayed) or by a special CT scan called a CT colonography or virtual colonoscopy.

Whichever method is used, the colon will need to be flushed out

COLOSTOMY

The type of stoma known as colostomy is when an opening is made in the large intestine and abdominal wall so that faeces can be collected in a colostomy bag outside the abdomen before they enter the anal canal. A colostomy is usually a temporary surgical procedure to enable the colon to heal, or other corrective surgery to be undertaken, but in some cases it can be permanent.

the day before using strong laxatives so that the lining of the colon can be clearly seen. Colonoscopy is the most commonly used technique of these three methods.

If you have colorectal cancer and no symptoms, it may be picked up when you are having other tests, for example if you have a family history of the disease and are being routinely screened.

MY TREATMENT OPTIONS

If cancer is diagnosed, you'll be advised to have further tests. You may need to have a CT scan of your chest and abdomen to check if the cancer has spread and to identify the stage it has reached. If you have rectal cancer, you will usually also need an MRI or ultrasound scan. Your treatment will depend on the stage of the disease. When discussing your options, ask your doctor about any possible side effects.

Colon or rectal surgery Part of your treatment will usually be surgery to remove the tumour from your colon or rectum. Sometimes you will also need a stoma – an opening in your abdomen for faeces to leave your body, bypassing the colon – either temporarily or permanently. If you need this procedure, your surgeon and a specialist stoma nurse will discuss it with you in advance.

Medication and radiotherapy

Sometimes chemotherapy (treatment with anticancer drugs) or with X-rays (radiotherapy) is advised before or after surgery to improve your overall outcome.

HOW CAN I HELP MYSELF?

There are several lifestyle changes you can make that may help to improve your health and reduce your risk of developing colorectal cancer:

Eat a healthy, balanced diet that includes plenty of fibre (roughage) (see pp52–5).

Maintain a healthy weight within the normal range for your height (see pp58–9).

Take regular exercise For more information, see pp56–7.

Avoid or give up smoking For more information, see p64.

Limit your alcohol intake For more information, see p65.

See your doctor if you have a family history of colon cancer. He or she will advise you if you need to be screened.

Take part in your national bowel cancer screening programme.

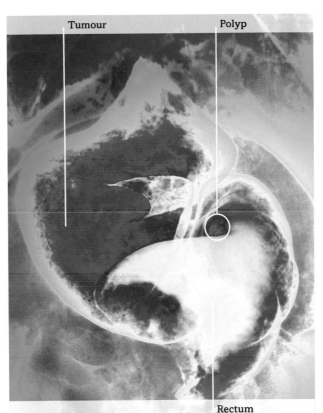

Tumour　　　Polyp

Rectum

Colon cancer and polyp

This X-ray shows a tumour at the junction of the rectum (lower right) and the colon. The patient also has a polyp – the dark circle in the bright part of the colon just to the right of the tumour.

INTESTINAL POLYPS

In many cases, colorectal cancer develops from polyps – growths in the lining of the colon and rectum. Most polyps are not malignant, but some have the potential to develop into a cancer if they aren't removed. Polyps can range in size from a millimetre to several centimetres ($\frac{1}{16}$–2in), and you may have just one or several hundred. You are more likely to develop polyps as you get older. You often don't have any symptoms from them and they are then detected only when your colon is examined for other symptoms, such as diarrhoea, or when they are detected during screening for colorectal cancer. Some people have bleeding from the rectum, which may be caused by polyps. The time between a polyp first developing and later turning into cancer can take months or years. Once a polyp is completely removed from the colon, the risk of cancer in that polyp is also removed, and it won't grow back.

If you have had polyps removed, you will usually be asked to return for a further colonoscopy (see opposite) several months or years later (depending on the type and size of the polyp) to check that no more polyps have developed.

Inflammatory bowel disease

Inflammatory bowel disease (IBD) is an umbrella term that includes two separate conditions: Crohn's disease and ulcerative colitis. Often affecting young adults, both disorders can cause distressing symptoms. But once diagnosed, these conditions can be successfully treated in most cases.

Often similar in terms of the symptoms they cause, ulcerative colitis and Crohn's disease have different causes and treatment.

WHAT IS IT?

Both of these conditions cause inflammation and ulceration in the intestine. One person in every 400 has IBD, and women are as likely to be affected as men. It's most likely to be first noticed between the ages of 10 and 40, but symptoms of the condition can appear at any age.

WHAT NEXT?

IBD can often be confirmed by a colonoscopy (see p308). During this procedure, the doctor will usually take biopsies of your colon to decide which type of inflammation you have. If your doctor suspects that your small intestine is affected, you may be given a barium X-ray, where you drink a thick white solution of barium that reveals the outline of your small intestine on an X-ray. Alternatively, you may have video capsule endoscopy; in this, you swallow a capsule-like camera that produces pictures of your small intestine. These are captured on a data recorder that you wear as a belt for 24 hours. You excrete the capsule with your stools. Sometimes ultrasound, CT, or MRI scans are advised.

HAVE I GOT THE SYMPTOMS?

The symptoms of ulcerative colitis are:
● Diarrhoea with or without blood
● Tiredness and lethargy.
Symptoms of Crohn's disease usually include:
● Diarrhoea with or without blood
● Weight loss
● Abdominal pain.
Both diseases can also cause inflammation in the eyes, joints, and skin.
See your doctor if you have one or more of these symptoms.

ULCERATIVE COLITIS OR CROHN'S DISEASE?

Ulcerative colitis only affects the colon (large intestine). Inflammation always begins in the lower colon (rectum) and spreads round the colon in a continuous pattern. Crohn's disease can affect any part of the intestine, but most commonly affects the end of the small intestine and the colon. Inflammation is patchy. Crohn's disease also causes narrowing of the bowel, which can cause abdominal pain.

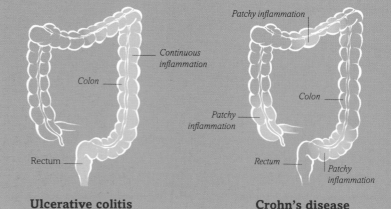

Ulcerative colitis — Continuous inflammation — Colon — Rectum

Crohn's disease — Patchy inflammation — Colon — Rectum — Patchy inflammation

MY TREATMENT OPTIONS

If you have ulcerative colitis, your doctor may advise one or more of the following treatments.

Medication Your doctor may try one or more of the following drug treatments, depending on your condition and symptoms. Ask about any possible side effects.

- 5-ASA (5-aminosalicylate) medicines: drugs such as mesalazine are often used to treat and prevent flare-ups.
- Steroids can be given to treat more serious flare-ups, and then tailed off when symptoms subside. If you have a very severe flare-up, they may be given intravenously in hospital. If inflammation is confined to the lower part of your colon, these drugs can be administered as suppositories or enemas.
- Immune-system suppressants: these drugs are used to prolong your symptom-free periods if you continue to have frequent attacks despite ASA treatment.

IBD AND PREGNANCY

Most women with IBD do not have reduced fertility or any difference in the progress of their pregnancy. Although most IBD drugs are safe, you should consult your doctor if you are planning a pregnancy, or if your partner has IBD, because a few of the drugs are best avoided in the months before conception and during pregnancy.

AM I AT RISK?

The exact cause of IBD is uncertain, but a combination of three factors is thought to be responsible: having a family predisposition (genetic factors), having an abnormal immune response in the intestine, and environmental triggers.

- Family predisposition means that there's a greater chance of developing the disease if your brother, sister, either of your parents, or your child is affected. The inherited risk is greater with Crohn's disease than with ulcerative colitis, and overall you're 10 times more likely to develop IBD if you've got one close relative with the condition; your risk is greater if two or more relatives are affected
- An abnormal immune response occurs as a result of oversensitivity of your immune system, Normally activated as a response to invading bacteria in your intestine, the activated immune cells release special proteins that not only kill the virus or bacteria but also give you some of the symptoms of infection, mainly fever and tiredness. In IBD your over-sensitive immune system attacks the beneficial bacteria that normally live in the intestine, causing inflammation and ulceration of your intestine
- Environmental factors play a part. Smoking, for example, has a role in Crohn's disease; smokers have a higher risk of developing the disease, have more frequent attacks, and respond less well to treatment. Stress may also trigger the IBD and also increases the chances of a relapse in those who have had the condition before.

Surgery The colon may need to be removed if drugs don't offer enough relief (see Colostomy, p308).

If you have Crohn's disease, medication options are similar to those for ulcerative colitis. In addition, a new range of drugs has recently been introduced, which deactivate the immune response. Methotrexate – used in the treatment of autoimmune disease – is sometimes prescribed.

Other treatments for Crohn's disease may include surgery to remove the affected part of the intestine, which may be advised if drugs fail to control your symptoms.

HOW CAN I HELP MYSELF?

You can increase the effectiveness of any treatment for IBD by making simple lifestyle changes:

Stop smoking This is particularly important if you have Crohn's disease because of its adverse effect on this form of IBD. For advice on giving up, see p64.

Eat a healthy, well-balanced diet with plenty of nutrients and vitamins (see pp52–5). In Crohn's disease a simple liquid diet may be recommended for a time.

Learn to manage stress, perhaps by attending relaxation classes or by doing yoga (see also pp62–3).

Diverticular disease

Diverticular disease is one of those complaints that you are more likely to experience as you get older. As with many other conditions affecting the bowel, you can reduce your chances of developing the disease in later life by making sure that you eat a healthy, high-fibre diet.

This condition is mainly a problem in industrialized societies, where diets that are high in processed food are more common. It occurs in over half of people in their 80s in the West, but it is rare in most parts of Asia and Africa.

WHAT IS IT?

In diverticular disease, small pouches, known as diverticula (singular diverticulum), develop in the wall of your colon. The exact

HAVE I GOT THE SYMPTOMS?

It is common for diverticula to cause no obvious symptoms. Some sufferers, however, have the following:

● Crampy abdominal pain
● Altered bowel habits such as diarrhoea or constipation
● Bleeding from the rectum.

If the diverticula become inflamed (diverticulitis), you may experience:

● Intense pain on the left side of the lower abdomen
● Fever.

See your doctor if you have any of these symptoms.

WHAT HAPPENS IN DIVERTICULITIS

In diverticular disease, small pouches form in the wall of the colon. If these pouches become infected, diverticulitis, a serious condition that causes abdominal pain and fever, is the result.

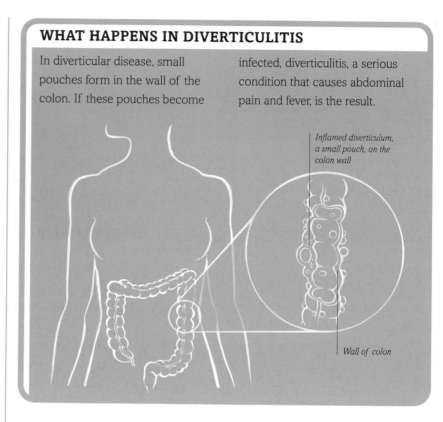

Inflamed diverticulum, a small pouch, on the colon wall

Wall of colon

cause is not known, but it's thought that a low-fibre diet and the constipation you're likely to experience as a result creates increased pressure in the colon. This increased pressure may force the inner lining (mucosa) through the outer muscle layer, leading to the formation of diverticula.

Diverticula can exist in the bowel without causing any symptoms, and this is known as diverticulosis.

But occasionally, diverticula can become inflamed – a condition known as diverticulitis – and this can lead to intense abdominal pain and a fever. In rare cases, an inflamed diverticulum can burst, which can lead to an abscess, peritonitis (inflammation of the lining of the abdominal cavity), or the formation of an abnormal connection (fistula) with the bladder or another section of intestine.

WHAT NEXT?

If your doctor suspects you've got diverticular disease, you will probably be advised to have some investigations, such as a barium enema (see p308) or colonoscopy (see p308). In some cases a CT scan may be recommended.

MY TREATMENT OPTIONS

If your diverticular disease isn't causing symptoms or if the symptoms are mild, you are unlikely to be offered medical treatment. Instead, you'll probably be advised to adopt a high-fibre diet (see How can I help myself?, below right). The following may be recommended in certain situations. Ask your doctor about possible side effects of any medication prescribed:

Antispasmodics if you're suffering from cramping pains in the abdomen.

Laxatives if you are suffering from severe constipation.

Antibiotics are often used to treat diverticulitis. In mild cases, you can take these by mouth, but for more severe diverticulitis, you may be admitted to hospital so that antibiotics and fluid can be given via an intravenous drip.

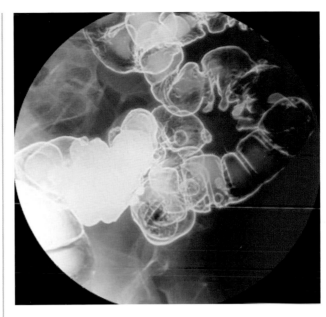

Colon affected by diverticular disease
This coloured X-ray shows several diverticula (in blue) protruding from the wall of the colon in a person with diverticular disease.

Surgery may occasionally be necessary to drain an abscess or repair a fistula. If you have diverticula that are bleeding, you may need to stay in hospital for observation and in severe cases, you may need a blood transfusion.

If part of your bowel is especially badly affected by the disease, you may be advised to have that part removed surgically. After the operation, the healthy sections of the intestine will be joined together.

HOW CAN I HELP MYSELF?

There are plenty of non-medical measures you can take, mainly to reduce any tendency to constipation. These can help to minimize your risk of getting diverticular disease and – if you have it already – can reduce the severity of your symptoms:

Eat a high-fibre diet that contains plenty of fruit, pulses, and vegetables. Choose wholegrain cereal products, such as wholemeal bread and pasta. See pp52–5 for further advice on a healthy diet.

Drink plenty of fluid, up to 1.5– 2 litres (2½ –3½ pints) a day to help keep your bowel movements soft.

Take regular exercise (see pp56 7) to maintain a regular bowel action.

For pain relief take paracetamol, if necessary, and avoid non-steroidal anti-inflammatory drugs (for example, ibuprofen and indomethacin). These medications have been linked to an increased risk of developing complications of diverticular disease.

AM I AT RISK?

The likelihood of developing diverticular disease is increased if:
- You're over 50
- You've suffered from constipation for long periods.

"In the industrialized West, diverticular disease affects over half of those in their 80s."

Haemorrhoids and anorectal conditions

Haemorrhoids (piles) and other minor problems of the anal region are extremely common conditions, but people are often too embarrassed to talk about them to anyone. The problems are rarely serious, but the symptoms can be irritating and can take a long time to clear up.

Haemorrhoids

Haemorrhoids (commonly called piles) are enlarged veins, similar to varicose veins, around the anus. Although they are a common problem for both sexes, they are a particular problem for women during pregnancy.

WHAT ARE THEY?
Haemorrhoids form when the blood in the veins around the anus slows down or stops flowing. This is often caused by constipation and straining when you go to the toilet.

When you are pregnant, you are particularly susceptible to haemorrhoids because of the increased pressure on the pelvic veins caused by enlargement of the uterus. Pregnancy also brings an increase in the amount of blood circulating through your body and hormonal effects on the walls of the veins make them weaker. In addition, your hormones have a relaxing effect on the muscles of the intestine and slow down the movement of food residue through the gastrointestinal tract, which can lead to constipation.

Although haemorrhoids are usually only a minor complaint, they can become very painful if a blood clot (thrombosis) forms within the vein.

WHAT NEXT?
Your doctor will examine you with a proctoscope (a hollow tube with a light source), which is passed into the anus. Some haemorrhoids protrude from the anus and can be seen without the proctoscope.

HAVE I GOT THE SYMPTOMS?

Symptoms range from temporary and mild, to persistent and painful (some people do not have any symptoms):
- Rectal bleeding, usually a small amount of bright red blood in the toilet or on toilet paper after wiping
- Anal itching
- Pain
- Awareness of a lump in the anus.

See your doctor if the bleeding or pain is persistent, or if there is altered (dark red or black) blood.

THE SITE OF HAEMORRHOIDS

Haemorroids form in the anus – either just inside or around the outside of the opening.

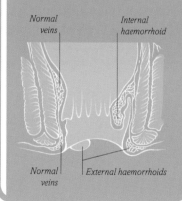

Normal veins

Internal haemorrhoid

Normal veins

External haemorrhoids

MY TREATMENT OPTIONS
Mild cases require no treatment.
Creams You can buy over-the-counter creams and suppositories to reduce the discomfort.

In more severe cases, you may be advised to have haemorrhoids removed by one of these methods:
Band ligation A rubber band is placed around the base of the haemorrhoid, cutting off the blood supply to the swollen vein.
Infrared light or laser in which the haemorrhoids are destroyed by

the burning action of the rays. **Injection of a sclerosant solution** into the haemorrhoid, which makes the vein wither away. **Surgery** to remove haemorrhoids is reserved for those whose symptoms persist in spite of these treatments, or when a haemorrhoid has become clotted with blood.

HOW CAN I HELP MYSELF?
Follow your doctor's advice and most importantly, avoid constipation and straining (see p303) when you go to the toilet.

Anal fissure

Like many other bowel conditions, anal fissure is associated with constipation and a low-fibre diet.

WHAT IS IT?
An anal fissure is a tear in the lining of the anal canal. Most are caused by local trauma, such as passing hard stools. The sphincter muscle may then go into spasm and pull the edges of the fissure apart, preventing healing.

WHAT NEXT?
Your doctor will make a diagnosis based on an external examination. Most fissures are not serious.

HAVE I GOT THE SYMPTOMS?

Typical symptoms include:
- Tearing pain on opening the bowels
- Rectal bleeding
- Itching around the anus.

See your doctor if you experience any of these symptoms.

MY TREATMENT OPTIONS
Simple treatment is effective in most cases. Ask your doctor about any possible side effects.
Laxatives These soften the stools and prevent constipation.

Local treatment The two most commonly used preparations are glyceryl trinitrate and diltiazem cream. These help to relax the sphincter muscle and prevent spasm. Some specialists recommend an injection of botulinum toxin (Botox) into the sphincter, which has a similar relaxing effect on the sphincter.
Surgery Only in rare cases is surgery needed.

HOW CAN I HELP MYSELF?
The most important measures you can take are those to help you avoid constipation and straining on the toilet, as described for haemorrhoids (see above).

Pruritus ani

A minor condition affecting the anal area, pruritus ani can usually be relieved by simple measures.

WHAT IS IT?
Pruritus ani is itching and irritation around the anus. It may be due to fissures and haemorrhoids (see above and opposite), to skin problems, such as eczema, in the anal area, or infection with thrush or threadworms. Often no definite cause can be identified.

WHAT NEXT?
Your doctor will make a diagnosis based on your symptoms, and will perhaps do a physical examination.

MY TREATMENT OPTIONS
Having eliminated any treatable cause, your doctor will probably advise self-help measures (below) and may recommend that you use a steroid cream.

HOW CAN I HELP MYSELF?
The following self-help measures are usually effective:

Avoid irritants Remove all possible irritants, such as soap, from the skin around the anus.
Keep clean Rinse the anal area thoroughly after you have opened your bowels. Use non-irritant aqueous cream instead of soap when you wash yourself.
Keep dry Dry the skin gently without rubbing after bathing and going to the toilet.
Avoid scratching
Stay cool Wear loose-fitting underwear made of a natural fibre such as cotton.

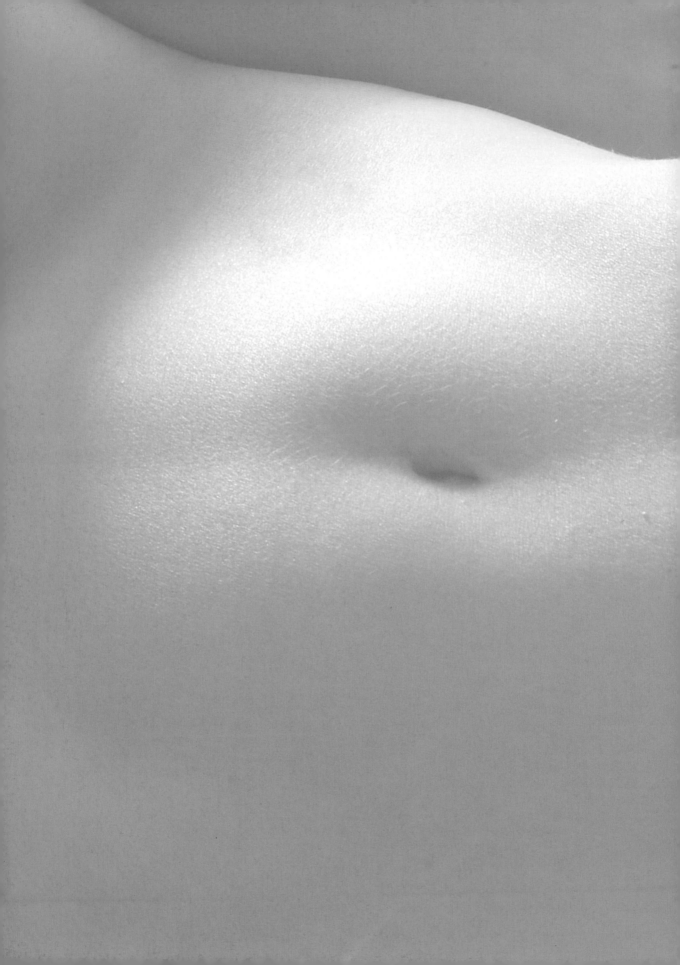

Hormones and metabolism

Dr Sarah Jarvis MA BM BCH DRCOG FRCGP

Your hormones and metabolism

Much of the way in which your body functions depends on your hormones. These are chemical messengers that initiate and regulate many of your bodily functions, including your fertility, growth, and energy needs. They are produced in glands situated throughout the body, known collectively as the endocrine system, and are released into the bloodstream, where they are carried to the various cells and tissues on which they have a specific influence.

There are a number of hormones that are produced in very different amounts in women and men. Sex-specific hormones are discussed in Chapter 5 (see pp86–141), but this chapter deals with hormones and any problems related to their production, which are common to both men and women. However, some of these disorders can have a different incidence in women, or they may affect women in a different way from men.

Your body produces several hormones that control the way that the body burns fuel for energy, lays down fat, and influences the rate at which many chemical processes occur. The umbrella term that is used to describe this complex collection of functions is metabolism – and many of the disorders in this chapter affect metabolic processes.

CAUSES OF HORMONAL PROBLEMS

Many hormone problems are related to autoimmune disease, in which the body's own immune system, which normally fights off infection, turns against

GLANDS AND HORMONES

The glands shown here produce some of the important hormones that are responsible for your wellbeing. Other hormone-producing glands are discussed in Chapter 5 (see pp86–141). The pancreas, which is an organ rather than a gland, also secretes many different hormones, including insulin. This helps to control blood-sugar levels (see p320).

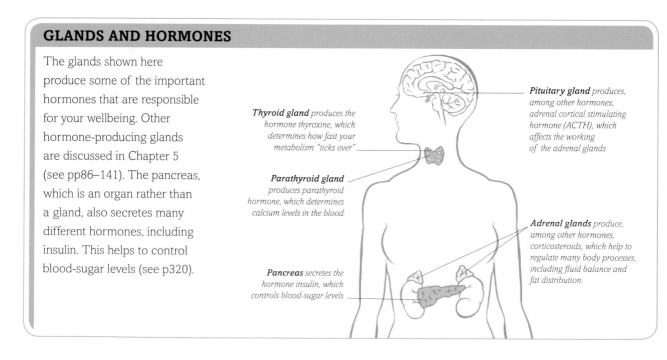

Thyroid gland produces the hormone thyroxine, which determines how fast your metabolism "ticks over"

Parathyroid gland produces parathyroid hormone, which determines calcium levels in the blood

Pancreas secretes the hormone insulin, which controls blood-sugar levels

Pituitary gland produces, among other hormones, adrenal cortical stimulating hormone (ACTH), which affects the working of the adrenal glands

Adrenal glands produce, among other hormones, corticosteroids, which help to regulate many body processes, including fluid balance and fat distribution.

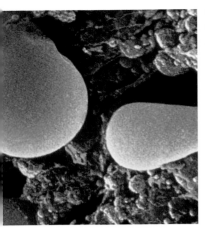

Thyroid gland
The tissue of the thyroid gland secretes thyroglobulin (coloured orange), from which the hormones thyroxine and triiodothyronine are produced. These hormones control your body's metabolism.

I'M EXHAUSTED!

Complaints of being "tired all the time" are one of the most common problems that doctors come across, and women present with it far more often than men.

Tiredness is an extremely vague diagnosis, and it's often not clear what's causing it. However, in women, the most common causes include thyroid problems (see pp326–9), and also anaemia (see p248).

Other hormone problems that cause tiredness are diabetes (see pp320–5) and Addison's disease (see p331). Although simple exhaustion, lack of sleep, stress, or depression can often be an underlying cause in our multi-tasking, fast-moving world – making it a requirement to take time out for yourself and relax – consult your doctor if you are consistently tired and lack energy.

one or more of its own organs (see p259). Hormonal disorders that have an autoimmune cause include underactive and overactive thyroid glands (see pp326–8) and Type 1 diabetes (see pp320–1). With the notable exception of Type 1 diabetes, women are much more prone than men to most of these disorders, although we don't yet know why this is so. These disorders are often linked and may run in families, so if you or other members of your family suffer from a hormonal problem, your risks of developing other, similar problems are increased.

HORMONES AND FERTILITY

Given how crucial your female hormones are in determining whether and when you ovulate, it's hardly surprising that the other hormones your body produces can have an impact on your fertility. Even a slightly over- or underactive thyroid gland can reduce your chances of conceiving. So if you have a known thyroid problem, you will be referred for fertility treatment more quickly than usual if you're having trouble getting pregnant. Likewise, if you have diabetes, you're likely to be referred if you've been trying to get pregnant unsuccessfully for a year. If you have such a condition, it's crucial to talk to your doctor in advance about your plans to become pregnant.

PREVENTING HORMONAL DISORDERS

Type 2 diabetes is the most preventable of the hormone disorders that are discussed in this chapter. It is almost exclusively a problem among people who carry excess weight, so it can usually be avoided by paying attention to particular aspects of your lifestyle, for example, making sure that you exercise regularly, ensuring that your weight is within the recommended limits for your height, and being sure that you have healthy eating habits (for more advice on a healthy lifestyle, see Chapter 3, pp48–69).

Unfortunately, you can't reduce your chances of developing most other types of hormonal disorder. However, you can be aware of the symptoms, especially if you're at particular risk of a specific disorder. It's always worth explaining your symptoms to your doctor if you think you might have a hormone problem. He or she may be able to rule it out with a blood test, or explain to you why you don't need to worry. Smoking may increase your risk of developing some hormone problems, and it can greatly increase your risk of developing the complications that are often associated with hormonal diseases..

> "Women are more prone than men to hormonal disorders, although we don't know yet why this is so."

Diabetes

"Sugar" diabetes, or diabetes mellitus, is one of the best-known hormone disorders. There are two main forms of the condition and although both have serious risks, the good news is that these risks can be greatly reduced if you stick carefully to your treatment plan and make lifestyle changes.

The key feature of diabetes mellitus is excess glucose in the blood. When we eat, food is broken down in the gut into sugars. The main sugar is glucose. This passes from the gut into the bloodstream. The pancreas responds to increased levels of glucose in the blood (blood sugar) by releasing the hormone insulin, which helps the body absorb the glucose and turn it into energy. In the two main types of diabetes mellitus – type 1 and type 2 – either the pancreas produces insufficient amounts of insulin or body cells are resistant to insulin's effect.

THE LONG-TERM RISKS OF DIABETES

If diabetes of either type is not diagnosed or properly controlled, you risk several serious conditions:

- Raised levels of cholesterol
- High blood pressure
- Heart attack. In particular, in women, the protection given by female hormones against heart disease is reduced
- Diabetic retinopathy (damage to the back of the eyes which can cause blindness)
- Kidney damage
- Poor circulation in the extremities, leading to damage to the nerves and a loss of sensation, and an increased risk of leg ulcers.

To make sure that any of these potential complications are picked up, it is important that anyone suffering from any form of diabetes has the following regular checks:

- Blood pressure checks
- Cholesterol level checks
- Examination of the retina (the back of your eyes) at least once a year
- Kidney function tests
- Foot examination.

Type 1 diabetes

This form of diabetes mellitus used to be known as "insulin-dependent diabetes", because everyone who gets it needs to take insulin every day. It usually first develops in childhood, adolescence, or young adulthood.

WHAT IS IT?

Type 1 diabetes develops when the insulin-producing cells in your pancreas stop producing insulin. It's an "autoimmune" condition (see p259) with several possible causes; it's probably a combination of genetic susceptibility and triggers in the environment. In this form of diabetes, the insulin-producing cells of the pancreas are totally destroyed. Once insulin production stops, you are likely to develop the symptoms described in the panel (opposite). You may also develop a condition called ketoacidosis. This is caused by the release of toxic chemicals, which occurs when – because of the lack of insulin – your body is forced to burn fat for energy rather than the sugars in your blood. Ketoacidosis causes nausea and vomiting, abdominal pain, and confusion, and often leads to your breath smelling of acetone (like nail-polish remover). This condition requires urgent medical help.

WHAT NEXT?

If your symptoms suggest type 1 diabetes, your doctor is likely to arrange for tests to determine the

In Type 1 diabetes, symptoms tend to come on over days rather than weeks or months. These symptoms include:

- Intense thirst
- Passing water very frequently
- Tiredness and lack of energy
- Blurry vision
- Rapid weight loss
- Poor concentration and sometimes collapse.

See your doctor if you have any of the above symptoms.

levels of sugar in your blood and urine to confirm the diagnosis. Blood tests may also indicate how much insulin is being produced by your pancreas.

MY TREATMENT OPTIONS

If you have type 1 diabetes, you'll certainly need insulin injections.
Medication There are both short- and long-acting forms of insulin. You'll be taught how to inject yourself and how to monitor your blood sugar levels. This is important, as it enables you and your doctor to see if the treatment is controlling your blood sugar effectively. You may need extra medication to treat any complications, such as high blood pressure or raised cholesterol.
Surgery In rare cases, a pancreas transplant may be offered, but unfortunately it carries a high risk of organ rejection.

HOW CAN I HELP MYSELF?

You must regulate your food intake to minimize blood-sugar level fluctuations. Much of the advice on diet for type 2 diabetics (see pp324–5) will also help you.

Monitor your blood sugar

When you're on insulin treatment, you must check your blood sugar, usually daily. Use a digital meter to painlessly prick your finger to release a drop of blood that you smear onto a test strip. Inserted into the meter, this shows your current blood-sugar level. The results will tell you if you need to adjust your insulin dose. Be sure to learn to recognize symptoms of excessively low blood sugar (hypoglycaemia). This can occur if your food intake, insulin levels, and energy output get out of balance. Always have readily absorbed sugar available (such as glucose tablets or sweet drinks) in case this happens.

AM I AT RISK?

The risk factors for type 1 diabetes, include:

- A family history of type 1 diabetes: you are at greater risk of developing it if your father suffered from it than if your mother did.
- Your sex: males and females are diagnosed at about the same rate under the age of 15. Over the age of 15, men are about 50 per cent more likely to be diagnosed with type 1 diabetes than women.

INSULIN SELF-TREATMENT

These days, there are lots of convenient and almost painless ways of injecting yourself with insulin, including devices no bigger than a fountain pen. The highlighted areas below show the best places for safely injecting insulin. You will need to change site every few days.

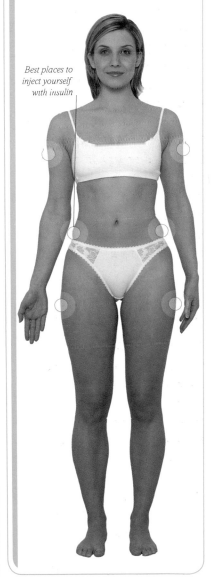

Best places to inject yourself with insulin

Type 2 diabetes

Type 2 diabetes accounts for 90–95 per cent of cases of diabetes in the UK today. It tends to be diagnosed later in life than Type 1 diabetes – almost always in adulthood – and the vast majority of those affected are overweight.

WHAT IS IT?

Type 2 diabetes occurs when your body gradually stops responding normally to insulin – a condition known as insulin resistance – so your pancreas needs to release higher and higher "doses" to keep your blood sugar at a normal level. Eventually, the insulin-producing cells in your pancreas are unable to keep up with your body's need for insulin. When you have a combination of insulin resistance and decreasing production of insulin, your body's blood-sugar levels can no longer be controlled and you develop the symptoms of type 2 diabetes.

WHAT CAUSES IT?

Type 2 diabetes is usually linked to obesity: four out of five people diagnosed with it are overweight or obese. Obesity is traditionally measured using the BMI, or body mass index, which is a ratio of your weight to height (see p59). This doesn't mean that everyone who is obese will develop diabetes, but they are at much greater risk. As a woman, if your BMI is over 35, you're 90 times more likely to develop diabetes than someone with a BMI of only 22.

These days, we've also learnt that it's not just how much you weigh, but where that weight sits that matters. Your abdominal circumference could be the key to your risk of developing diabetes. Those who tend to lay down fat in the abdominal area are at far greater risk of developing type 2 diabetes (as well as a number of other disorders) than those who tend to put on weight on their hips, bottoms, and thighs.

Nowadays, men are slightly more likely to be diagnosed with type 2 diabetes than women. This may be linked to their tendency to store excess fat around their abdomens. Smoking is a risk factor for type 2 diabetes that seems to affect women more than men. Women who smoke heavily are up to 75 per cent more likely to develop diabetes than those who've never smoked; in men, that figure is just under 50 per cent. And if you do have diabetes, smoking amplifies the risks associated with the disease.

WHAT NEXT?

Diagnosing diabetes at an early stage is crucial if you want to avoid the serious complications it causes; as long as diabetes is undiagnosed, your body is living with damagingly

---

HAVE I GOT THE SYMPTOMS?

The symptoms of Type 2 diabetes are easily overlooked. They tend to come on gradually and can include:

- Needing to pass urine often (including needing to get up at night)
- Constant thirst
- Recurrent thrush, boils or minor skin infections
- Feeling generally tired and run down.

See your doctor if you have any of the above symptoms.

AM I AT RISK?

The risk factors for type 2 diabetes, include:

- A family history of developing type 2 diabetes
- A past history of developing "gestational diabetes" in pregnancy (see pp127, 324)
- Being overweight or obese (particularly if you tend to put on weight mainly in your abdominal area)
- Your ethnic background (being of South Asian or Afro-Caribbean origin)
- Taking certain medications (including long-term treatment with steroids and some types of blood pressure medication)
- Having polycystic ovary syndrome (see p95).

"Smoking is a risk factor for Type 2 diabetes that seems to affect women more than men."

high levels of blood sugar, and probably raised cholesterol and blood pressure as well. The early symptoms of type 2 diabetes are often very mild and non-specific; sadly, this means that all too many people ignore the early symptoms, or put them down to stress.

MY TREATMENT OPTIONS

Your doctor will advise on lifestyle changes (see p324). In addition to such changes, a number of drugs can help regulate blood-sugar levels:

Antidiabetic medications

The drug metformin increases the sensitivity of tissues in the body to insulin. Drugs from a family of medicines called sulphonylureas may be prescribed as an alternative, or together with metformin. These stimulate the pancreas to produce increased levels of insulin. Other families of drugs that may be prescribed include the "glitazones", the prandial glucose regulators, and the "gliptins". Your doctor will explain the possible side effects of each of these options and work with you to find a drug-treatment regime that is best-suited to your circumstances and condition.

Other forms of medication

Further drug treatment is aimed at treating possible complications of your condition.

- If you have raised blood pressure, the level for treatment is anything over 140/90 for diabetes. Your doctor will want your blood pressure kept to a level of 130/80 or below. If you have high blood pressure, two groups of related drugs called the ACE inhibitors (see p170) and the ARBs, or sartans, can also help to protect your kidneys from damage if you have diabetes.

- If you have raised cholesterol levels, you are likely to be prescribed statins (see p170), though you may need to stop taking them before you consider getting pregnant (see p324). A healthy lifestyle can delay or even prevent the need for this medication. If you're over 40, you'll probably be prescribed a statin as a matter of course.

- To help you lose weight, your doctor may consider prescribing you a drug that helps you to control your weight.

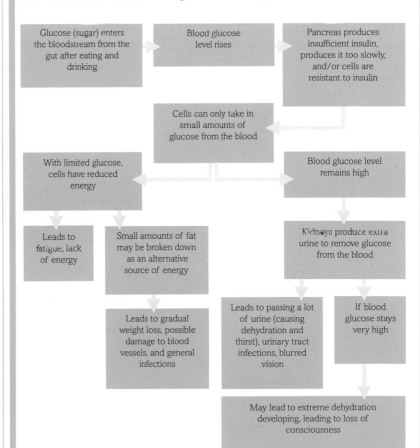

TYPE 2 DIABETES: HOW YOUR BODY USES GLUCOSE

In type 2 diabetes, your pancreas doesn't produce sufficient insulin, produces it too slowly, or your body cells are resistant to it. As the diagram below illustrates, this in turn affects the body's ability to use blood glucose (sugar) properly, resulting in a range of health problems.

Glucose (sugar) enters the bloodstream from the gut after eating and drinking

Blood glucose level rises

Pancreas produces insufficient insulin, produces it too slowly, and/or cells are resistant to insulin

Cells can only take in small amounts of glucose from the blood

With limited glucose, cells have reduced energy

Blood glucose level remains high

Leads to fatigue, lack of energy

Small amounts of fat may be broken down as an alternative source of energy

Kidneys produce extra urine to remove glucose from the blood

Leads to gradual weight loss, possible damage to blood vessels, and general infections

Leads to passing a lot of urine (causing dehydration and thirst), urinary tract infections, blurred vision

If blood glucose stays very high

May lead to extreme dehydration developing, leading to loss of consciousness

"Reduce your weight to a healthy level through regular exercise and diet."

HOW CAN I HELP MYSELF?

Being diagnosed with diabetes is always a shock but it's important to keep things in perspective. There's a lot you can do to help yourself, alongside taking any medication your doctor may prescribe for you.

Lose weight One of the most important things you can to is to reduce your weight to a healthy level through regular exercise and a healthy diet. This will help you to avoid the complications of diabetes. There's plenty advice on healthy eating and losing excess weight on pp52–9.

Control your blood sugar

Keeping blood-sugar levels stable helps the effectiveness of any medication you are taking and reduces the risk of complications. Tips for regulating your blood sugar include:

- Eat regularly – don't go more than four hours between meals
- Choose foods that release their energy slowly (see opposite)
- Avoid high-sugar, high-fat foods such as sweets and pastries
- Be aware that your female hormones, levels of which vary with your menstrual cycle, can affect your blood-sugar control. In particular, you may be more prone to both low blood sugar and raised blood sugar around the time of your period.

Lower your cholesterol level

The risks of high cholesterol levels are discussed in Chapter 7. These risks are much higher for women with diabetes than for men. That makes reducing your levels of cholesterol even more crucial than it is for a man. Fortunately, diet and exercise can make a big difference (see pp52–7).

DIABETES AND PREGNANCY

Pregnancy can cause gestational diabetes. It affects up to one in 25 women. In most cases, you'll need insulin treatment until your baby is born. However, having a history of gestational diabetes increases your risk of developing type 2 diabetes in the future, so you'll probably need a blood test for diabetes once a year for the rest of your life (see also p127).

If you're already taking drugs for type 2 diabetes, you may need to change medication before getting pregnant. Insulin, though, is perfectly safe during pregnancy, and is likely to be recommended as a substitute.

Your abdominal fat (see p322), has a huge impact on your cholesterol levels. Reducing your weight by just 10 per cent can reduce your abdominal fat by a massive 30 per cent. Your doctor may also recommend that you take medicine that will reduce your cholesterol (see p323).

Control your blood pressure

After raised cholesterol, raised blood pressure (see p161) is one of the most important risk factors for heart disease, and particularly for stroke. This is especially true if you have diabetes, so it's crucial to get your blood pressure checked at least twice a year. You may need to take a blood-pressure lowering drug (see p170).

METABOLIC SYNDROME

Also known as insulin resistance syndrome, metabolic syndrome is a cluster of risk factors that significantly increase your risk of both diabetes and heart disease. The problem centres around excess fat that is laid down in the abdominal area. This fat affects the way your body metabolizes fat and sugar. It predisposes you to the following conditions:

- Insulin resistance and diabetes
- Higher levels of "bad" cholesterol, lower levels of "good" cholesterol
- Raised blood pressure.

Metabolic syndrome itself doesn't usually cause any symptoms, but because of the health risks it's important to know if you might be at risk. If you think you might have abdominal obesity (see pp58–9), it is essential to seek medical advice.

Slow energy-release foods

If you have either type of diabetes, controlling your blood glucose (blood sugar) will be much easier if your diet consists mainly of foods that release their energy slowly. These are sometimes called "low GI" foods. Some examples of these foods are shown below.

Pulses

Pulses are the ideal low GI food. They supply a steady release of energy, with protein and plenty of fibre, and are low in fat.

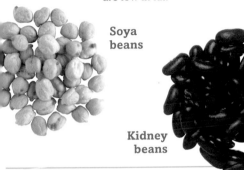

Soya beans

Kidney beans

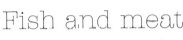

Mackerel

Fish and meat

If you have diabetes you need about 10–15% of your daily calorie intake to be low-fat protein, such as fish and white meat (chicken and turkey).

Sardines

Vegetables

Vitamin-rich vegetables are broken down slowly into glucose by the body, so they supply higher levels of energy for longer. Fresh fruit (not juices) works in a similar way.

Broccoli

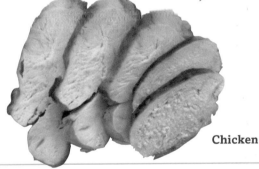

Chicken

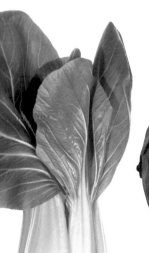

Pak choi

Cabbage

Bread and cereals

White bread and many wheat- or corn-based cereals are high GI: they raise your blood sugar quickly, making it harder to control your overall sugar levels. Whole grain bread and cereals based on whole grains, like oats, are much better.

Rolled oats

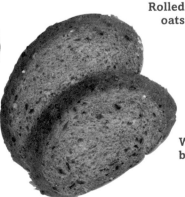

Wholegrain bread

Disorders of the thyroid gland

The hormone thyroxine is produced by the thyroid gland, which is located at the front of your neck. This hormone plays a major part in determining how fast your metabolism (the body's chemical processes) "ticks over". Problems can occur if the body produces either too much or too little of this hormone.

The thyroid gland is one of the main glands in the endocrine system, which helps to regulate the body's energy levels. With up to ten times as many women as men affected by thyroid problems, the thyroid is a gland that every woman should be aware of.

Many of the cells and tissues in our bodies need sufficient amounts of thyroxine if they are to work correctly. If your thyroid gland produces too little thyroxine, many of your body's natural functions slow down; if it produces too much, many aspects of your metabolism speed up. Normally, your body's production of thyroxine is controlled by a feedback mechanism of interacting hormones (see left). Some types of thyroid imbalances are caused by disruption to this process resulting from problems with the pituitary gland.

Disorders of the thyroid gland usually come on slowly, and it is possible to overlook the symptoms for months or even years. However, once your doctor suspects you have a problem with the proper functioning of your thyroid, the initial diagnosis is usually easily made through a blood test. Sometimes further tests may be needed in order to determine the underlying cause of the problem. Once over- or underactivity of the thyroid gland is confirmed, the condition is usually easily treated with drugs, which often produce a rapid improvement in symptoms. Sometimes, however, treatment needs to continue indefinitely.

THYROXINE PRODUCTION

The hypothalamus, situated at the base of the brain just above the pituitary gland, secretes the thyrotropin-releasing hormone (TRH), which triggers the pituitary gland into producing a thyroid-stimulating hormone (TSH). This in turn tells the thyroid gland to start secreting thyroxine into the bloodstream. When levels are high enough, the hypothalamus and pituitary glands reduce their output of TRH and TSH until the thyroxine levels drop again. The hypothalamus, pituitary, and thyroid glands work together to ensure the right levels of thyroxine are produced.

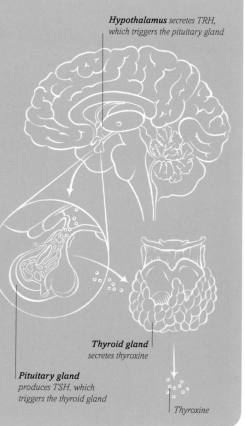

Hypothalamus *secretes TRH, which triggers the pituitary gland*

Thyroid gland *secretes thyroxine*

Pituitary gland *produces TSH, which triggers the thyroid gland*

Thyroxine

Underactive thyroid

This highly treatable condition is ten times more common in women than in men, and particularly affects the over 50s.

WHAT IS IT?

When you have an underactive thyroid (hypothyroidism), it does not produce enough of the hormone thyroxine. This causes a general slowing down of many processes in the body, resulting in many of the symptoms described in the panel (right).

Worldwide, the most common cause of hypothyroidism is a lack of iodine (one of the components of thyroxine) in the diet. In most of the Western world, however, the main cause is inflammation of the thyroid, often caused by an autoimmune response (see p259). It can raise your blood cholesterol and therefore your risk of heart disease.

HYPOTHYROIDISM IN PREGNANCY

It's particularly common for women to develop hypothyroidism in pregnancy – it affects up to one in 40 pregnant women. If it's not treated, it can increase the risk of certain complications of pregnancy, including premature labour, raised blood pressure, anaemia, stillbirth, and serious bleeding after the birth.

This is one of the few types of hypothyroidism that can get better by itself. However, it can recur later in life, so if you've suffered from

---

HAVE I GOT THE SYMPTOMS?

The most common symptoms of hypothyroidism include:
- Tiredness and sleeping longer
- Weight gain without overeating
- Susceptibility to the cold
- Constipation
- Dry skin and coarse hair
- Depression
- Mental slowness
- Fluid retention.

Less common symptoms of the condition include:
- Irregular or heavy periods
- Problems getting pregnant
- Hoarse voice
- Forgetfulness
- Enlargement of the thyroid gland (see Goitre, p329).

See your doctor if you have two or more of these symptoms.

---

hypothyroidism in pregnancy, you should have your thyroid levels checked once a year for the rest of your life.

WHAT NEXT?

Your doctor will arrange for your blood to be tested to check the levels of thyroxine in your body.

MY TREATMENT OPTIONS

Once you're diagnosed with hypothyroidism, you'll be treated with thyroxine tablets. Be sure to discuss any potential side effects with your doctor. You'll probably be

started on a low dose to see how your body responds. The dose may be increased later.

In most cases, you'll be given a blood test every few weeks to check the blood levels of thyroxine. Once your levels are stable, you'll probably only need a blood test every year or so, but in most cases you'll need treatment for life.

HOW CAN I HELP MYSELF?

Follow your doctor's advice on your medication programme, and make sure you have a healthy lifestyle (see Chapter 3, pp48–69).

AM I AT RISK?

Apart from being a woman, risk factors for hypothyroidism include:
- Being over 50 years old
- Pregnancy
- A history of hypothyroidism in the family
- A history of an overactive thyroid gland (see pp328–9) due to an autoimmune cause
- Having another autoimmune disease (see p259)
- Having certain inherited conditions, such as Down's syndrome or Turner's syndrome
- Taking certain medications such as amiodarone (to treat heart rhythm disorders) and lithium (to treat bipolar disorder).

Overactive thyroid

Hyperthyroidism, or an overactive thyroid gland, is also known as thyrotoxicosis. It affects about ten times more women than men. This manageable condition is most likely to develop between the ages of 20 and 40.

WHAT IS IT?

Hyperthyroidism affects up to one in 50 women. In up to four out of five of those women affected, the malfunction of the thyroid gland has an autoimmune cause, in which the body's antibodies stimulate excessive production of thyroxine. Graves' disease (see opposite) is a common cause of overactivity of the thyroid gland.

The course of hyperthyroidism is highly variable. In many of those affected, the condition settles by itself within one and half to two years. If this happens in your case, you'll still need to make sure you get your thyroid function checked regularly, since the condition can recur. However, for others, treatment needs to continue for many years.

WHAT NEXT?

Hyperthyroidism is diagnosed with blood tests to check your body's levels of thyroxine (which are high in hyperthyroidism) and TSH (which are low). Sometimes, hyperthyroidism is associated with an irregular swelling of the thyroid gland (see Goitre, opposite), in which case you may be sent for an ultrasound of your thyroid gland.

MY TREATMENT OPTIONS

You'll need to be referred to a specialist at the hospital to discuss the options. Your doctor will suggest

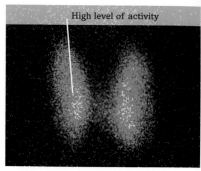

High level of activity

Scan of a normal thyroid gland
This scintogram shows hormone-producing activity in a healthy thyroid gland. The bright green areas are the most active, the blue areas are the least active.

one of several treatments to stop your body from producing too much thyroxine. These include:
- Medication
- Surgery
- Radioactive iodine.

Each of these treatments is appropriate in different circumstances, and each has its pros and cons. Your doctor will work with you to choose the best treatment for your circumstances; be sure to discuss any side effects.

Medication The most common antithyroid medication used in the UK is carbimazole. This takes four to eight weeks to work, because it cuts down the amount of thyroxine your body makes, but doesn't affect the thyroxine your body has already stored.

While you're waiting for the carbimazole to take effect, you may need to take other drugs, such as beta blockers, to help control your symptoms. You'll also need to seek urgent medical advice if you develop any other symptoms of infection, such as a fever or sore

> "1 in 50 women develops overactivity of the thyroid gland."

HAVE I GOT THE SYMPTOMS?

Symptoms of hyperthyroidism may include some or all of the following:
- Irritability and anxiety
- Weight loss, despite increased appetite
- Poor sleep
- Palpitations
- Diarrhoea
- Shortness of breath
- Light or absent periods
- Tremor (especially of the hands)
- Dislike of heat, and excess sweating
- Itching
- Thinning of the hair or patchy hair loss
- Enlarged thyroid gland (called a goitre), causing a visible swelling in the throat
- Bulging eyes.

See your doctor if you have two or more of the above symptoms.

GRAVES' DISEASE

This is an autoimmune disease that accounts for at least two thirds of cases of hyperthyroidism. The condition occurs when your body starts producing antibodies that stimulate your pituitary gland to produce TSH, even when your body's levels of thyroxine are normal or high. About half of those who have Graves' disease develop prominent, bulging eyes, dryness and soreness of the eyes, and/or double vision. Unfortunately, lowering your thyroid levels doesn't reverse the eye changes. Some people notice the onset of eye symptoms even after starting treatment for the disease.

For most people affected, using artificial tears, wearing sunglasses, and using eye protectors when asleep control the symptoms adequately. However, if you have severe eye changes, you'll need to have regular checks in hospital. Sometimes fatty tissue builds up behind the eyeballs, and this may need to be removed by surgery. Alternatively, your specialist may recommend X-ray therapy or steroid tablets.

throat. This is because very occasionally (in less than one in 200 people taking it), carbimazole can adversely affect the white blood cells in your blood, which help to combat infection. After about 12–18 months, your doctor will probably recommend tailing off your dose of carbimazole to find out if your condition has settled on its own. However, you may need to take further courses of the drug in the future if the condition flares up again. If the condition doesn't correct itself naturally, your doctor may suggest one of the other recommended treatment options.

Surgery Some kinds of hyperthyroidism cause a large swelling of your thyroid, called a goitre (see below). In these cases, surgery, which has a 98 per cent success rate, is an option. There is a small risk of complications, such as bleeding and problems with your vocal cords. It's also common to develop hypothyroidism after surgery, but this can be treated in the same way as other causes of hypothyroidism.

Radioactive iodine In this form of treatment, you simply swallow a liquid or capsule of radioactive iodine. The radioactive iodine concentrates in your thyroid gland, reducing its ability to make thyroxine. One treatment is usually sufficient to improve your symptoms. In the long term, between half and three quarters of those treated with radioactive iodine develop hypothyroidism, but this is easily treated with supplements of thyroxine.

HOW CAN I HELP MYSELF?

There is no specific self-help advice for those who have an overactive thyroid gland. Be sure to follow the treatment programme prescribed by your doctor and be vigilant for any complications.

GOITRE

A goitre (swollen thyroid gland) in the throat can range in size from a small lump to a large swelling. It indicates an under- or overactive thyroid.

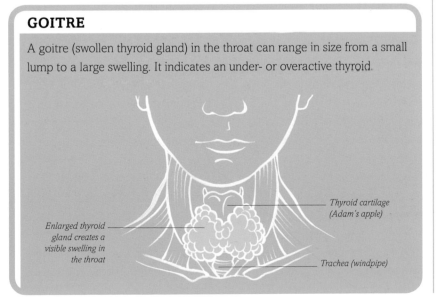

Enlarged thyroid gland creates a visible swelling in the throat

Thyroid cartilage (Adam's apple)

Trachea (windpipe)

Disorders of other glands

The parathyroid, pituitary, and adrenal glands may be less well known than some other hormone-producing glands, such as the thyroid gland, but the hormones they produce are nevertheless vital. Over- or underproduction of any of these hormones can occur, but fortunately such conditions are rare.

Parathyroid gland disorders

Situated in the neck behind the thyroid gland, the parathyroid gland produces parathyroid hormone. Sometimes too much is produced (hyperparathyroidism), or too little (hypoparathyroidism).

WHAT IS IT?

Parathyroid hormone determines the calcium levels in your body. Overproduction can lead to excess calcium in the blood, which can cause the formation of calcium-rich "stones" in the kidneys (see pp346–7) and fragile bones.

WHAT NEXT?

You may need a blood test to check your levels of parathyroid hormone.

MY TREATMENT OPTIONS

Parathyroid underactivity is treated with surgery to remove excess glandular tissue, while overactivity of the gland is usually treated with dietary supplements of calcium and vitamin D.

HOW CAN I HELP MYSELF?

There is no self-help advised to complement medical treatment.

HAVE I GOT THE SYMPTOMS?

An overactive parathyroid gland may cause:
- Abdominal pain,
- Nausea
- Constipation
- Loss of appetite and weight
- Tiredness and depression.

An underactive parathyroid gland may cause:
- Muscle spasm
- Numbness or tingling.

See your doctor if you have any of the above symptoms.

Pituitary gland disorders

HAVE I GOT THE SYMPTOMS?

A problem with the pituitary gland can cause a wide variety of different symptoms that can include:
- Headaches
- Disturbances in vision
- New onset squint
- Irregular periods.

See your doctor if you have any of the above symptoms.

The tiny pituitary gland is situated deep inside the brain. It is often called the master gland because the hormones it releases govern many different body processes. Many of these hormones regulate the levels of other hormones in the body. For example, it produces adrenal cortical stimulating hormone (ACTH), which acts on the adrenal glands (see opposite). The pituitary gland also produces several hormones involved in the reproductive processes.

WHAT IS IT?

Pituitary gland disorders are rare. Growths may, however, occur within the gland. Such tumours may be benign (non-cancerous) or malignant (cancerous), but either type can make the gland grow, leading to pressure on surrounding parts of the brain.

One of the most common effects of a pituitary tumour is that too much prolactin – the milk-producing hormone – is produced. The result of this is that women who aren't pregnant produce milk as though they were.

WHAT NEXT?

If your doctor suspects a pituitary gland problem from an account of your symptoms, the diagnosis can be confirmed by blood tests and possibly MRI or CT scans. In some cases you could be asked to undergo tests on your field of vision, if a tumour is thought to be creating pressure on the part of the brain that governs vision.

MY TREATMENT OPTIONS

Tumours of the pituitary gland are commonly treated with surgery and radiation (X-rays). Many pituitary tumours can be treated with drugs.

HOW CAN I HELP MYSELF?

There are no adjustments to your lifestyle that can prevent or treat pituitary problems.

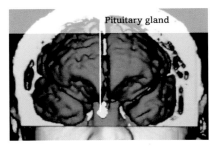

Pituitary gland

Pituitary gland
The location of the pituitary gland in the brain, as shown on a coloured 3-D CT scan. The gland is about the size of a pea.

Adrenal gland disorders

The adrenal glands produce corticosteroids (often called steroids), which help to maintain muscle and fat structure and fluid balance, as well as influencing blood pressure, blood-sugar levels, and bone density.

WHAT IS IT?

Adrenal gland disorders include:
Cushing's disease This results from excess production of corticosteroid hormones by the pituitary gland. It may be caused by a tumour.
Addison's disease This is usually the result of an autoimmune problem (see p266) and causes adrenal underactivity.

WHAT NEXT?

Levels of adrenal hormones can be assessed through a blood test. Further tests may then be needed.

HAVE I GOT THE SYMPTOMS?

Cushing's disease may cause symptoms that include:
- Weight gain around the abdomen
- Reddening and rounding of the face
- Increased hairiness of the face and body.

Addison's disease may cause:
- Tiredness
- Weight loss
- Irregular periods.

See your doctor if you have any of the above symptoms.

STEROIDS – THE RISKS FOR WOMEN

Steroid drugs are given by mouth to treat a wide variety of medical problems. But high levels of steroids in your body, especially over more than a few months, can bring a variety of unwanted effects and make you prone to:
- High blood pressure
- Raised blood sugar (see Diabetes, pp322–5)
- Wasting of the muscles of the arms and legs
- Easy bruising
- Thinning of the skin and stretch marks
- Laying down of fat around the stomach
- Filling out of the cheeks, resulting in a "moon faced" appearance
- Frequent infections of all kinds.

In addition, prolonged steroid treatment makes you more prone to osteoporosis (see pp260–2). If you have to take steroid tablets in the long term, talk to your doctor about measures to prevent osteoporosis.

MY TREATMENT OPTIONS

Treatment for Cushing's disease may involve surgery to remove excess adrenal tissue. Steroid tablets are usually given for Addison's disease.

HOW CAN I HELP MYSELF?

Follow the treatment programme prescribed by your doctor.

Bladder and urinary tract

Miss Tamsin Greenwell MD FRCS (Urol)

Bladder & urinary tract

Your urinary tract consists of a pair of kidneys, a pair of ureters, a bladder, and a urethra. Its main functions are to get rid of the waste products that accumulate in your body, regulate water levels, and make sure your bodily fluids are kept in balance. The key organs are the kidneys, which actually carry out the process of filtering out wastes and excess water from the blood to produce urine. The urine then flows down the ureters to the bladder and is passed out of the body through the urethra.

THE FEMALE URINARY SYSTEM

Your kidneys are situated on either side of the spine, at the back of the abdomen just below the diaphragm. Each adult kidney is a reddish-brown bean-shaped organ about 12cm (4¾in) long and 7cm (2¾in) wide. Each kidney is connected to a ureter, a muscular tube about 25cm (10in) long that carries urine to the bladder. Essentially a muscular bag, the bladder stores urine until it is passed out of the body through the urethra, a tube about 4cm (1½in) long.

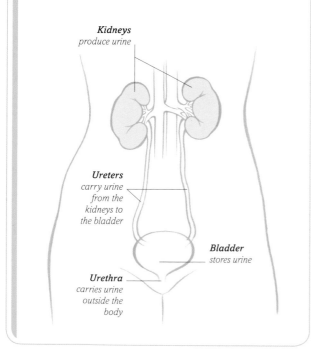

Kidneys
produce urine

Ureters
carry urine from the kidneys to the bladder

Bladder
stores urine

Urethra
carries urine outside the body

THE URINARY TRACT

Your kidneys are designed to filter your blood but they do so selectively, removing waste products and excess water but retaining useful substances, such as glucose (blood sugar). (The liver has a similar waste-removal function, but it removes different waste products.) The filtered waste products and water are what make up your urine. Together, the kidneys produce a minimum of 30ml (1fl oz) of urine every hour, and this amount increases the more you drink. By regulating the amount of water lost from the body in the urine your kidneys keep your body fluids balanced so you don't get dehydrated or overhydrated. Your kidneys also play an important role in the production of red blood cells and in making vitamin D. If your kidneys stop working, you will become overloaded with fluid, anaemic, and be very ill due to the build-up of waste products in your body. You may also develop other problems, such as high blood pressure and osteoporosis (thinning of the bones).

The ureters are muscular tubes that carry (in fact, they squeeze) the urine from your kidneys into your bladder. They run alongside the bones of your spine and then turn inwards at the level of your pelvis to pass obliquely into your bladder. The tunnel formed by the oblique passage of the ureters acts as a one-way valve. This stops urine flowing back up into the kidneys when your bladder contracts to empty out the urine.

The bladder is a muscular bag that is lined with specialized waterproofed cells. It is designed to store urine and to let it out when required. Usually we pass about 450–500ml (14–18fl oz) each time, although this varies according to how big you are – small people have smaller bladders! It's normal to pass urine about every four hours during the day, but this becomes more frequent the more you drink and even more frequent if you drink diuretic fluids (fluids that increase urine flow), such as alcohol (and coffee and tea in excess). Before you are 50 years old, it isn't normal to have to get up to go to the toilet during the night, but as you get older it becomes increasingly common. In fact, it is considered normal to get up in the night once in your 50s, twice in your 60s, and three times in your 70s.

DIFFERENCES BETWEEN WOMEN AND MEN

Up to the bladder, the urinary tracts of men and women are the same. It is the structure beyond that point – the urethra, which carries urine from the bladder to outside the body – that differs. In women, the urethra is relatively short – about 4cm (1½in) long – and is surrounded by a muscle called the urethral sphincter. It passes into the front wall of the vagina and exits in the midline between the clitoris and vagina.

In men, the urethra is longer – about 25cm (10in) long – and S-shaped. It has a sphincter (ring of muscle) both where it joins the bladder and below the prostate gland, and passes through the penis. Both ejaculate (the fluid produced by men during orgasm) and urine leave the body via the urethra.

DISORDERS OF THE URINARY TRACT

The most common urological disorders that affect women are urinary tract infection (cystitis), kidney infections (pyelonephritis), urinary incontinence, and bladder pain syndrome. Other conditions include urinary tract cancers, especially those of the bladder and kidneys, and stones in the urinary tract.

> "Your kidneys not only remove waste products and excess water from the body, but also help in the production of red blood cells."

KIDNEY CROSS-SECTION

The kidney has an outer cortex that filters blood to produce urine, which passes into the medulla, then the pelvis, and then out through the ureter.

Cortex *produces urine*

Medulla *collects urine from the cortex*

Pelvis *collects urine from the medulla*

Renal artery *brings blood to the kidney*

Renal vein *takes blood from the kidney*

Ureter *carries urine to the bladder*

FEMALE AND MALE URETHRAS

The female urethra runs from the bladder to leave the body between the vaginal opening and the clitoris. The male urethra runs from the bladder, through the prostate gland, and exits via the penis.

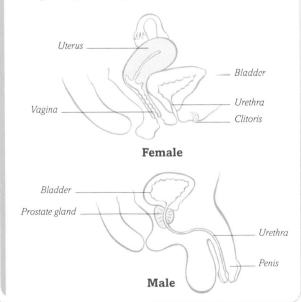

Uterus

Bladder

Vagina

Urethra

Clitoris

Female

Bladder

Prostate gland

Urethra

Penis

Male

Urinary tract infection

About half of all women get a urinary tract infection (UTI) at least once in their lives, and some women suffer repeated infections. However, it is usually easily treated with a short course of antibiotics. You will only need further investigation and treatment if you keep getting infections.

HAVE I GOT THE SYMPTOMS?

The most common symptoms of UTI are a sudden onset of:
- Burning pain when you pass urine
- Needing to pass urine very frequently
- Passing only small amounts of urine
- Difficulty in delaying urination
- Blood in urine
- Pain or discomfort just above your pubic bone.

See your doctor if your UTI doesn't clear up using self-help measures (see What Next?, right). Seek urgent medical help if you think that you might have PN (see p338).

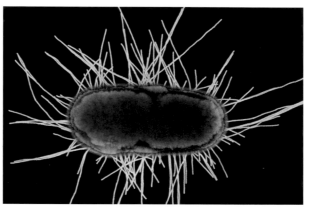

E. coli bacterium
This usually harmless inhabitant of the intestine is the cause of most urinary tract infections.

WHAT IS IT?

The term "UTI" is usually used to refer to cystitis (a bacterial infection of the bladder), but it may be used to talk about an infection anywhere in your urinary tract, from your kidneys to your urethra. Urine is normally sterile so the presence of any bacteria in it is abnormal. A UTI is diagnosed when the urine contains a significant number of bacteria. The bacteria – usually the ones living in your intestine, such as *Escherichia coli* (usually known simply as *E. coli*) – may enter your urinary tract through your urethra. This most commonly happens during sex.

WHAT NEXT?

When you first develop symptoms, you should increase the amount you drink – try drinking 600ml (1 pint) of water immediately, then 300ml (10 fl oz) every 30 minutes. This will increase your production of urine and the number of times you pass urine.

If you have mild UTI, there's a good chance it will then clear up within a few days. You should also avoid having sex until the infection has cleared up.

If your symptoms persist for longer than a few days, you should see your doctor. He or she will test your urine for infection, either with a urine dipstick test or by sending a sample to the laboratory for a culture test to see if there's any infection present.

If there's a delay before you can see the doctor, then you can try over-the-counter urine alkalizers, such as potassium citrate and

> "Eating live yoghurt can help to encourage more 'friendly' bacteria into your intestine, reducing the chance of getting a UTI."

sodium citrate, and painkillers such as ibuprofen to help relieve symptoms. A word of caution, though. If you're pregnant, breast-feeding, or are taking any other medications, ask your doctor or pharmacist before trying these over-the-counter remedies.

If your UTI doesn't respond to treatment, or it recurs more than three times in six months, then your doctor will refer you to an urologist for further investigation.

MY TREATMENT OPTIONS

If your infection hasn't cleared up by itself or with self-help measures (see right), your doctor will probably prescribe medication.
Medication Your doctor will prescribe a short (3–5 day) course of antibiotics. Ask your doctor about any side effects and make sure you tell him or her if you are pregnant or breast-feeding.

Further treatment If your UTI recurs, your doctor may prescribe for you a six-week course of vaginal oestrogen cream or pessaries plus a further course of antibiotics.

For some women who suffer from recurrent UTIs, the doctor may recommend dilation (stretching) of the urethra to help with emptying the bladder, a month-long course of antibiotics together with a short course to treat your partner, or a course of six weekly instillations of sodium hyaluronate (Cystistat) into your bladder to improve the protective layers of the lining of the bladder (see also p344).

HOW CAN I HELP MYSELF?

To help prevent a UTI:
Drink more Increase your fluid intake to 1.5–2 litres (about 2½–3½ pints) per day.
Sex Make sure you pass urine within about an hour of sex, to flush out any bacteria.
Contraception Avoid using spermicidal gel.
Drink cranberry juice A large glass of cranberry juice per day may reduce the number of UTIs you have if you get them often.
Eat yoghurt Eating a pot of live yogurt once a day encourages the replacement of the aggressive bacteria in the intestine with more "friendly" bacteria.

AM I AT RISK?

All women are at risk of UTI because they have relatively short urethras (see p335), but you may be at risk if:
- You are sexually active
- You use spermicidal gel as part of contraception
- You are pregnant
- You are postmenopausal
- You have problems with urinary incontinence (see pp339–41)
- You have a family history of UTIs.

DEALING WITH AN ACUTE ATTACK OF UTI

If you are suffering from an acute attack of UTI, even if it's during the night, then try the following:
- Immediately drink 600ml (1 pint) of water, then drink 300ml (10fl oz) every 30 minutes
- If you're in pain, fill two hot water bottles, wrap them in towels, and put one on your lower back and one between your thighs
- Mix 1 teaspoon of bicarbonate of soda with some water and drink it; repeat every three hours. If you have high blood pressure, you should talk to your doctor before you take bicarbonate of soda. Alternatively, if you've had UTI attacks in the past, keep a supply of cystitis-relief sachets

from your pharmacist at home and take one as soon as an episode starts
- Take one or two painkillers, such as ibuprofen, to help with the pain. However, if you are pregnant, you should talk to your doctor before taking any painkillers
- Try to relax by reading or watching TV, either in bed or in a comfortable armchair.

You may find that the symptoms start to subside after about three hours of this routine, but you should see your doctor if the attack continues for longer than a day, if you're pregnant, or if you notice any blood in your urine.

Pyelonephritis

Painful urination, together with intense pain in your lower back, could mean you have the common kidney disorder known as pyelonephritis (PN). This condition is usually treated easily and can clear up in a few days. But prompt attention is needed, as untreated pyelonephritis can lead to kidney damage.

WHAT IS IT?

PN, which is an inflammation of one or both of kidneys, is usually caused by a bacterial infection. The disorder often follows on from a urinary tract infection (see pp336–7). More rarely, pyelonephritis may occur if there is a blockage in the urinary tract, such as a kidney stone (see pp346–7). Occasionally, PN can become a long-term disorder, especially if it is associated with abnormalities of the bladder. Recurring inflammation (chronic PN) can result in scarring of the kidney tissues and possibly kidney failure later on.

WHAT NEXT?

If you have the symptoms of PN, consult your doctor the same day. He or she will test your urine for an infection and start treatment (see below). If PN persists, your doctor will refer you to an urologist. This specialist may carry out blood tests, an ultrasound scan of your kidneys, and a micturating cystourethrogram (MCUG), a test which checks for backflow of urine from the bladder to the kidneys.

MY TREATMENT OPTIONS

PN needs immediate treatment to prevent kidney damage.

Medication A 7–14 day course of antibiotics is usually effective in clearing the infection. Ask your doctor about possible side effects.

Hospital If you are very unwell, you may be admitted to hospital for emergency treatment with intravenous antibiotics.

HOW CAN I HELP MYSELF?

If you develop the symptoms of PN, start drinking plenty of water. For long-term protection, you need to drink at least 1.5–2 litres (2½–3½ pints) a day – more in hot weather or if you are particularly active.

Drink cranberry juice In people who suffer from recurrent PN, drinking a large glass (over 350 ml/12fl oz) of cranberry juice per day may reduce the frequency of attacks.

HAVE I GOT THE SYMPTOMS?

The symptoms of PN tend to appear suddenly and include:
- Intense pain in your back or side, or the area of your waist
- Fever
- Uncontrollable shivering
- Nausea and vomiting
- Blood in your urine
- Strong-smelling urine
- Pain when you pass urine
- Increased frequency of passing urine.

See your doctor immediately if you think you have PN. It is important not to delay treatment.

AM I AT RISK?

Women are more likely to get pyelonephritis than men, because bacteria can travel rapidly up their shorter urethras. If you suffer from a malformation of the ureter that allows urine backflow, then you are at a significantly increased risk.

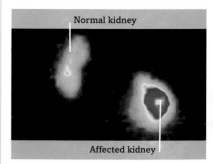

Normal kidney

Affected kidney

Pyelonephritis
This scan shows the inflamed area (red) in a kidney affected by PN. Recurrent and/or prolonged PN may cause serious damage.

Urinary incontinence

The loss of bladder control – urinary incontinence (UI) – is extremely common in women, yet many are too embarrassed to talk to anyone about it. Left untreated, UI can seriously affect your quality of life, but there's no need to suffer in silence, there are many effective treatments available.

HAVE I GOT THE SYMPTOMS?

The most common symptoms of urinary incontinence are:

- Involuntary leakage of urine following a cough, sneeze, or during strenuous exercise
- Frequent, sudden urges to pass urine
- Difficulty in delaying urination
- Complete inability to control urination once the flow of urine has started.

See your doctor as soon as possible if you think that you may have UI.

WHAT IS IT?

Urinary incontinence (UI) is the involuntary loss of urine from the bladder. This very common problem affects between 25 and 45 per cent of women of all ages.

There are different types of UI, which occur for a variety of reasons. These include:

Stress incontinence Leakage of small amounts of urine when you cough, sneeze, or exercise. This is the most common type of UI. It is caused by weak pelvic floor muscles failing to hold the bladder in the correct position. Stress incontinence may follow pregnancy or pelvic surgery, or occur in older women who have lost muscle tone.

Urge incontinence The sudden urge to pass urine, often followed by uncontrollable emptying of the bladder. In most cases, urge incontinence occurs without any identifiable underlying cause.

Mixed incontinence This disorder is a combination of urge and stress incontinence.

Overflow incontinence When blockage effectively prevents normal urination, so urine continually overflows.

Vesicovaginal fistula An abnormal connection between the bladder and vagina which allows

SOME COMMON TYPES OF UI

Urge incontinence, the feeling that you won't "make it" to the toilet in time, is caused by uncontrollable contractions of the bladder muscles. This is usually because the bladder wall has become overactive. Stress incontinence, the involuntary leakage of urine when you cough, sneeze, or exercise, is the result of weak pelvic floor muscles. Lack of support causes the neck of the bladder to sag down, which makes it impossible for the muscles that control urine flow to close properly.

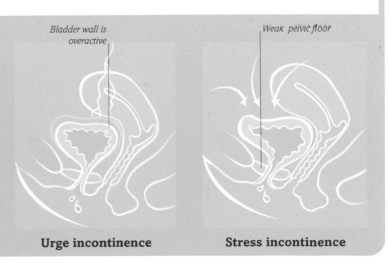

Bladder wall is overactive

Weak pelvic floor

Urge incontinence

Stress incontinence

> "There are a number of excellent treatments
> available that can either greatly improve or
> even cure urinary incontinence."

AM I AT RISK?

There a number of risk factors for developing stress UI:

- Pregnancy and childbirth, with each pregnancy increasing the risk
- Family history of stress UI
- Surgery to the lower spine or in the pelvic area
- Hysterectomy.

You may be at increased risk of urge UI if you are:

- Past the menopause
- Suffer from diabetes mellitus (see pp320–5).

If you do develop mild UI it may be made worse by:

- Smoking
- Drinking alcohol or caffeinated drinks
- Taking sleeping tablets and sedatives
- Taking diuretic medication to treat high blood pressure.

urine to escape into the vagina. A fistula may be caused by injury (during childbirth or surgery) or disease.

WHAT NEXT?

If you develop UI you should see your doctor to discuss the problem. Don't let embarrassment prevent you from getting the help you need. Your doctor will assess the type and severity of your incontinence and check for any associated symptoms that may need further investigation. You may be referred to a continence therapist, who will examine your abdomen and do an internal examination to assess the strength of your pelvic floor muscles. He or she may carry out tests to measure the flow-rate of your urine and to check whether you are completely emptying your bladder. You may also have an ultrasound scan of your bladder, and a sample of your urine may be tested for evidence of bleeding or infection.

MY TREATMENT OPTIONS

Treatment depends on what type of UI you have. Some options involve surgery. Your doctor will be able to advise you on the relative effectiveness and possible side effects, if any, of each treatment. To treat stress UI:

Pelvic floor exercises The initial treatment for all uncomplicated stress UI is 3 months of regular pelvic floor exercises (see right).

Injections A silicone paste is injected into the bladder neck to bulk up the tissues and improve closure of the outlet.

Tension-free vaginal tape A piece of special tape is placed around your urethra. Insertion of the tape involves a relatively simple operation that may be carried out under local anaesthetic.

Pubovaginal sling In this operation, tissue from another part of the body, such as the abdomen, is wrapped around the neck of the bladder to form a supporting sling.

Colposuspension This operation involves lifting up the vagina and attaching it behind your pubic bone.

PELVIC FLOOR MUSCLES

The pelvic floor muscles act as a supportive sling that holds the bladder, vagina, uterus, and rectum in place. Loss of muscle tone, often due to overstretching during childbirth but also because of ageing, can cause the pelvic floor to become slack. If this happens, the pelvic organs sag down, and problems such as incontinence occur. Exercises can help to restore the strength of the pelvic floor muscles (see opposite).

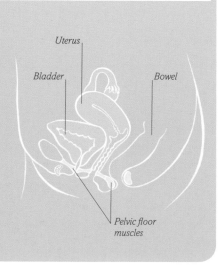

Uterus

Bladder

Bowel

Pelvic floor
muscles

PELVIC FLOOR EXERCISES

Also sometimes called Kegel exercises, pelvic floor exercises help to strengthen the muscles and tighten the ligaments at the base of the abdomen. This is a proven method of helping to reduce stress urinary incontinence (SUI), although there is less evidence that it helps with urge incontinence.

Pelvic floor exercises can be done standing, sitting, or lying down and don't need any special equipment, although some women find that using a vaginal cone (a small weight shaped like a tampon that is placed in the vagina) is helpful. The exercises should be done every day, and it may take several months before you notice any benefit. To perform pelvic floor exercises, you should do the following:

Identify the muscles Tighten the muscles around your vagina and anus and lift upwards and inwards. Alternatively, try to stop the flow of urine when you are on the toilet. To check you're using the right muscles, put two fingers in your vagina when trying to tighten the muscles; you should feel a gentle squeeze.

Contract the muscles Having found the right muscles, you need to carry out both fast and slow contractions.

Ideally, you should do a set of slow contractions, plus a set of fast contractions, six times every day. Some women find that using biofeedback while doing the exercises helps them make sure the correct muscles are being used. The exercises should not be done while passing urine as this may lead to urinary retention.

To do slow contractions, slowly tighten the pelvic floor muscles to a count of 10, hold them contracted for 10 seconds, then relax and rest for 10 seconds. Do this sequence 10 times to complete one set.

To do fast contractions, tighten your pelvic floor muscles quickly, hold them contracted for one second, then relax and rest for one second. Do this sequence 10 times to complete one set.

Alternatives to pelvic floor exercises Some people have found that electrical stimulation helps to improve bladder control. A probe is inserted into your vagina to the muscles around the bladder and a weak electric current is passed through the probe. This causes a tingling sensation but is not painful. It may take daily sessions of up to an hour each for several months to produce noticeable results.

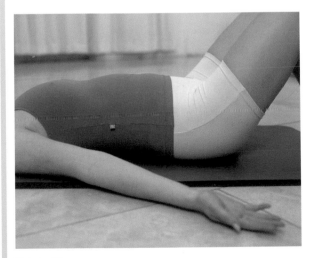

Pelvic tilts
Step 1 This simple exercise is another way to strengthen your pelvic floor muscles, while also toning your lower abdominal muscles. Lie on your back, and take a big breath in.

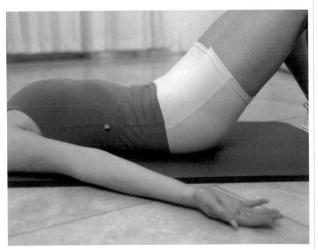

Step 2 Breathe out, squeeze your pelvic floor muscles and draw your lower abdominal muscles towards your spine – think "navel to spine" – as you curl your buttocks slightly off the floor. Keep your buttocks relaxed. Repeat 5–10 times.

The top of the vagina stretches across the bladder opening to form a sling.

Artificial urinary sphincter Used only as a last resort, this method employs an inflatable cuff that wraps around the neck of the bladder to keep it closed. This is connected to a pressure-regulating balloon placed in the abdominal cavity and a tiny pump implanted in the labia majora. Pressing the pump with a finger releases the cuff to let urine flow out.

To treat urge UI:

Bladder training The initial treatment is bladder training (see below) with some lifestyle changes.

Medication Your doctor may give you antimuscarinic tablets, which help reduce involuntary contractions in the bladder muscles. If these don't work or you can't tolerate the side effects you'll be referred to a specialist for further treatment.

Botulinum toxin (Botox) injections Injected into the lining of your bladder, these drugs block muscle contractions.

Sacral neuromodulation An implant is inserted near to your bladder. This sends out mild electrical impulses that stimulate the nerves to the bladder and give you better bladder control.

Clam cystoplasty A patch of tissue taken from the intestine is inserted into the bladder to lessen the impact of muscle contractions.

HOW CAN I HELP MYSELF?

If you have a mild form of UI, there are a number of self-help measures that you can take to improve your condition:

> "Practising pelvic floor exercises regularly, stopping smoking, and eating a healthy diet may help to prevent urinary incontinence."

Adjust your lifestyle Eat plenty of fibre-rich foods, such as bran, wholemeal bread, wholegrain cereals, fruit, leafy vegetables, beans, and lentils, and keep active to prevent constipation (see also pp52–7). Straining the bowels puts stress on the pelvic muscles.

Drink more To stop your urine becoming too concentrated and irritating the bladder, aim to drink about 1.5–2 litres (2½–3½ pints) of fluid a day.

Cut down on caffeine and carbonated drinks Reduce or eliminate these types of drinks as they tend to overstimulate both the bladder and the kidneys.

Stop smoking This irritates the bladder lining and makes UI worse.

BLADDER TRAINING

If you suffer from urge incontinence, you may be able to improve your bladder control with a method known as bladder training. This technique needs perseverance – you will not see results overnight – but many women find it very effective.

Set times Bladder training involves visiting the toilet only at fixed intervals. The idea is to train yourself to delay emptying your bladder for gradually extended periods.

Starting with an empty bladder, decide on an interval during which

you will resist the urge to urinate. At first, try to "hold on" for five minutes before going to the toilet. When you can manage this, gradually extend the interval – to 10 minutes, 15 minutes and so on – until you can delay urinating for three or four hours. At first, leakages will be inevitable, but as your bladder is re-educated, these will occur less often. It may take several weeks, or even months, to achieve your goal.

Distraction techniques You can try various ploys to keep your mind off

wanting to "go" during intervals between toilet visits. Some women use relaxation techniques, such as deep breathing, to control their urges. You could also take the opportunity to do some pelvic floor exercises to help things along.

Getting help Your doctor or incontinence nurse will help you to work out a personal bladder training schedule. They will probably suggest that you monitor your progress by keeping a diary of both successes and leakages.

Bladder pain syndrome

This long-term bladder problem causes pain in the lower part of the abdomen and a frequent urge to pass urine. As these symptoms are shared by various other urinary tract disorders, such as cystitis, bladder pain syndrome is difficult to diagnose. Treatment is aimed at relieving discomfort, rather than cure.

HAVE I GOT THE SYMPTOMS?

The symptoms of bladder pain syndrome vary from person to person, but the most common are a sudden or gradual onset of:

- Pain on passing urine
- Increased frequency of urination
- Pain, sometimes severe, in the lower abdominal area, just above the pubic bone
- Blood in the urine
- Pain or discomfort felt in the urethra or vagina
- Pain during sexual intercourse

See your doctor as soon as possible if you experience any of the above symptoms.

WHAT IS IT?

Bladder pain syndrome (BPS) generally refers to a collection of symptoms affecting the pelvic area. The disorder is also known as bacterial cystitis, interstitial cystitis, chronic pelvic pain syndrome, and painful bladder syndrome. Its symptoms are similar to those of some UTIs (see p336), but bacteria aren't involved.

Little is known about the causes of BPS, but it's thought to occur as a result of a severe bacterial infection. The bladder has a coating of mucus to protect it, and the joins between the cells of the bladder lining are very tight to prevent urine damage. Sometimes these defences are damaged by a UTI and then urine will inflame and irritate the wall of the bladder.

WHAT NEXT?

If you develop symptoms of BPS you should see your doctor who will send a urine sample to the laboratory for testing to exclude infection and cancer, and to look for cells in the urine, such as white blood cells, which indicate inflammation. If your samples don't grow any bacteria, you will be sent to an urologist for further examination. He or she will examine your abdomen and pelvis, and perform an internal vaginal examination to ensure that there aren't any other possible causes for your symptoms.

The urologist will also send a urine sample to look for cancer cells, and a blood sample to check you are not diabetic and have normal kidney function. You will also have an X ray, an ultrasound scan of your urinary tract, and an ultrasound scan of your bladder after you have passed urine to ensure you have no other urinary problems. You will be asked to keep a diary to see how often you pass urine and how much you pass.

MY TREATMENT OPTIONS

There are many treatments available – each having about a 50 per cent success rate. Your doctor

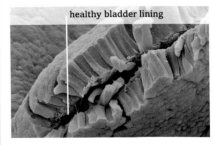

healthy bladder lining

The lining of the bladder
A section of the lining of a healthy bladder. The cells are very tightly packed to prevent damage from the urine.

> "Stress may aggravate your symptoms so try and make sure you have plenty of relaxation time in your life."

> **"A number of treatments are often used at the same time to tackle successfully the different symptoms associated with bladder pain."**

will work with you to find the best treatment for you personally. Ask your doctor about any side effects if you are prescribed medication.

Tests The initial treatment is, while you are anaesthetized, to look into your bladder via your urethra with a cystoscope – a type of viewing instrument. The doctor may gently stretch your bladder by filling it with sterile liquid to see how much fluid it will hold, to see whether there are any signs of discomfort, and to look for evidence of inflammation when your bladder is emptied after the gentle stretch. The doctor may also take a biopsy of your bladder to rule out cancer and to look for inflammatory cells, and may also gently stretch your urethra. If you have urethral discomfort, the doctor may also inject a local anaesthetic and steroid around your urethra. This procedure is performed primarily for diagnosis but provides 6–12 months' relief of symptoms in about 50 per cent of women. You'll be reviewed about six weeks afterwards to see how you are – and additional treatment will be started as required.

Medication If you still have symptoms then antihistamine medication will be started for a minimum of six weeks to reduce the inflammation in your bladder. If this fails, or simultaneously, you

may also be given a nerve-blocking painkiller along with an anti-inflammatory painkiller. If frequent urination is a particular problem, antimuscarinic tablets are added. You may be also given antibiotics to try to eliminate any bacteria that may be present and contributing to the BPS.

Pain specialist You may be referred to a pain specialist. He or she will help to manage the pain with strong nerve-blocking painkillers, intravenous lidocaine injections, local and spinal nerve-block injections, and superficial neuromodulation (TENS). This uses electrical stimulation to confuse nerves into not sending pain signals. If your pain is very bad, the specialist may also involve a psychologist, who can offer you techniques to help cope with it.

Bladder instillations If you don't respond to oral medication, your bladder may be filled with a solution containing the drug RIMSO. This is done via a catheter. The catheter is then removed and the drug stays in the bladder for 20 minutes and is then passed out as though you were passing urine. If this fails, instillations of sodium hyaluronate (Cystistat) may be tried.

Acupuncture If the bladder instillations fail or if they aren't acceptable, then a course of acupuncture (see below) may help.

Injections Botulinum toxin injections into your bladder lining may help. This procedure needs you to be able to insert a catheter into your own bladder in order to empty it if needed.

Electrical stimulation If these treatments fail sacral neuro-modulation (see p342) can be used.

Surgery If all these treatments fail, and the pain is very severe, then surgery might be suggested. The possibilities are clam

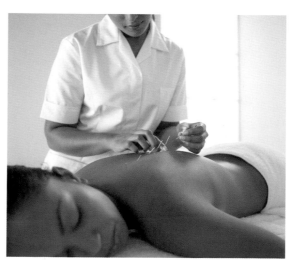

Acupuncture
This traditional Chinese practice uses needles inserted in the skin to relieve pain and to treat a wide range of disorders. It is thought that the needles stimulate the release of endorphins, the body's natural painkillers.

cystoplasty (see p342), diversion of the urine into a special bag (stoma, or urostomy, bag) that is worn outside the body on the abdomen, or the surgical removal of the bladder with or without the urethra.

Reconstruction of a new bladder from bowel tissue may be suggested.

HOW CAN I HELP MYSELF?
The following may help:
Keep a food diary (see below).

Avoid stress Stress exacerbates the problem, so it's wise to try to de-stress your life (see pp62–3).
Try acupuncture This may be help both the symptoms and to aid relaxation and de-stressing.

Foods and drinks that may trigger bladder pain

Many women who suffer from bladder pain syndrome agree that certain foods and drinks can irritate a sensitive bladder. Some of the most common triggers are detailed below. Keep a diet and symptom diary over a few weeks to try to identify dietary factors that may be triggering your symptoms. Avoiding these foods and drinks may help ease your symptoms.

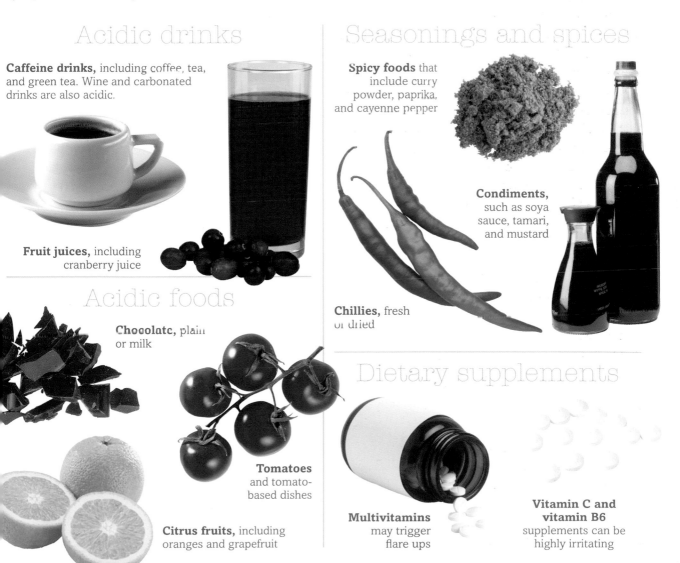

Acidic drinks

Caffeine drinks, including coffee, tea, and green tea. Wine and carbonated drinks are also acidic.

Fruit juices, including cranberry juice

Acidic foods

Chocolate, plain or milk

Tomatoes and tomato-based dishes

Citrus fruits, including oranges and grapefruit

Seasonings and spices

Spicy foods that include curry powder, paprika, and cayenne pepper

Condiments, such as soya sauce, tamari, and mustard

Chillies, fresh or dried

Dietary supplements

Multivitamins may trigger flare ups

Vitamin C and vitamin B6 supplements can be highly irritating

Urinary tract stones

The most noticeable symptom of a stone in the urinary tract is excruciating pain in the back – many women say it's far worse than childbirth! These stones are a problem that tends to affect men more frequently than women, but it's now becoming increasingly common in women, too.

WHAT IS IT?

Urinary tract stones are small solid masses – some are as small as a grain of sand, others are much larger – that form in one or both of your kidneys. They are caused by substances in your urine turning into crystals.

The stones may either stay in your kidney and in the top end of the ureter or they can travel down into your bladder. Most stones are small, less than 5mm (¼in) across, and stones this small usually pass out of your body in the urine without causing problems.

However, if a stone is large, it is more likely to get stuck and cause symptoms (see Have I got the symptoms?).

WHAT NEXT?

If you develop the symptoms of a urinary tract stone you should first take a simple over-the-counter non-steroidal painkiller, such as ibuprofen, and then consult your doctor immediately.

Your doctor will test your urine for blood and to check for infection. If he or she suspects a stone, you will be referred to a urologist – as a matter of urgency if simple painkillers are not controlling your pain and/or if you have a high temperature.

The urologist will also carry out tests, including a blood test to check kidney function, and urine tests to look for any blood in the urine and to check for the possibility of a UTI (see p336). A specialized X-ray will also be done to look for stones in your kidneys, ureters, and bladder; this X-ray may be a CT scan, KUB (a type

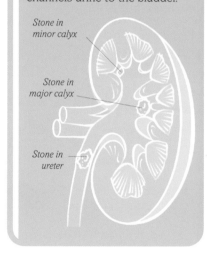

SITES OF URINARY TRACT STONES

The most common sites of stones are the major and minor calyces (the urine-collecting areas) and the ureter, which channels urine to the bladder.

Stone in minor calyx

Stone in major calyx

Stone in ureter

of abdominal X-ray), or an intravenous urogram (IVU). An IVU involves a series of X-rays taken before and after you have had an injection of a special dye. If you pass any stones, the urologist will also examine these to identify the precise type of stone.

HAVE I GOT THE SYMPTOMS?

The symptoms of a urinary tract stone are a sudden onset of:
● Severe colicky pain on one side of your back, often radiating to the front of the abdomen towards the groin
● Nausea and vomiting
● Blood in urine
● Increased frequency of passing urine.
See your doctor immediately if you have any of these symptoms.

"Stones can be as small as a grain of sand and pass out of your body naturally."

MY TREATMENT OPTIONS

There are a number of treatment options available depending on the size and type of your kidney stone. If the stone is small, you may require only pain relief; you will also be advised to drink plenty of fluids to help flush out the stone. Larger stones or stones that have become stuck in the urinary tract may need lithotripsy or surgery to break up the stones so that they can be passed out naturally. Very rarely, drainage of the kidney may be needed.

Pain relief Medication for pain relief is the first treatment you will be offered. The most effective pain relief comes from prescription anti-inflammatory drugs, such as diclofenac.

Lithotripsy Also known as external shock wave lithotripsy (ESWL), this is the most common method of treating larger stones or those that are stuck in the urinary tract, although it is not suitable in all cases. Lithotripsy is a non-surgical procedure in which focused sound waves are used to break up the stones into small fragments that can be passed out naturally when you urinate. Painkillers are usually given before the procedure, as it may cause some discomfort. For a few days afterwards you may have blood in your urine and there may be tenderness over the treated area.

Surgery If a stone is stuck in your ureter, a small viewing tube (called a ureteroscope) is inserted into your ureter via your urethra and bladder, and a laser is used to break up the stone so that it can be passed out naturally. If a stone is stuck in your kidney, a viewing tube (called a nephroscope) is inserted into your kidney and upper ureter through an incision in your back. The stone is pulled out or broken up via the nephroscope. Most urinary tract stones that require surgical treatment can be treated using these minimally invasive techniques. Only rarely is it necessary to remove stones by open surgery.

Drainage Very rarely, a stone-related blockage can cause a serious infection in the kidney. Such an infection may be life-threatening and requires emergency drainage of the kidney. Drainage may be carried out under local anaesthesia using a tube inserted through your skin. Alternatively it may be done via the bladder, in which case general anaesthesia is used.

HOW CAN I HELP MYSELF?

You can help prevent stones by eating a healthy diet and by avoiding becoming dehydrated. It is generally advised that you should drink 1.5–2 litres (about 2½–3½ pints) a day if you've never had a stone, or 2–3 litres (about 3½–5 pints) a day if you have had stones before.

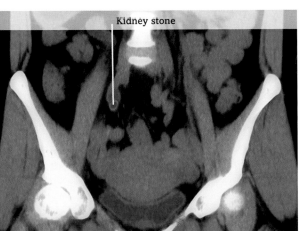

A kidney stone
This CT scan clearly shows the presence of a kidney stone (red) in the woman's right ureter (the tube that channels urine from the kidney to the bladder).

> ### AM I AT RISK?
>
> You may be at risk of urinary tract stones if you have:
>
> - A diet that is high in protein and low in fibre
> - A sedentary lifestyle
> - High calcium levels in your blood, which may be associated with parathyroid gland problems
> - Other metabolic abnormalities, such as hyperuricaemia (associated with gout) and an inherited condition called cystinuria
> - An untreated long-term urinary tract infection.

Urinary tract cancer

Although serious, there's a good chance that urinary tract cancer can be treated successfully, particularly if it's detected early. The crucial thing is to see your doctor as soon as possible if you notice any symptoms. There may well be nothing to worry about, but you should get a medical check to make sure.

WHAT IS IT?

Urinary tract cancer refers to cancer of your bladder, kidney, and ureters. Bladder cancer usually starts in the lining of the bladder, and it ranges from small wart-like growths to large tumours. There are several types of kidney cancer, but the most common is renal cell cancer, which affects the cells that make up the main body of the kidney. Cancer of the ureter affects the tube that carries urine from the kidney to the bladder. In all types, there are often no symptoms in the early stages. If you do have any symptoms, make an urgent appointment to see your doctor.

Of the three types of urinary tract cancer, bladder cancer is the most common in women and ureter cancer the least common. The causes of urinary tract cancer aren't known, but it's thought that smoking and exposure to certain chemicals may increase the risk of developing it. The risk also increases with increasing age.

WHAT NEXT?

Your doctor will ask about your symptoms and examine your abdomen and pelvis. He or she will do an internal examination to make sure your symptoms aren't due to a gynaecological problem, and will also do a dipstick test on a urine sample to check for blood. If these tests indicate cancer may be a possibility, you'll be referred to a urologist specializing in cancer.

The urologist will send a urine sample to the laboratory to see if there are any cancer cells, and a blood sample to check your kidney function. The urologist may look into your bladder using a flexible viewing instrument (called a cystoscope) that is passed through your urethra into the bladder. This is done under a local anaesthetic. If abnormalities are found, you'll be given a general anaesthetic and a rigid cystoscope will be used to take a tissue sample from your bladder and to remove any small tumours. You'll also have an X-ray taken of your kidneys, ureters, and bladder (called a KUB) and an intravenous urogram (IVU; see p346) of your urinary tract. You may also have a CT scan of your urinary tract, and an X-ray of your lungs to see if cancer has spread.

HAVE I GOT THE SYMPTOMS?

You may not have any symptoms but the most common ones are:

- Blood in your urine
- Needing to pass urine frequently
- Pain when you pass urine
- Difficulty in delaying passing urine
- A constant feeling of needing to pass urine.

If you also have either or both of the following symptoms, this may be an indication of kidney cancer:

- Pain in your side that won't go away
- A lump in your abdomen.

See your doctor as soon as possible if you have any of these symptoms.

AM I AT RISK?

You may be at increased risk of urinary tract cancer if:

- You smoke
- You are over the age of 60
- You are obese
- You have a poor diet
- You have been exposed to any cancer-causing chemicals, such as asbestos.

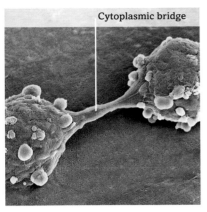

Cytoplasmic bridge

Bladder cancer cells dividing
This colour-enhanced scanning electron micrograph (SEM) shows the final stage of a bladder cancer cell dividing. The two cells that are produced are attached by a cytoplasmic bridge (thin thread).

THE RISK OF BLADDER CANCER FROM SMOKING

The biggest risk of developing bladder cancer comes from smoking. The more cigarettes you smoke and the more deeply you inhale, the greater the risk. This graph shows the number of times (on a scale of 1–6) by which your risk is increased the more you smoke.

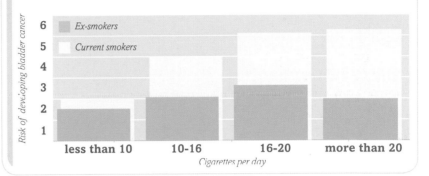

Risk of developing bladder cancer

☐ Ex-smokers
☐ Current smokers

less than 10   10-16   16-20   more than 20

Cigarettes per day

MY TREATMENT OPTIONS

Treatment will depend on the type of urinary tract cancer:

Surgery If you have bladder cancer and it's in the early stages the tumour can usually be removed using a cystoscope. However, if the cancer is more advanced, you'll need surgery to remove the bladder. If you have kidney or ureter cancer and the tumour hasn't spread, then you'll usually have surgery to remove the tumour.

You may also have all or part of your kidney removed. However, if you have only a small tumour in your ureter, it may be possible to remove only the affected part and rejoin the ureter.

Laser therapy If you have a tumour on the surface of your ureter and it's in the early stages, then it may be possible to remove it by laser therapy.

Radiotherapy If surgery isn't an option or the cancer has spread, then radiotherapy may be recommended. Ask your doctor about any potential side effects.

After surgery Depending on the type and severity of your cancer, other treatments may be given after surgery, including chemotherapy, radiotherapy, and immunotherapy (treatment to stimulate your immune system to destroy cancer cells).

Follow-up After treatment you'll have regular check-ups to monitor your recovery.

HOW CAN I HELP MYSELF?

You can reduce the chance of developing urinary tract cancer with the following lifestyle changes:

Stop smoking if you smoke (see p64 for advice)

Eat healthily (see pp52–5 for advice on eating a healthy diet)

Take regular exercise (see pp56–7) to prevent yourself from becoming obese.

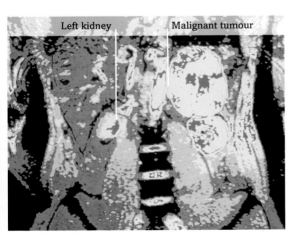

Left kidney   Malignant tumour

Cancer of the kidney
This colour-enhanced MRI (magnetic resonance imaging) scan of the abdomen shows a large malignant tumour on the right kidney. The pelvic area is at the bottom and parts of the arms are upper left and right. The the central black areas are the lower part of the spinal column.

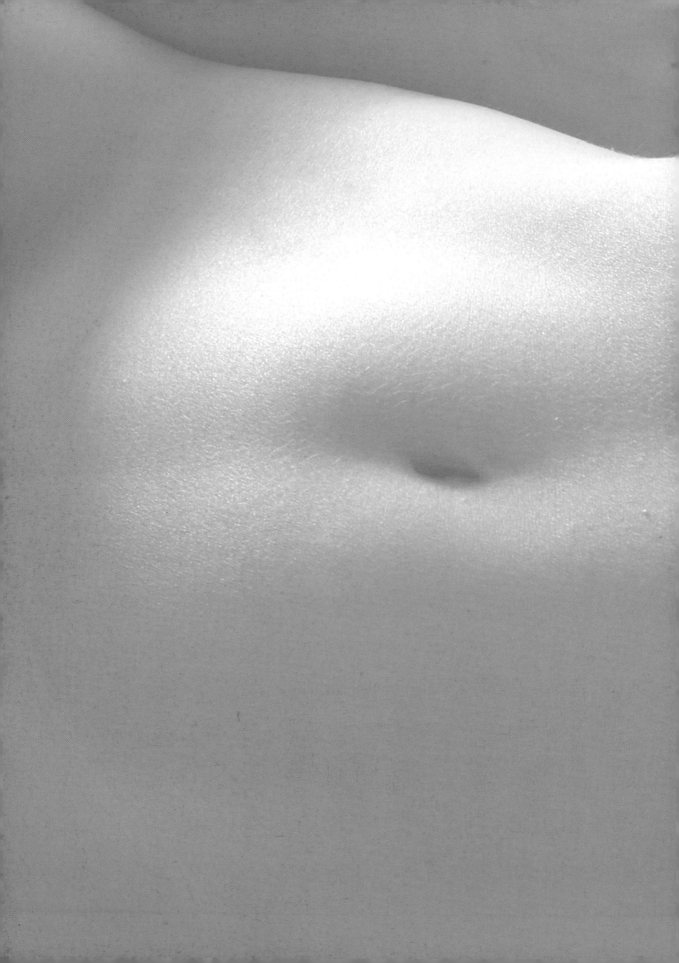

Skin and hair

Dr Nerys Roberts MD FRCP MRCPCH BSc

Your skin and hair

Think of your skin and hair as an accurate reflection of your health and lifestyle. If you are full of zest for life and are looking after yourself, eating well, being active, and making sure you have some "you time", then your skin will be radiant and your hair will be lustrous. Neglect yourself or indulge in bad habits, such as smoking or crash-dieting, and your skin will pay the price in the form of accelerated ageing and premature wrinkles, and your hair may well start falling out in clumps. So, start a good skin and hair care regime (see pp66–7).

WHAT IS SKIN MADE OF?

The skin is the largest organ in the body, covering, on average, 2sq m (2½sq ft). This physical barrier – even at just 6mm (¼in) thick – protects our bodies from the outside environment. The base ingredient for skin is the fibrous protein keratin, which is made by the keratinocyte skin cells in the epidermis (the uppermost skin layer).

The skin's dermis lies beneath the epidermis and houses the cells that make elastin and collagen to give skin its plumpness and elasticity. This layer also contains blood vessels, nerve endings, hair follicles, and the other elements that are needed in order to maintain healthy skin.

Skin cells, along with hairs, follow a cycle: growth, no-growth, and then shedding. Disruptions or upsets to the cycle can cause conditions such as psoriasis (see p356) or alopecia (hair loss, see p368).

HOW SKIN CHANGES AS WE AGE

The major cause of ageing is ultraviolet light from the sun. You probably know that UV light produces extra pigmentation in terms of a sun tan but were you aware that it can also result in sunspots, broken

WHAT LIES BENEATH THE SURFACE?

In this cross-sectional view through the skin, you can see the myriad elements contained within the two basic layers of the epidermis and the dermis.

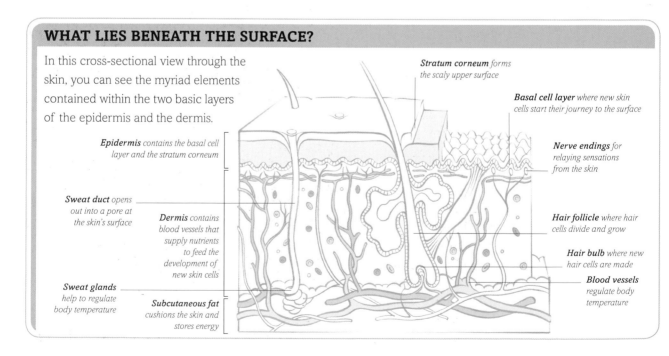

Stratum corneum *forms the scaly upper surface*

Basal cell layer *where new skin cells start their journey to the surface*

Nerve endings *for relaying sensations from the skin*

Hair follicle *where hair cells divide and grow*

Hair bulb *where new hair cells are made*

Blood vessels *regulate body temperature*

Epidermis *contains the basal cell layer and the stratum corneum*

Sweat duct *opens out into a pore at the skin's surface*

Dermis *contains blood vessels that supply nutrients to feed the development of new skin cells*

Sweat glands *help to regulate body temperature*

Subcutaneous fat *cushions the skin and stores energy*

blood vessels, and wrinkles, as well as drying out the skin generally? Super-hydrated skin appears to be firm and youthful, so if you want to appear younger, make sure that you use an effective moisturizer and reapply it frequently.

HOW ARE WOMEN DIFFERENT?

Some small anatomical differences explain why women's skin is different from men's.

Women's skin tends to secrete a little less oil from the sebaceous glands than men's, due to the effects of oestrogen. Having less oily skin has its benefits; you're less likely to have acne and other blemishes. However, drier skin is more prone to wrinkles.

Overall, women have thinner skin than men and so are more susceptible to the damaging effects of the sun's ultraviolet rays. The thickness of skin starts to decline after the menopause. Collagen content is lower to start with and collagen degradation occurs to a greater extent in women's skin, meaning that women often look older than men of the same age.

WHAT IS HAIR MADE OF?

As with skin, the base ingredient for hair is the protein keratin. Each strand of hair consists of three concentric layers:

- The cuticle – this thin, colourless outer layer protects the inner layers
- The cortex – this thick layer contains melanin, which gives hair its colour. Eumelanin produces brown or black hair; pheomelanin produces red hair. Blonde hair results from low amounts of melanin
- The medulla – this innermost layer reflects light, giving hair its various tones of colour.

HOW HAIR CHANGES AS WE AGE

The most obvious sign of getting older is greying hair. Over time hair follicles stop making melanin and white or grey hairs start to appear. Much of how you age is genetically determined, so think about how your parents aged in terms of their hair. What's more, your hair becomes thinner and may even become quite sparse in places (female-pattern baldness, see p371).

SKIN THROUGH THE AGES

Genetics, hormonal changes, and the sun all play a part in how your skin changes through the decades. So what can you expect from your skin as you get older? Read on to find out.

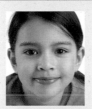

Under 11

This near-perfect skin has a smooth overall texture with small pores. Hydration is good, the activity of the sebaceous glands is low, and healing capability is excellent.

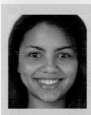

11–25

Sebaceous gland activity is high, helping to cause bouts of acne that can affect the texture and colour of the skin. Later, the first fine lines start to appear and pore size increases.

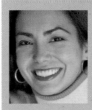

25–45

A noticeable drop in skin hydration causes more fine lines, and even first wrinkles, to appear. There are early signs of the skin sagging around the eye area as it loses some of its elasticity.

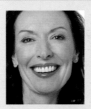

45–55

The skin is drier and the epidermis thins. The texture of the skin becomes rougher and pores enlarge as the skin loses elasticity. Age spots appear and the skin sags near the eyes and cheeks.

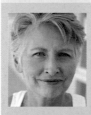

55–65

Wrinkles and fine lines are abundant. Skin colour is uneven and sagging worsens. Oil production is low and the skin's ability to repair itself after injury is diminished.

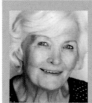

Over 65

The skin is more transparent and fragile as collagen diminishes. Numerous wrinkles are now apparent and sagging is pronounced. Skin growths and pigment spots are more noticeable.

Dermatitis

Substances in perfumes, cosmetics, detergents, jewellery, and clothes can irritate your skin or even, if you are abnormally sensitive, prompt an allergic reaction. In many cases, once the offending substance has been identified, avoiding it and using simple treatments will be enough to solve the problem.

WHAT IS IT?

Dermatitis, literally meaning "inflamed skin", is a common skin condition. It's very likely that you'll know of someone with dermatitis: 19 per cent of primary care consultations and 17 per cent of new referrals to dermatologists are for dermatitis. It is also known as eczema and the terms can be used interchangeably. While it's not dangerous, it can cause you a lot of discomfort.

The two main types of dermatitis are classed as exogenous (caused by contact with a chemical, irritant, or allergen) and endogenous (the causes are within your body rather than from any external factors). The latter type includes atopic dermatitis.

WHAT NEXT?

More often than not, your doctor will be able to identify dermatitis based on the pattern of redness and the appearance of the rash.

Next, your doctor will probably ask some questions about your skincare regime as well as prompting you to remember anything new that you've used or worn in the past weeks or months since you've noticed the change in your skin – costume jewellery, perfume, and soaps, for example.

If nothing obvious springs to the fore, your doctor may then arrange a patch test to find the allergen (the substance that is causing your allergic reaction), done either in the surgery or by referral to a dermatologist. This very simple test is safe and effective. A series of chemicals on small discs is taped to your back and left in place for 48 hours. After this time, your doctor examines the skin on your back, looking for any area that has turned red, indicating that your skin is sensitive and you're allergic to that particular chemical.

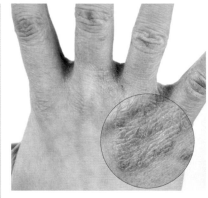

Checking for dermatitis
Early signs of dermatitis often occur between the fingers, encroaching down the tops of the hands.

HAVE I GOT THE SYMPTOMS?

The following symptoms may occur as a result of coming into contact with an irritant, or they may be an allergic reaction to a substance:

- Dry, red, itchy patches of skin (commonly between the fingers and beneath rings)
- Scaling or blistering skin
- Swollen eyes (if the dermatitis is very severe, your eyes may be swollen shut).

A common symptom of internal (endogenous) dermatitis is:

- Red, itchy, swollen patches of skin, especially in the elbow and knee creases, neck, and face.

See your doctor if you have any of the above symptoms.

"It's possible you may have developed an allergy to a product you have used without problem for a long time."

In many cases, your doctor will be able to give you a list of products that the offending chemical is in. Common allergens include:

- Nickel, which is often found in costume jewellery
- Fragrances, which are used in perfume, skincare products, soaps, air fresheners, and a wide range of other household products
- Latex, which is present in disposable gloves and condoms.

The best test for atopic dermatitis is a RAST (radioallergosorbent) test, done by checking the blood for allergies to foods (such as chocolate, eggs, milk, and peanuts), latex, pet dander (the skin that is shed from pets and their fur), and dust mites. The results of the RAST test can be compared with the skin prick tests to confirm the findings.

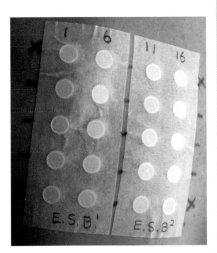

Allergy grid
To test for allergies, a grid consisting of discs with chemicals applied to them will be taped to your back for 48 hours. Reddening of your skin will identify your chemical sensitivities.

> ## ATOPIC DERMATITIS
>
> Atopic dermatitis, also known as eczematous dermatitis, is a condition in which there is an inherited tendency towards sensitive skin. Such sensitivity usually occurs early in life and is often associated with hayfever and asthma (see pp238–9). Atopic dermatitis can be exacerbated by excessive bathing with hot water, detergent soaps, and irritating fabrics such as wool. It's best treated by keeping skin hydrated (use a humidifier or put saucers of water on the radiators), showering with warm rather than hot water, and using emollient foams and creams, and a steroid cream.

MY TREATMENT OPTIONS

It is essential in the long term to avoid the irritant or allergen causing your dermatitis, but you will also need short-term treatment to quell the inflammation.

Steroid ointments The reaction occurring in your skin needs to be treated with a steroid ointment.

Antihistamines Your doctor may also prescribe antihistamine tablets which will help you sleep and reduce itching until the steroids heal the problem.

Anti-inflammatories If your dermatitis is proving hard to treat, you may be given azathioprine, ciclosporin, methotrexate, or drugs called calcineurin inhibitors to reduce the inflammation.

Antimicrobials Secondary bacterial infection is common, in which case your doctor may also give you oral or topical antibiotics.

HOW CAN I HELP MYSELF?

There are several ways in which you can ease your dermatitis.

Check your beauty products Identify which of them may be responsible for your dermatitis and take them to the dermatologist when you are having your patch test so that he or she can test for all the possible culprit allergens and help you eliminate them. Be aware that you may have developed an allergy to a product you have used without problem for a long time.

Use fragrance-free products Fragrances are the most common cause of allergic skin reactions. Read the manufacturers' labels on your cosmetics and household products carefully. Note that even products that can legally claim to be unscented may contain "masking fragrances".

Keep your skin moist Ask your pharmacist to advise you on a medical moisturizer to reduce water loss from your skin.

For atopic dermatitis Clean your skin and use a medical moisturizer (see above) frequently, take warm not hot baths and showers, and keep your nails short to limit damage from scratching. Rinse clothes well – if necessary, use an extra rinse cycle.

Psoriasis

Cold, windy weather, or even central heating, can result in dry, red skin. But if your skin starts becoming red, thick and scaly, psoriasis rather than environmental issues may be the cause.

WHAT IS IT?

Psoriasis is a long-term condition, the exact cause of which isn't known, but both genetic and environmental influences play a role. In patches of skin affected by psoriasis, the skin cells are produced abnormally quickly, producing the characteristic thickness and scaling. This is accompanied by an immune response in which white blood cells proliferate and blood vessels dilate, causing the redness (see box below). Psoriasis can occur anywhere on the body, but the elbows, knees, and scalp are the most common sites.

Various environmental factors may trigger psoriasis in people who are genetically predisposed to it (see box opposite). For most people, the condition is persistent, although in some the disease comes and goes. A few people have arthritis associated with psoriasis. Often, only small joints such as knuckle, finger, and thumb joints, are affected, although sometimes the neck and back are affected. Psoriatic arthritis is rarely as troublesome as rheumatoid arthritis.

WHAT NEXT?

Your doctor will usually be able to diagnose the most common

HAVE I GOT THE SYMPTOMS?

Psoriasis symptoms can vary but generally include:

- Pinkish-red patches of skin covered with silvery scales
- Dry, cracked skin that may bleed
- As well as skin changes, you may notice thickened, pitted, or ridged nails. If your joints are swollen and painful, you may have psoriatic arthritis. A minority of people with psoriasis develop this inflammatory condition.

See your doctor if you have any of the above symptoms.

type of psoriasis (chronic plaque psoriasis) based on a physical examination of some affected skin. Rarely, he or she may want to take a small skin sample to send off for laboratory testing to confirm psoriasis. If your doctor suspects you have psoriatic arthritis, he or she will take a sample of blood to rule out other conditions.

MY TREATMENT OPTIONS

Unfortunately, it is not possible to cure psoriasis and the various treatments are aimed at reducing the proliferation of skin cells. Your doctor will work with you to find the best one for you personally. The traditional approach is to start with the mildest – creams and phototherapy – and progress to stronger ones as necessary.

CELL TURNOVER IN PSORIASIS

Cells in the epidermis change gradually as they move towards the surface where they are shed continually in a process that normally takes three to four weeks. In skin affected by psoriasis, the rate of cell turnover speeds up so that the process takes only three to four days. Dead skin can't slough off quickly enough and builds up in thick, scaly patches on the skin.

The epidermis is the outer layer of skin, through which cells move to the surface

Overproduction of skin cells causes scaly patches of dead skin

Inflammatory response causes redness

Skin affected by psoriasis

Creams, ointments and solutions If you have mild to moderate psoriasis your skin can often be improved with topical treatments alone. Some can also be combined with phototherapy.

- Vitamin D analogues are synthetic forms of vitamin D. They reduce inflammation and help to stop cells reproducing. They can be applied even to sensitive areas of the body, such as the armpits, face, and groin.
- Dithranol is an extract of tree bark. It slows down skin cell production and removes scales but stains everything it touches and can irritate unaffected skin.
- Coal tar is probably the oldest known treatment for psoriasis. How it works isn't known, but it's messy, stains clothing, and smells, although it can be very effective.
- Vitamin A analogues, such as tazarotene (Zorac), reduce skin cell production and may also help psoriasis on the nails. Tell your doctor if you plan to become pregnant as you will not be able to use tazarotene.
- Steroid creams are usually used only in combination with the other treatments above to reduce irritation, although they may sometimes be used alone to treat the genital area or other sensitive regions.

Phototherapy Many psoriasis sufferers have discovered that sunlight helps their psoriasis and this fact has been used by doctors, who use artificial ultraviolet (UV) light therapy, either alone or in combination with medication. UV treatment theoretically carries an increased risk of skin cancer but this is thought to be minimal.

- Narrowband UVB therapy uses controlled doses of UVB light and is mainly used for people whose psoriasis is extensive, has not responded to simple topical treatments, or who are having dithranol or coal tar applied in a day-care setting.
- PUVA is a combination of UVA light treatment and a psoralen, a chemical that makes the skin more sensitive to light. The psoralen is given, either topically or orally, before exposure to UVA light and sensitizes the skin to the UV light. PUVA is usually used only for people whose psoriasis has not responded to narrowband UVB therapy.
- Excimer laser is a beam of UVB light aimed at psoriatic skin to control scaling and inflammation.

Medication If you have severe psoriasis or it's resistant to other treatments, your doctor may prescribe drugs as tablets or as injections. Unfortunately, many come with serious side effects.

- Retinoids may be used alone or in combination with phototherapy. You should avoid getting pregnant for three years after receiving this therapy.
- Cytotoxic drugs, such as hydroxycarbamide and methotrexate, reduce skin cell production. You should not take these drugs if you are pregnant or plan to become so.
- Immunosuppressants, such as ciclosporin, are thought to act mainly by suppressing inflammation. They usually take effect quickly
- Immunomodulators, such as etanercept and infliximab, damp down the immune response. They are given by intravenous infusion or subcutaneous injection.

HOW CAN I HELP MYSELF?
A few simple measures can improve your skin.

Eat oily fish three times a week; studies have shown this can help.
Carefully expose your skin to small amounts of sunlight, which may help, but avoid sunbeds.
Apply moisturisers These can help to reduce the scaling.
Don't smoke and only drink alcohol moderately.

TRIGGERS FOR PSORIASIS

Environmental factors that may trigger psoriasis include:
- Infections, such as strep throat, HIV, and skin infections
- Injury to the skin, such as a cut, insect bite, severe sunburn, or from some chemicals
- Stress
- Smoking
- Heavy alcohol consumption
- Some medications, including lithium, beta-blockers, non-steroidal anti-inflammatory drugs, ACE inhibitors, and antimalarial drugs.

Skin cancer

In these days of sophisticated fake tans, there really is no excuse to bake in the sun and risk sunburn, which is actually a type of skin damage. Not only is it painful, but repeated sunburn can increase your risk of the different types of skin cancer: basal cell carcinoma, squamous cell carcinoma, and melanoma.

AM I AT RISK?

Risk factors for non-melanoma skin cancer include:

- Year-round sun exposure
- Childhood sunburns
- Fair skin, especially with blonde or red hair and freckles
- A large number of moles
- A suppressed immune system (e.g. due to HIV/AIDS or medication)
- Scars (burns, vaccinations) or leg ulcers are at risk of becoming cancerous
- Radiotherapy.

Risk factors for melanoma include:

- Fair skin, especially with blonde or red hair and freckles
- A history of blistering sunburn
- Use of sunbeds
- Excessive sun exposure
- More than 50 moles
- A family and/or personal history of melanoma
- A suppressed immune system (e.g. due to HIV/AIDS or medication)
- Exposure to environmental chemicals such as creosote
- Genetic diseases associated with sun sensitivity.

UV LIGHT AND YOUR SKIN

Skin cancer is mainly due to overexposure to ultraviolet (UV) light from the sun and other sources. There are three types of UV light: UVA, UVB, and UVC. The ozone layer in the earth's atmosphere screens out UVC but UVA and UVB rays penetrate the atmosphere and can damage your skin. UVA penetrates deep within the skin to damage DNA in skin cells, making them more susceptible to cancer. UVB rays cause sunburn and also increase the risk of skin cancer.

Weather forecasts often include a sun or UV risk index so you can take the action needed for the different categories:

Minimal You can safely stay outside with no protection.

Low to moderate You should limit exposure between 10am and 4pm. Wear protective clothing, including a hat and UVA/UVB sunglasses; an ordinary T-shirt has an SPF of approximately 6, but it is possible to buy T-shirts with an SPF of 30. You should use sunscreen of at least SPF15.

High to very high You should avoid the sun as far as possible between 10am and 4pm and cover up as above.

MY TREATMENT OPTIONS

Most skin cancers can be treated successfully by:

Excisional surgery The cancerous tissue is removed, plus a margin of healthy skin around it. This is the only safe treatment for melanoma.

For non-melanoma skin cancer, other options are:

Freezing Small, early skin cancers can be destroyed with liquid nitrogen (cryosurgery).

Anticancer creams Small, early skin cancers can also be treated with anticancer creams that "burn" off abnormal cells.

Mohs surgery This is used for cancers in certain locations, such as near the nose, upper lip, and eye, as well as for recurring or difficult-to-treat cancers.

Curettage Layers of cancer cells are scraped away using a curette (circular blade).

Radiotherapy If surgery isn't possible, radiation may be used.

Chemotherapy A cocktail of anticancer drugs is used to kill the cancer cells.

Basal cell carcinoma

This is the most common type of skin cancer, but fortunately it's also one of the most easily treated and least likely to spread around the body (metastasize).

WHAT IS IT?

Basal cell carcinoma (BCC) is thought to arise from immature cells in the epidermis of the skin, although its origin is not certain. It occurs most commonly on areas that are exposed to the sun, such as your face, neck, hands, and ears. BCC can sometimes look like other skin conditions such as eczema or psoriasis, so you should always have any skin complaints checked out to be on the safe side.

WHAT NEXT?

Your doctor may be able to make a diagnosis during the consultation, but it's likely that a biopsy will be necessary if he or she suspects BCC. A small sample of the affected skin may be taken or the whole area cut out (known as an excision biopsy).

MY TREATMENT OPTIONS

Basal cell carcinomas may be treated by freezing, chemotherapy, excisional surgery, or curettage; if they're in a difficult location, your doctor may recommend a Mohs procedure (see opposite). About 94–99 per cent of people with BCC are successfully treated, and this cancer is rarely life-threatening.

HAVE I GOT THE SYMPTOMS?

A basal cell carcinoma may appear as:
- A scab that bleeds from time to time but doesn't heal properly
- A flat, scaly red mark
- A shiny bump
- Or as a growth with elevated rolled edges, like a crater.

See your doctor if you notice any of the above.

HOW CAN I HELP MYSELF?

Check your skin regularly for any changes such as marks that are growing. Protect yourself from the sun (see opposite).

Squamous cell carcinoma

This less common skin cancer is a tumour of the squamous cells that lie just below the surface of the epidermis.

WHAT IS IT?

Squamous cell carcinoma (SCC) is more likely to spread to other parts of your body than basal cell carcinoma, but is easily treated if it's detected early. They can occur anywhere on the body but, like basal cell carcinomas, are most common in areas that get the most sun exposure: the face, neck, ears, and hands. They can also appear on scars, ulcerated skin, as well as in chronic wounds.

WHAT NEXT?

If you've noticed any unusual changes in the texture of your skin, visit your doctor. An immediate diagnosis may be possible, but you will probably need to have a small sample of the affected skin taken (a biopsy) or the whole area cut out (an excision biopsy) for examination under a microscope. When your doctor gets the results, he or she will be able to advise you on further treatment.

MY TREATMENT OPTIONS

These cancers are usually treated surgically; in some cases, if they're in a difficult location, your doctor may recommend a Mohs procedure (see opposite).

HOW CAN I HELP MYSELF?

Check your skin regularly for any changes such as a blemish that won't heal. Protect yourself from the sun (see opposite).

HAVE I GOT THE SYMPTOMS?

A squamous cell carcinoma typically appears as:
- A raised, rough, scaly lump that may sometimes bleed and doesn't heal properly.

See your doctor if you have such a lump.

Melanoma

Melanoma is the most serious form of skin cancer; if it's left untreated it can spread around your body and kill you. However, early treatment brings good results.

WHAT IS IT?

Malignant melanomas often develop in or near a mole, but they can appear anywhere on the skin. The cancerous cells then spread to the surrounding skin and possibly to the lymph nodes and other areas of the body.

WHAT NEXT?

If you've noticed any changes in a mole, consult your doctor as soon as possible. Unless he or she can rule out melanoma, you'll be sent to have the mole removed and examined under a microscope.

MY TREATMENT OPTIONS

If microscopic examination of the mole reveals that it is not cancerous, no further treatment is needed. However, if it turns out to be a melanoma, a larger area of skin around the site of the melanoma will be removed surgically (see excisional surgery, p358). If the cancer was deep, your lymph nodes will be examined, and you may also have an ultrasound or CT scan to check for any spread of cancer cells; if lymph nodes have been affected these may need to be removed as well. You may also need chemotherapy (see chemotherapy, p358) if the melanoma is very advanced and has spread.

HOW CAN I HELP MYSELF?

With early detection and treatment many cases of melanoma can be cured, so it is vital to make sure you check your skin every few months (get your partner or a friend to check your back for you). You should, of course, immediately report anything untoward to your doctor.

Most importantly, always protect yourself in the sun (see p358).

HAVE I GOT THE SYMPTOMS?

Symptoms may include:
- A mole that changes colour, size, or shape, or the appearance of what looks like a new mole
- If it is untreated, a melanoma may become lumpy and ooze or bleed.

See your doctor if you have any of the above symptoms.

WATCH OUT FOR WARNING SIGNS OF MELANOMA

Doctors have a simple way of remembering what to look for in a mole that could be undergoing cancerous changes – and it's as easy as ABCDE.

A is for asymmetry; if a mole grows on one side more than the other it warrants investigation as they are normally symmetrical.

B is for border; if the outer edge becomes irregular and not round, get your doctor to check it out.

C is for colour; if the colour becomes uneven or darker (even black), show it to your doctor.

D is for diameter; if a mole grows larger than 6mm (¼in) it needs medical examination.

E is for elevation; if a mole that was flat becomes raised or uneven on its surface, see your doctor.

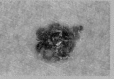

Asymmetry
A mole grows more on one side.

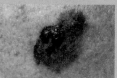

Border
The outer edge of a mole is irregular.

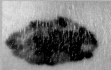

Colour
The colour varies from one shade to another.

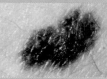

Diameter
The mole grows larger than 6mm (¼in).

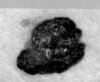

Elevation
A mole that was flat becomes raised.

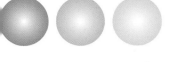

Pigmentation problems

Skin colour is determined by your genes and the amount of pigment – melanin – your skin makes and stores. Normally, skin is an even colour, but problems with pigment production turn patches of skin lighter or darker than usual. Two of the most common conditions are vitiligo and melasma.

Vitiligo

This patchy, often symmetrical, white discoloration commonly affects the face and hands.

WHAT IS IT?

In vitiligo the pigment cells malfunction. The cause isn't clear, but it is thought to be one of the autoimmune disorders that have a genetic component.

WHAT NEXT?

Your doctor will make a diagnosis usually based on your medical history and an examination.

MY TREATMENT OPTIONS

There is no cure, but there are some medical options you can try. **Steroid creams** can help halt further pigment loss if started early. **Repigmentation** Controlled exposure to sunlight or narrowband UVB (see p358) may cause pigment to return. **Depigmentation** This involves fading the rest of your skin to match the white areas.

HAVE I GOT THE SYMPTOMS?

The symptoms may include:
- Usually symmetrical white areas on the face, hands, armpits, groin, feet, elbows, and knees.
- Whitening of your hair.

See your doctor if you have any of the above symptoms.

HOW CAN I HELP MYSELF?

You can use camouflage make-up.

Melasma

This patchy brown discoloration that mainly affects women appears on various areas of the face.

WHAT IS IT?

Melasma is due to skin cells producing too much melanin. It's most likely to develop when you're pregnant and it usually appears on your cheeks, forehead, chin, and upper lip. It often develops gradually and may fade once the baby's born. It may also sometimes occur with the contraceptive pill or as a reaction to cosmetics.

WHAT NEXT?

Your doctor will make a diagnosis based on examining your skin.

MY TREATMENT OPTIONS

Consider stopping the pill and any causative cosmetics. If melasma doesn't fade after pregnancy, you may benefit from treatment. **Topical medication** Azelaic acid or retinoids are usually the first option. **Bleaching** Hydroquinone may be used, but its effects are permanent. **Light chemical peels** These remove the outer skin layers. **Non-ablative laser treatment** This blends back skin colour.

HOW CAN I HELP MYSELF?

Sun exposure worsens melasma, so sunblock with good UVA and UVB protection is vital (note that UVA can penetrate glass). It may help to avoid using cosmetics or anything else that may irritate your skin.

HAVE I GOT THE SYMPTOMS?

The symptoms may include:
- Dark irregular patches on your face.

See your doctor if you have the above symptoms.

Acne and rosacea

Many teenagers suffer from acne vulgaris, the most common form of acne, which is triggered by hormonal changes at puberty; it usually clears up as people reach their 20s, although it can come and go during adult life, too. Rosacea is a skin condition that usually affects people in middle age.

Acne vulgaris

WHAT IS IT?

Skin with acne vulgaris is very oily with blackheads, whiteheads, cysts, and pimples. Women have both oestrogen and testosterone, a male hormone that circulates in our bloodstream and that is partly responsible for acne. It seems that in women with persistent acne, some have abnormally high levels of testosterone in their bloodstream whereas others have normal testosterone levels but their skin's sebaceous (oil-producing) glands are particularly sensitive to the hormone. In both cases the result is excess production of waxy, oily sebum. Contrary to popular belief, there is no good evidence that foods such as chocolate or greasy foods cause acne or make it worse. However, a balanced diet is important in helping to keep your body, including your skin, healthy.

As if oily skin were not enough, skin with acne cannot exfoliate dead skin cells properly. This is known as faulty keratinization. Every day our skin makes new cells and we need to shed old or dead ones, otherwise they clog up the pores on our skin. Clogged pores appear as stubborn whiteheads and blackheads.

There is a bacterium called *Propionobacterium acnes* that lives and multiplies in the sebum on the skin, causing inflammation and redness. With the helping hand of colonies of this bacterium, your skin then develops not only the blackheads and whiteheads, but also pimples and pustules. Large acne cysts develop if there is a lot of inflammation. If you squeeze any of these "spots" you risk scarring your skin.

WHAT NEXT?

Your doctor will examine your skin carefully as the treatment depends on the combination of acne features predominant on your skin.

HAVE I GOT THE SYMPTOMS?

Acne vulgaris concentrates in areas with lots of sebaceous glands and appears as:

- Excessive oiliness of the face
- Tiny blackheads
- Small whiteheads
- Red pimples
- Painful large red lumps
- Tender lumps beneath the skin without any heads (cysts)
- Pus pimples.

See your doctor if a symptom causes you problems.

SAFETY OF RETINOID DRUGS

Retinoid drugs, which are derived from vitamin A, can potentially cause serious side effects. They should not be used during pregnancy because they may cause birth defects in the unborn baby. Any woman who is of childbearing age and is prescribed a retinoid must be monitored with blood tests to ensure that she is not pregnant and must use appropriate contraception. Retinoids may also cause dryness of the skin and may increase the skin's sensitivity to sunlight so a sunblock should be used at the same time as the retinoid medication. Isotretinoin may also cause raised blood cholesterol levels. Women with a history of depression should tell their doctor if he or she is considering prescribing isotretinoin.

HOW PIMPLES APPEAR

Your skin contains hairs that grow up through the epidermis from the dermis. A sebaceous gland around each hair produces sebum (oil) that waterproofs and lubricates the skin. When the gland is blocked, excess oil is trapped, the epidermis becomes inflamed, and a pimple results.

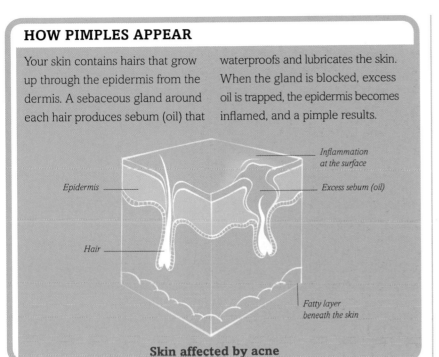

Skin affected by acne

MY TREATMENT OPTIONS

There are various treatments available for acne. Your doctor will work with you to find one that produces the best results with the least side effects for your particular form of acne. If you have had acne and it has left scarring, there are treatments available to help improve the appearance of your skin. Your doctor may be able to advise you about these or he or she may refer you to a cosmetic dermatologist.

Topical treatments If your acne consists predominantly of blackheads or whiteheads – known as comedonal acne – your doctor may recommend a gel, cream, or lotion containing benzoyl peroxide, a retinoid drug, or azelaic acid. Benzoyl peroxide and azelaic acid help destroy bacteria on your skin. Retinoids, such as retinoic acid, adapalene, and isotretinoin, help to unclog the pores by promoting the sloughing off of dead skin cells. However, they also have various potentially serious side effects (see Safety of retinoid drugs, left).

If your acne consists mainly of papules (small, solid spots) or pustules (pus-filled spots) and is of the inflammatory type – known as papulopustular inflammatory acne – your doctor may prescribe a topical antibiotic, such as clindamycin or erythromycin, a topical retinoid, such as adapalene or isotretinoin, or topical nicotinamide (a B vitamin).

Oral treatments If your acne is of the comedonal or papulopustular inflammatory type and hasn't improved with topical treatment alone, your doctor may prescribe oral antibiotics together with a topical retinoid; alternatively, he or she may prescribe an oral contraceptive or oral isotretinoin.

Oral contraceptives work by countering the effects of testosterone. Oral tretinoin works by blocking the effects of hormones on the skin and sebaceous glands, thereby unblocking the pores and preventing the glands from swelling and rupturing. Like topical isotretinoin, the oral form can have potentially serious side effects (see Safety of retinoid drugs, left). In a few cases, oral spironolactone, which reduces testosterone levels, may be prescribed. This may produce potentially serious side effects and may affect an unborn baby so it is essential that you do not become pregnant while taking this drug; careful monitoring with blood tests is also important.

If your acne consists mainly of nodules (small firm lumps) and/or cysts – known as nodulocystic acne – and has caused scarring or is likely to do so, your doctor may

> "Acne is a common problem, especially in the teenage years, but there are many effective treatments available."

prescribe oral isotretinoin. This is usually extremely effective – curing the acne in over 95 per cent of cases – and is the only treatment that can prevent further scarring but, as already mentioned, it may have serious side effects (see Safety of retinoid drugs, previous page).

Treatments for acne scarring

Various cosmetic procedures are available to help reduce the appearance of acne scars, such as chemical peels, dermabrasion, or laser treatment. All of these treatments work by removing the top layer of skin, leaving a more even skin surface. However, such treatments should not be done until your acne has been controlled or cured.

HOW CAN I HELP MYSELF?

In addition to following the medical treatment prescribed by your doctor, you may find it helpful to try one or more of the following self-help measures:

Keep your skin clean You should wash your skin with warm water and a gentle cleanser no more than twice a day on the problem areas.

Avoid irritating the skin Facial scrubs, astringents, face masks and even washing too much can irritate the skin and may make your acne worse.

Don't pick or squeeze spots Tempting though it may be, you should resist the urge to either pick or squeeze your acne spots because this can lead to infection or scarring.

Don't block the pores of your skin You should choose skincare products that are either water-based or non-comedogenic (non-pore-clogging). You should also always remove your make-up before going to bed as keeping make-up on all through the night means that the pores will become clogged.

Use lightweight make-up You should opt for powder cosmetics rather than cream versions because they are generally less irritating to the skin.

Keep your skin oil- and sweat-free You should take a shower after you have finished exercising or if you have become sweaty. Oil and sweat can trap dirt and bacteria on your skin.

Rosacea

WHAT IS IT?

This is a chronic skin condition affecting the face that starts with flushing on the cheeks, nose, and forehead then develops into more persistent redness of the face. The small blood vessels in the skin become broken, and there may be outbreaks of inflamed pimples and pus-filled spots. Rosacea is more common in women than men, often runs in families, and typically first appears in the over-30s.

WHAT NEXT?

Your doctor will usually be able to make a firm diagnosis after thoroughly examining your skin.

Sometimes a tiny skin biopsy (a small sample of skin) may be taken for tests to exclude other rare types of facial rash.

MY TREATMENT OPTIONS

Your doctor may recommend any of a number of treatments to help you combat rosacea:

Oral antibiotics The mainstay of treatment is tetracycline, but your doctor may also prescribe doxycycline or minocycline.

Antibiotic creams Creams with metronidazole reduce inflammation and improve the complexion.

Sunscreen Sunscreen containing zinc, which has anti-inflammatory properties, can reduce the inflammation of rosacea.

HAVE I GOT THE SYMPTOMS?

Rosacea affects more women than men and often runs in families. It first appears as red flushing on the cheeks, nose, and forehead. Other symptoms may include:

- Red, puffy skin
- Small red bumps
- Small pimples with white or yellow heads
- Tiny broken blood vessels
- If the rosacea affects the nose, the skin may thicken and turn a purplish-red colour.

See your doctor if you have any of these symptoms.

Laser treatment After the rosacea has cleared up, laser treatment can reduce any underlying redness and broken blood vessels on the nose and cheeks. The laser heat seals the blood vessels back together so that any red wiggly lines at the corners of the nose vanish. Laser treatment may also be helpful in reducing any thickening of the skin on the nose.

HOW CAN I HELP MYSELF?

There are a number of measures you can take to avoid making your rosacea worse:

Avoid trigger foods See below for a list of food that may trigger rosacea or make it worse.

Mild cleansers Only use gentle, non-irritating skincare products to avoid stripping your face of its essential oils.

Avoid excess heat Sessions in a sauna or steam room can aggravate the redness.

Avoid excess cold Exposure to cold temperatures and wind can worsen redness, so use a scarf to protect your face.

Avoid exposure to sun Cover up when you're in the sun as exposure can make your skin condition worse.

Foods that may trigger rosacea

Keep a diary of what you eat and drink, and then figure out which are your particular triggers and steer clear of them. Some of the known trigger foods are shown below. Other potential food triggers include dairy products, such as pasteurized milk, yoghurt and cream, as well as chocolate, wheat and wheat products, white flour, sugar, garlic, and eggs.

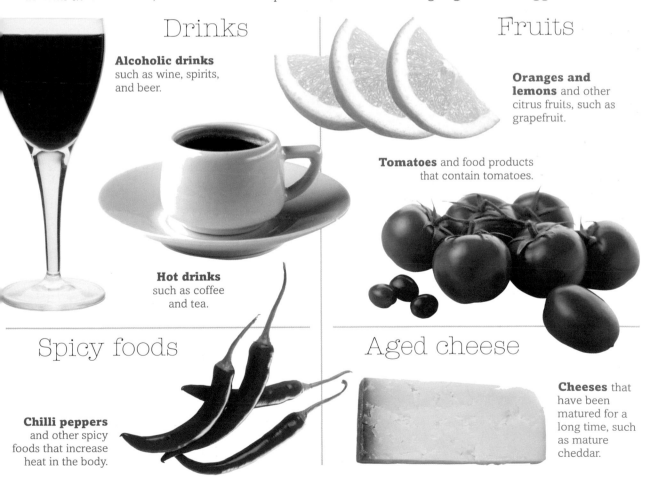

Drinks

Alcoholic drinks such as wine, spirits, and beer.

Hot drinks such as coffee and tea.

Fruits

Oranges and lemons and other citrus fruits, such as grapefruit.

Tomatoes and food products that contain tomatoes.

Spicy foods

Chilli peppers and other spicy foods that increase heat in the body.

Aged cheese

Cheeses that have been matured for a long time, such as mature cheddar.

Skin infections

When the protective barrier of the skin is breached by a microorganism, an infection is the result. Good hygiene routines help you to stay free from infection, and occasional invasions by a virus, bacterium, or fungus can normally be quickly and simply remedied to restore your skin's equilibrium.

Folliculitis

WHAT IS IT?

Infection of a hair follicle is likely to be the result of a cut inflicted while shaving your legs, allowing bacteria to enter. If you have repeated bouts of folliculitis it may be best to use a different method of hair removal.

WHAT NEXT?

Your doctor will probably be able to diagnose the problem from an examination of the affected area.

MY TREATMENT OPTIONS

Your doctor may prescribe a topical antibiotic to put on the affected area. If a large area is affected, you may also be offered oral antibiotics. Ask your doctor about any side effects.

HOW CAN I HELP MYSELF?

Treat razors hygienically Soak reusable razors in an antiseptic solution for five minutes before use, and never share razors.
Get wet first Shaving after showering, when your hair is softer, makes it less likely that you will cut yourself while shaving.

HAVE I GOT THE SYMPTOMS?

In folliculitis you may have:
- Small, yellow, pussy pimples
- Itching.

See your doctor if you have the above symptoms and are at all worried.

Warts

WHAT ARE THEY?

These skin growths come and go, and it can be difficult to eliminate them forever. They are caused by human papilloma viruses and can occur anywhere. Verrucas are warts on the soles of the feet.

WHAT NEXT?

Most warts disappear without treatment, but this can take some time. If you have a persistent wart, visit your doctor or buy one of the over-the-counter wart treatments.

MY TREATMENT OPTIONS

Salicylic acid This is the active ingredient in many over-the-counter wart treatments.
Removal Your doctor may freeze off the wart with liquid nitrogen (cryotherapy) or burn it off using acid or electrodesiccation.

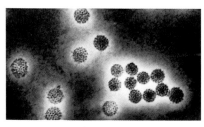

Human papilloma virus
There are over 100 different types of human papilloma virus. Most are harmless, but some cause warts.

HAVE I GOT THE SYMPTOMS?

There are three types of wart:
- Common warts on the hands, dotted with black spots
- Plantar warts on the soles of the feet (verrucas); these are dotted with black spots
- Flat warts on the wrists, backs of the hands, and face.

See your doctor if these are bothering you.

HOW CAN I HELP MYSELF?

Apply over-the-counter salicylic cream to the warts.

Impetigo

WHAT IS IT?

Impetigo is commonly seen on the face as honey-coloured crusts. It is the result of a bacterial infection through broken skin, such as a cut, cold sore, or dermatitis (see p354).

WHAT NEXT?

Your doctor will probably be able to diagnose the problem from close examination of the area. He or she may also take a skin swab and send it for laboratory investigation to identify the offending bacterium. Over 90 per cent of cases involve *Staphylococcus* but, rarely, *Streptococcus* may be the culprit. Impetigo is extremely contagious and is spread by direct contact.

MY TREATMENT OPTIONS

If detected very early, your doctor may prescribe a topical antibiotic but if new blisters appear within 48 hours, you will also be prescribed an oral antibiotic.

HOW CAN I HELP MYSELF?

To prevent infection, avoid direct contact with others who are infected. If you are infected, see your doctor.

HAVE I GOT THE SYMPTOMS?

The symptoms often develop in a typical sequence:
- Red skin and tiny fluid-filled blisters appear
- The blisters burst and release a yellow fluid
- The skin under the blisters becomes red and weeping
- The blisters dry out to form an itchy, honey-coloured crust.

See your doctor if you experience the symptoms described above.

Cold sores

WHAT IS IT?

Cold sores have a habit of appearing at the most inopportune of times, often presaged by a telltale tingle. The result of infection with herpes simplex virus type 1, cold sores can come and go throughout life. The virus is contagious and is passed on by direct skin contact. Most people have been infected with the virus by the time they reach adulthood, but only about 25 per cent experience symptoms.

WHAT NEXT?

Self-help is sufficient provided you act in time (see below). If not, visit your doctor.

MY TREATMENT OPTIONS

Your doctor will be able to prescribe an antiviral drug such as aciclovir, famciclovir, or valaciclovir.

HOW CAN I HELP MYSELF?

When you feel the characteristic tingling on your lip make sure you have some remedies to hand.
Antiviral medications Apply one of the over-the-counter topical antiviral medications. For this cream to be effective, you must apply it as soon as the first symptoms develop.

Trigger factors To prevent cold sores recurring, try to steer clear of these well-known trigger factors: stress, tiredness, cold winds, and sunburn.

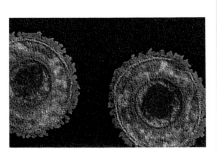

Herpes simplex virus
This is the virus that causes cold sores. It invades skin cells then lies dormant in the roots of the nerves.

HAVE I GOT THE SYMPTOMS?

Cold sores most commonly occur around the lips. Symptoms tend to appear in a certain order:
- The first indication is often a tingling in the affected site
- About six hours later, clusters of tiny, painful blisters begin to develop
- A day or so later, the blisters burst and then become crusty
- The blisters subside after 10–14 days.

See your doctor if you are bothered by these symptoms.

Hair loss

Losing hair can be extremely distressing. For many women, having a full head of hair is an integral part of feeling feminine, sexy, and healthy. However, a bad diet, stress, or overstyling can cause hair to fall out, though the good news is that most hair loss is only temporary – your hair will grow back in time.

If you're suffering from some form of hair loss, the first thing to do is carry out a hair count – that is, count all the hairs from your hairbrush and the plug hole each day. If, after a week of counting, you have over 700 hairs, it's time to see your doctor.

POSSIBLE CAUSES

To start with, he or she will want to ask some questions to find out if any new medications (such as lithium, isotretinoin, or heparin) or life events (such as illness requiring surgery, a bereavement, or crash weight loss) could be to blame. In addition, your doctor will want to take a blood sample to screen for other conditions that can cause your hair to fall out, including an underactive thyroid gland (see p327), lupus (see p269), and iron-deficiency anaemia (see pp248–9).

BOOST HAIR GROWTH

Your treatment will depend on what type of hair loss you have. Hair can often regrow, but it just takes time. In the meantime, boost your hair-growing power by eating some key foods (see p370).

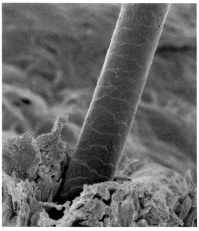

From root to tip
Overlapping scales cover the outside of each hair, the cuticle, to protect its central core of the fibrous protein keratin.

HOW YOUR HAIR GROWS

Each hair grows from a hair follicle within the dermis of the skin. In the hair bulb, or base of the follicle, cells divide rapidly to make each strand of hair. Each follicle follows a cycle of growth and rest, but not all follicles are synchronized, so every day some hairs grow while others fall out.

Your scalp has approximately 100,000 hairs and most are in the growing phase (the anagen phase). Hairs remain in this phase from two to seven years, though the exact time depends on your genetic inheritance.

The anagen phase is followed by an intermediate catagen phase, then a resting, or telogen, phase. At the end of the resting phase, the hair falls out and a new one starts to grow. It's quite normal to lose hair every day (on average, you lose about 100 telogen hairs daily) because hairs are being constantly renewed and replaced.

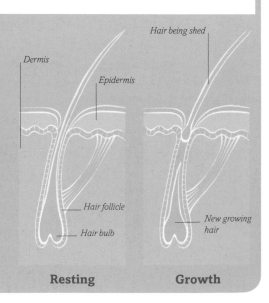

Hair being shed

Dermis

Epidermis

Hair follicle

Hair bulb

New growing hair

Resting   **Growth**

Traction alopecia

WHAT IS IT?
Alopecia is the medical term for hair loss and traction refers to a persistent tug on the hair follicle over time, eventually causing the hair to fall out, This is usually caused by certain severe hairstyles, such as tight buns, chignons, ponytails, and close braiding, tugging too harshly on the hair follicles themselves. This constant strain on the follicles, over time, can lead to scarring of the scalp and permanent damage to the hair root, which can mean that the hair doesn't grow back.

WHAT NEXT?
The good news is that hair usually does grow back if the pulling on the follicles ceases.

HAVE I GOT THE SYMPTOMS?

In traction alopecia, hair loss is associated with:
- Wearing bands in your hair that are too tight
- Always wearing a ponytail
- Wearing braided hair.

See your doctor if self-help measures don't work

MY TREATMENT OPTIONS
If you have tried changing your hairstyle and your hair is still not growing back, see your doctor. Bear in mind that Afro hair is more fragile than Caucasian hair, so if you braid your hair, take time out between braidings to let your follicles recover.

HOW CAN I HELP MYSELF?
Consider cutting your hair; if you always wear it up or back perhaps it's time to try a different style. If you want to keep it long, avoid wearing it tightly all the time – pinning your hair back while preparing food is fine, but wear it loosely the rest of the time.

Telogen effluvium

WHAT IS IT?
Telogen effluvium is a temporary hair loss that can be alarming since quantities of growing hairs shift into the telogen phase, and your hair starts falling out in clumps.

This type of hair loss is usually due to a change in, or interruption to, your hair's normal cycle. This often occurs after pregnancy – the post-pregnancy "moult" – and is nothing to worry about. At other times, it may be related to a physical or emotional shock, such as an illness in which you had a fever; undergoing surgery that required general anaesthesia; sudden weight loss; or a stressful event such as a bereavement.

WHAT NEXT?
If you have persistent hair shedding, your doctor may want to exclude conditions such as hyperthyroidism.

MY TREATMENT OPTIONS
No treatment is required. Typically, the hair follicles become active again in two or three months and your hair soon grows back.

HAVE I GOT THE SYMPTOMS?

In telogen effluvium:
- Handfuls of hair fall out while washing, handling, or brushing your hair
- There is overall hair thinning.

See your doctor if you have the above symptoms.

HAIR BREAKAGE

One type of hair loss that is on the rise is from the resurgence in hair straightening. Hairs lost from excessive straightening tend to break off in pieces, so you end up with short strands of hair. Treat your hair kindly and don't choose a hairstyle that involves daily straightening with irons or periodic chemical straightening. Your hair will thank you for it.

HOW CAN I HELP MYSELF?
Avoid breaking your hair through straightening (see above). If your hair loss occurred after pregnancy or is due to illness or stress, your hair will grow back in time. If it doesn't, see your doctor as there may be another cause for the loss.

How to eat to keep your hair healthy

If you don't eat a good balanced diet, say you're trying to lose a few kilos and aren't following your usual good habits, then your hair is the first part of your body to reflect this. For full, lustrous locks, make sure your diet includes the following ingredients.

Zinc

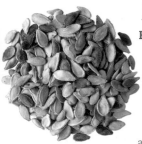

Pumpkin seeds, beef, and chickpeas are all zinc-rich foods, which are vital for hair growth. It helps to oil your scalp and ward off dandruff. In dietary supplement form, you should not take more than 40mg a day.

B vitamins

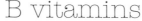

Bananas are rich in B6, essential for healthy hair, and also contain B3, B5, and folic acid (B9). All the B vitamins contribute to good skin and hair. Avocados are another good source of B vitamins.

Iron

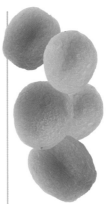

Dried apricots, liver, eggs, and wholemeal bread are all iron-rich foods that contribute to healthy hair growth. Loss of hair can be a sign of iron-deficiency anaemia (see p248–9).

Protein

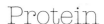

Fish, meat, eggs, tofu, and pulses are all good sources of protein. Eat protein at every meal; healthy hair growth requires a reasonable amount of protein to be able to manufacture the hair protein keratin.

Biotin

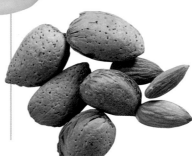

Almonds and other nuts contain biotin (100g/4oz of almonds = approx. 64mcg biotin), which helps to keep hair and nails thick and healthy. The recommended daily intake is 100–200mcg.

Alopecia areata

WHAT IS IT?

The cause of alopecia areata is not known, although many doctors believe that it's an autoimmune disease (see p259), in which your body sees your hair as "foreign" and attacks the hair follicles.

WHAT NEXT?

If you are worried, see your doctor.

MY TREATMENT OPTIONS

After examination and testing, your doctor will discuss what treatments are available to you, along with any potential side effects.

Steroids The aim of these drugs is to stop the immune system from attacking your hair. The drugs can be applied as ointments or injected directly into the scalp. Injections are usually done every month for three to six months. Steroid treatment is usually effective and typically yields results within about three months. Early hair regrowth may be with grey hairs but don't be alarmed by this as your normal colour usually returns eventually.

Other treatments If steroids don't work, your doctor may suggest treatment with topical immunotherapy, topical minoxidil, or phototherapy (see p357).

HOW CAN I HELP MYSELF?

See your doctor and follow their advice and/or treatment.

> ### HAVE I GOT THE SYMPTOMS?
>
> In alopecia areata:
> - Hair loss usually appears as small, round bald patches all over the scalp.
>
> **See your doctor** if you have the above symptom.

Female-pattern baldness

It is common for men to lose hair in a certain way as they get older – they go thin on top and the hairline recedes. Few of us expect women to be similarly affected.

WHAT IS IT?

Female-pattern baldness (also known as androgenetic alopecia) differs from the classic male pattern (although both are related to testosterone levels in the body): women usually have thinning of the hair at the front, sides, or crown, and rarely go completely bald.

As we age, hair thins naturally and this is more apparent in some women: if you have lots of thick hair you'll fare better than those with less abundant, finer hair.

In female-pattern baldness, the growing phase of the hairs shortens and the hairs become fine and more fragile. With each cycle, the hairs become rooted more superficially and fall out more easily. Female-pattern baldness often runs in families. And heredity will also influence the age at which you start to experience hair loss, as well as the pattern of your baldness, how fast your hairline changes and hair falls out, and how much falls out.

WHAT NEXT?

Because hormones play a part in female-pattern baldness, hair loss may first become apparent during the menopause, so if you are worried, make an appointment with your doctor.

MY TREATMENT OPTIONS

When discussing treatments, ask your doctor about any potential side effects.

Minoxidil lotion This comes in two strengths (2% and 5%) and is used either twice daily (2%) or once daily (5%). This treatment is beneficial in up to half of affected women. However, to continue the success you must use it each and every day otherwise the new hairs that have grown will fall out within a few months.

Spironolactone This drug blocks the actions of testosterone and can be taken as a tablet, but it can have adverse effects on a fetus so you must avoid getting pregnant while taking this medication.

Oral cyproterone This needs to be taken with oral contraceptives, with or without oestrogens.

HAVE I GOT THE SYMPTOMS?

In female-pattern baldness:
● Hair is fine and fragile
● Hair falls out more easily than normal for you.
See your doctor if you have the above symptoms.

Hair transplants If the hair loss can be stabilized then hair transplanting can be effective. Transplanting single follicular units works best rather than multiple follicles. The hair takes three months to grow back.

HOW CAN I HELP MYSELF?

There's nothing you can do to stop the hair loss, but many women find that changing their hairstyle, hair extensions, or wigs help improve their appearance.

HAIR-LOSS PATTERNS

Female-pattern baldness can be inherited from either side of your family. Women's hair loss tends to follow a different pattern from men's: it becomes thinner overall, especially at the front, sides, and crown. Doctors assign a category to the amount of hair left from grade 1 (mild loss) to grade 3 (marked loss).

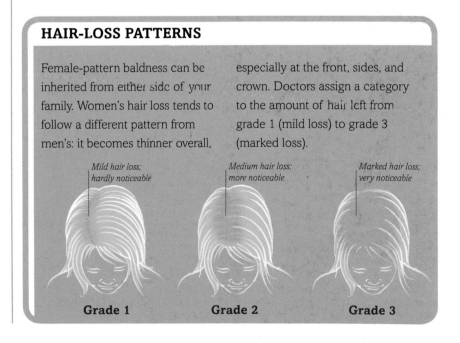

Mild hair loss; hardly noticeable

Medium hair loss; more noticeable

Marked hair loss; very noticeable

Grade 1　　**Grade 2**　　**Grade 3**

Cosmetic dermatology

As we get older we tend to worry more about skin changes – noticing every new wrinkle or blemish. Many women are anxious to improve their complexion and retain a more youthful appearance. Whether it's achieving a more even skin tone or plumping up some laughter lines, there are plenty of options available.

HAVE I GOT THE SYMPTOMS?

Cosmetic dermatology can help hide the effects of a wide range of skin symptoms, including:

- Lines and wrinkles
- Uneven pigmentation
- Non-cancerous moles
- Sun-related ageing
- Acne scars.

Laser treatment
A targeted laser beam is used to treat a very precise area. Laser skin resurfacing can remove brown spots and melasma (see p361) and fade prominent or broken blood vessels.

WHAT IS IT?

Cosmetic dermatology is treatment of the skin, for example laser treatment or chemical peeling. These techniques help to improve the physical appearance of the skin, such as acne scarring or skin discoloration. The treatment may or may not include healing a medical condition.

WHAT NEXT?

When assessing what procedures to use to improve your overall complexion, your cosmetic dermatologist will consider:

- The texture of your skin
- The tone (firmness) of your skin
- The evenness of colour
- How much laxity there is (that is, how your skin drapes and sags)
- The size of the pores
- Any lumps and bumps
- Any clogged pores or cysts.

Many studies show that when people evaluate age they think someone is older than they really are if they have brown spots. It seems that anything that mars the surface makes us appear older.

MY TREATMENT OPTIONS

Your cosmetic dermatologist will talk you through the most common procedures and advise you on which is best for your skin problem. Each treatment is usually delivered over several sessions. Be sure to ask about any potential side effects. You may feel that your skin needs time to settle before you go out in public.

Bleaching If you have brown spots or melasma (see p361), your doctor may suggest bleaching.

Chemical peels Your doctor will apply an acid to the area. It can target brown spots or fade blood vessels. The depth of skin removed by a peel can be varied. Superficial peels remove only a portion of the epidermis, whereas a medium-depth peel removes the whole epidermis and a tiny part of the underlying dermal tissue too. Peels stimulate the fibroblasts in the skin and new skin forms to replace peeled-off skin. Your skin will have some redness, which can last a while. After a series of peels, your skin will look smoother and less wrinkled, and your complexion more even.

> "Between ages 25 and 30, collagen-making slows, yet collagen breakdown continues."

Microdermabrasion This removes surface skin, but uses tiny crystals instead of acid. It is a more refined technique, removing only a fine layer of skin. A targeted stream of aluminium oxide crystals "sandblasts" your skin. You may notice a slight redness, but this fades quickly; several sessions two to four weeks apart result in younger-looking skin. This procedure is not suitable for those with eczema (see pp354–5) or acne rosacea (see pp364–5) as it can cause flare-ups.

Laser skin resurfacing Your dermatologist uses a laser beam to destroy the epidermal layer and heat the underlying dermis. This stimulates the fibroblasts to produce new collagen fibres, to make skin appear smoother. The laser destroys tissue, which then repairs itself with new cells. This treatment is harsher than others, so can take a few months to heal fully.

There are less intense lasers available, called non-ablative lasers and radiofrequency devices. These treatments heat up the dermis, but without causing any damage to the epidermis. Recovery time is shorter, but you'll need more treatments to make your skin appear younger.

Laser resurfacing can remove brown spots and melasma (see p361) and fade prominent or broken blood vessels. About six sessions are necessary.

Botox is short for botulinum toxin type A. When injected into specific muscles, this neurotoxin blocks nerve impulses and paralyses and relaxes muscles. The skin flattens and smooths. Each treatment lasts three to six months, so repeat injections are needed. Botox works well on deep, upper-face lines, especially frown lines, horizontal forehead lines and crow's feet.

Injectable dermal fillers can plump up and smooth out lines and folds. Such fillers can be based on fat, collagen, hyaluronic acid, or calcium hydroxyapatite. These plumping agents give only temporary effects and the procedure needs to be repeated every few months. You may experience temporary redness, swelling, and bruising. The week before treatment you should not take aspirin or vitamin E, or drink any alcohol, to reduce the chances of bruising. You may have needlemarks or swelling afterwards.

There is some research to suggest that products based on

COSMECEUTICALS – THE FUTURE?

Products once restricted to the use of qualified medical practitioners are making their way into over-the-counter products. The dermal filler hyaluronic acid, for example, is now an ingredient of some over-the-counter anti-wrinkle creams. The effectiveness of many such products is unproven, but it will be interesting to see how many dermatological therapies you will be able to try yourself in the comfort of your own home.

hyaluronic acid may stimulate your body to make its own collagen, so long after treatment your skin may still look younger.

HOW CAN I HELP MYSELF?
Reduce the need for cosmetic dermatology by protecting yourself against potential sun damage. Use a high-factor sunscreen and avoid excessive sunbathing. This will reduce the build-up of lines and wrinkles and the possibility of unsightly skin discoloration.

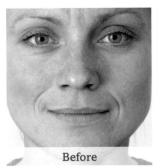
Before

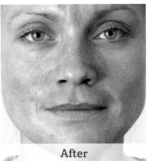
After

Disappearing wrinkles
Injectable dermal fillers can smooth out deep frown lines and wrinkles. After treatment, the wrinkles between nose and mouth and under the eyes are less prominent.

Resources

CHAPTER 2: UNDERSTANDING THE CHANGES

Menopause Matters

www.menopausematters.co.uk
Email: info@menopausematters.co.uk
An independent, clinician-led website that provides easily accessible, up-to-date, accurate information about the menopause, menopausal symptoms and treatment options.

NHS Cancer Screening Programmes

Fulwood House
Old Fulwood Road
Sheffield S10 3TH
Tel: 0114 271 1060
www.cancerscreening.nhs.uk
E-mail: info@cancerscreening.nhs.uk
For information about the nationally coordinated cancer screening programmes in England.

Women's Health Concern

4–6 Eton Place
Marlow
Buckinghamshire SL7 2QA
Tel: 01628 478 473
Confidential advice line: 0845 123 2319
www.womens-health-concern.org
Email: info@womens-health-concern.org
Provides an independent service to advise, reassure and educate women about their health concerns, to enable them to work in partnership with their own medical practitioners and health advisers.

CHAPTER 3: STAYING WELL

Food Standards Agency

Aviation House
125 Kingsway
London WC2B 6NH
Tel: 020 7276 8829
www.food.gov.uk
Email: helpline@foodstandards.gsi.gov.uk
An independent Government department set up by an Act of Parliament in 2000 to protect the public's health and consumer interests in relation to food.

NHS Choices

Tel: 0845 4647
www.nhs.uk
NHS website that helps you make choices about your health, from lifestyle decisions to the practical aspects of finding and using NHS services when you need them.

Wellbeing of Women

27 Sussex Place
Regent's Park
London NW1 4SP
Tel: 020 7772 6400
www.wellbeingofwomen.org.uk
Email: wellbeingofwomen@rcog.org.uk
A charity devoted to raising money to invest in medical research and the development of specialist doctors and nurses working in the field of reproductive and gynaecological health.

CHAPTER 5: REPRODUCTIVE SYSTEM

Infertility Network UK

Charter House
43 St Leonards Road
Bexhill on Sea
East Sussex TN40 1JA
Tel: 0800 008 7464
www.infertilitynetworkuk.com
Email: admin@infertilitynetworkuk.com
Povides support and information for anyone affected by infertility issues.

International Community of Women Living with HIV/AIDS

International Support Office
Unit 6, Building 1
Canonbury Yard
190a New North Road
London N1 7BJ
Tel: 020 7704 0606
www.icw.org
Email: infor@icw.org
An international network for HIV+ women. Members receive a newsletter, can chat with other HIV+ women, and can join message forums.

Royal College of Obstetricians and Gynaecologists (RCOG)

27 Sussex Place
Regent's Park
London NW1 4RG
Tel: 020 7772 6200
www.rcog.org.uk
Its charter states that its objectives are "the encouragement of the study and the advancement of the science and practice of obstetrics and gynaecology". The website offers patient information, explains medical terms and provides links to many other useful organisations.

Terence Higgins Trust

314–320 Gray's Inn Road
London WC1X 8DP
Tel: 020 7812 1600
Helpline: 0845 12 21 200 (10am–10pm, Monday–Friday, 12 noon–6pm, Saturday and Sunday)
www.tht.org.uk
Email: info@tht.org.uk
Provides support, advice and information on sexual health and HIV.

CHAPTER 6: BREAST HEALTH

Breast Cancer Care

5–13 Great Suffolk Street
London SE1 0NS
Telephone helpline: 0808 800 6000
www.breastcancercare.org.uk
Email: info@breastcancercare.org.uk
Offers information, practical assistance and emotional support for anyone affected by breast cancer.

NHS Cancer Screening Programmes

See entry under Chapter 2

CHAPTER 7: HEART AND CIRCULATION

British Cardiac Patients Association

2 Station Road
Swavesey
Cambridge CB24 5QJ
Telephone helpline: 01223 846845
Enquiries: 0195 420 2022
www.bcpa.co.uk
Email: Enquiries@BCPA.co.uk
Offers support, reassurance and practical advice for cardiac patients, their families and carers.

British Heart Foundation

14 Fitzhardinge Street
London W1H 6DH
Tel: 020 7935 0185
Heart information line: 08450 70 80 70
www.bhf.org.uk
Email: via the website
Funds research projects, supports and cares for heart patients and aims to educate the public about heart disease and how to deal with an emergency.

HEART UK

7 North Road
Maidenhead
Berkshire SL6 1PE
Helpline: 0845 450 5988
www.heartuk.org.uk
Email: ask@heartuk.org.uk
Committed to raising awareness about the risks of high cholesterol, lobbying for better detection of those at risk, funding research into improved treatment and supporting health professional training.

Her at Heart

www.heratheart.org.uk
Email: via the website
This scientific initiative is aimed at raising awareness among healthcare professionals and the general public on the under-recognition of heart disease in women. The website gives useful information on the prevention, risk factors, symptoms, and treatment of cardiovascular disease.

CHAPTER 8: BRAIN AND NERVES

Alzheimer's Society

Devon House
58 St Katharine's Way
London E1W 1JX
Tel: 020 7423 3500
Dementia Helpline: 0845 300 0336 (usually open 8.30am–6.30pm, Monday–Friday)
www.alzheimers.org.uk
Email: enquiries@alzheimers.org.uk
This website is really comprehensive, with lots of useful information, from advice for people worried about their memory, to information on the various types and causes of dementia and sections for carers. The site has hundreds of downloadable factsheets on a huge variety of aspects and issues, with often very practical advice given.

Mayo Clinic

www.mayoclinic.com/health/tension-headache
This website give lots of sensible advice for people suffering from tension-type headaches, including drug therapies, lifestyle and home remedies, and advice on coping and support.

Migraine Trust

55–56 Russell Square
London WC1B 4HP
Tel: 020 7436 1336
Helpline: 020 7462 6601 (Monday–Friday, 10am 5pm)
www.migrainetrust.org
Email: info@migrainetrust.org
A national charity giving support to people who suffer migraine and promoting research into the disorder. The website lists excellent factsheets available to download on many aspects of migraine, ranging from triggers, medication, and migraine in pregnancy, through to migraine and stroke.

Motor Neurone Disease Association

PO Box 246,
Northampton
NN1 2PR
Tel: 01604 250505
Helpline 08457 62 62 62 (normal opening hours Monday–Friday, 9.00am–5pm; people affected by MND can also phone outside of normal office hours: Monday–Friday, 7pm–10.30pm).
www.mndassociation.org
Email: mndconnect@mndassociation.org
The main national UK organisation dedicated to the support of people with MND and their carers. The website provides practical information on how to access care services in addition to information on equipment loan, financial support, and current research.

Multiple Sclerosis Society

MS National Centre
372 Edgware Road
Staples Corner
London NW2 6ND
Tel: 020 8438 0700
Helpline: 0808 800 8000
www.mssociety.org.uk
Email helpline@mssociety.org.uk
Lots of good information on how the diagnosis is made, coming to terms with the diagnosis, accessing care and support, and evaluation of new treatments. Particularly good literature on MS and women's health available to download.

National Institute of Neurological Disorders and Stroke

National Institutes of Health
9000 Rockville Pike
Bethesda, Maryland 20892
www.ninds.nih.gov
This is a very comprehensive website of the section of the US National Institute of Health that deals with neurological disorders and strokes. If you know your diagnosis, this site will give you good information about your condition.

National Society for Epilepsy (NSE)
Chesham Lane
Chalfont St Peter
Bucks SL9 0RJ
Tel: 01494 601300
Helpline: 01494 601400
(10am–4pm, Monday–Friday)
www.epilepsynse.org.uk
A useful website with lots of
information about the condition and an
extensive frequently asked questions
section.

Parkinson's Disease Society
PDS National Office
215 Vauxhall Bridge Road
London SW1V 1EJ
Tel: 020 7931 8080
Helpline: 0808 800 0303 (Monday–
Friday, 9.30am–9pm, Saturday, 9.30am–
5.30pm)
www.parkinsons.org.uk
Email: enquiries@parkinsons.org.uk
In addition to information about the
disease, treatments and support, this
site has recently added a forum section
where people can ask questions and
share experiences of living with the
condition.

Stroke Association
Stroke House
240 City Road
London
EC1V 2PR
Tel: 020 7566 0300
Stroke helpline: 0845 3033 100
(Monday–Friday, 9am–5pm)
www.stroke.org.uk
Email: info@stroke.org.uk
The website has a very clear and
comprehensive information area, with a
particularly good section on "When a
stroke happens", and what to expect in
the first hours, days and weeks
afterwards. Good explanation of the
various tests and assessments that are
likely to be performed. Excellent
downloadable information leaflets.

CHAPTER 9: MENTAL HEALTH

Institute of Psychiatry
King's College London
De Crespigny Park
London SE5 8AF
Tel: 020 7836 5454
www.iop.kcl.ac.uk
A postgraduate research and teaching
institution devoted to the understanding
and treatment of mental disorders and
related disorders of the brain. Its
website provides links to some useful
organisations.

Royal College of Psychiatrists
17 Belgrave Square
London SW1X 8PG
Tel: 020 7235 2351
www.rcpsych.ac.uk
Email: rcpsych@rcpsych.ac.uk
Primarily a professional organisation,
but the website offers a large number of
downloadable information leaflets in
several languages on a range of mental
health issues, as well as many useful
weblinks.

CHAPTER 10: BREATHING AND RESPIRATION

British Lung Foundation
73-75 Goswell Road,
London EC1V 7ER
Helpline: 08458 50 50 20
www.lunguk.org
Email: via the website
Provides support and information for
people with a variety of lung diseases,
as well as providing funding for research
projects.

British Thoracic Society
17 Doughty Street
London WC1N 2PL
Tel: 020 7831 8778
www.brit-thoracic.org.uk
Email: bts@brit-thoracic.org.uk
The website contains information of
interest to people who have respiratory
diseases, as well as links to dedicated
sites run by lung charities.

CHAPTER 11: BLOOD DISORDERS

Circulation Foundation
The Vascular Society Office
The Royal College of Surgeons of
England
35–43 Lincoln's Inn Fields
London WC2A 3PE
Tel: 020 7304 4779
www.circulationfoundation.org.uk
The Foundation merged with the
Vascular Society in 2004. It carries out
fundraising activities and supports
research projects and grants, and its
website contains lots of useful
information for people suffering from
vascular complaints.

Lifeblood: The Thrombosis Charity
The Thrombosis & Haemostasis Centre
Level 1, North Wing
St Thomas' Hospital
London SE1 7EH
Tel: 020 7633 9937
www.thrombosis-charity.org.uk
Email: via the website
A charity that promotes awareness
about thrombosis and aims to increase
understanding of its causes, effects and
the treatment available. The website
provides a large number of
downloadable factsheets.

CHAPTER 12: BONES AND JOINTS

Arthritis Care
18 Stephenson Way
London NW1 2HD
Tel: 020 7380 6500
Helpline: 0808 800 4050 (10am–4pm,
weekdays)
www.arthritiscare.org.uk
Email info@arthritiscare.org.uk
Provides support and information about
all types of arthritis and publishes
Arthritis News, a bi-monthly magazine.

Arthritis Research Campaign
Copeman House
St Mary's Court
St Mary's Gate
Chesterfield
Derbyshire S41 7TD

Tel: 0870 850 5000
www.arc.org.uk
Email: info@arc.org.uk
Provides reliable information on arthritis and a variety of conditions such as carpal tunnel syndrome, fibromyalgia and neck pain.

British Society for Rheumatology
Bride House
18–20 Bride Lane
London EC4Y 8EE
Tel: 020 7842 0900
www.rheumatology.org.uk
Email: bsr@rheumatology.org.uk
A professional medical society "committed to advancing knowledge and practice in the field of rheumatology". It offers weblinks to useful patient support associations.

CHAPTER 13: DIGESTIVE SYSTEM

British Liver Trust
2 Southampton Road
Ringwood BH24 1HY
Helpline: 0800 652 7330 (Monday–Friday, 9am–5pm)
www.britishlivertrust.org.uk
Email: info@britishlivertrust.org.uk
Offers support to sufferers of liver disease and produces leaflets and factsheets on a range of liver disorders.

CORE (Digestive Disorders Foundation)
3 St Andrews Place
London NW1 4LB
Tel: 020 7034 4972
www.digestivedisorders.org.uk
Email: info@corecharity.org.uk
Provides information leaflets and factsheets online or by post on a range of digestive disorders.

CHAPTER 14: HORMONES AND METABOLISM

Diabetes UK
Macleod House
10 Parkway
London NW1 7AA

Tel: 020 7424 1000
Careline 0845 120 2960 (Monday–Friday, 9am–5pm)
www.diabetes.org.uk
Email: info@diabetes.org.uk
Provides information and advice on all aspects of diabetes.

Heart UK
See entry under Chapter 7

CHAPTER 15: BLADDER AND URINARY TRACT

Bladder and Bowel Foundation
SATRA Innovation Park
Rockingham Road
Kettering
Northamptonshire NN16 9JH
Tel: 0153 653 3255
Helpline: 0845 345 0165
www.bladderandbowelfoundation.org
Email: info@bladderandbowelfoundation.org
Provides information on incontinence and help for those living with bladder and bowel disorders.

British Association of Urological Surgeons
35–43 Lincoln's Inn Fields, London WC2A 3PE
Tel: 020 7869 6950
www.baus.org.uk
Email: admin@baus.org.uk
A professional association that will direct enquiries from the public to the appropriate organisation. The website offers a number of useful weblinks.

Cystitis & Overactive Bladder Foundation
76 High Street
Stony Stratford
Buckinghamshire MK11 1AH
Tel: 01908 569169
www.cobfoundation.org
Email: info@cobfoundation.org
Provides support and information about variety of bladder problems.

EdRenINFO
Renal Medicine
Royal Infirmary
Little France
Edinburgh EH16 4SA
Scotland
Tel: 0131 242 1233
http://renux.dmed.ed.ac.uk/edren/
Website of the Royal Infirmary of Edinburgh Renal Unit offreing information about a range of kidney problems.

CHAPTER 16: SKIN AND HAIR

British Association of Dermatologists
Willan House
4 Fitzroy Square
London W1T 5HQ
Tel: 0207 383 0266
www.bad.org.uk
Provides a lot of information for people suffering from skin disease and a list of all the patient support groups in the UK.

Skin Treatment and Research Trust (START)
Chelsea & Westminster Hospital
Fulham Palace Road
London SW10 9HH
Tel: 020 8746 8174
www.start-skin.org
Email: via the website
A charity founded by a group of dermatoilogists with the aim of funding research into all aspects of skin disease, including eczema, psoriasis and skin cancer.

SunSmart
Cancer Research UK
PO Box 123
London WC2A 3PX
Tel: 020 7121 6699
Helpline: 0808 800 4040
http://info.cancerresearchuk.org/healthyliving/sunsmart/
Email: cancer.info@cancer.org.uk
Part of Cancer Research UK, SunSmart provides support and information on skin protection and skin cancer.

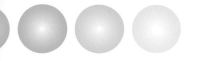

Index

and smoking 64
otitis externa 186
otitis media 187, 188
ovaries 13, 15, 88–9, 96
   disorders of 94–5, 145
   menopause 136–7, 138
   perimenopause 34
ovulation 89, 91, 112–13

P

palpitations 76, 167
pancreas 318, 320–3
panic attacks 63, 205
parathyroid gland 318, 330, 347
Parkinson's disease 42, 47, 192, 197
pelvic floor muscles 339–41
   exercises (Kegel) 223, 341
   weakened 303
pelvic inflammatory disease (PID) 98, 102
pelvis 14, 15
perimenopause 34, 136
perinatal depression 214, 215
personality 20–1
personality disorders 218–19
pharyngitis 237
phytoestrogens 141
pigmentation problems 361
piles 314–15
pimples 362–4
pituitary gland 318, 326, 330–1
placental disorders 128–9, 130
plasma 246, 254
platelets 246, 250
pneumonia 43, 234
Poland's syndrome 151
polycystic ovary syndrome (PCOS) 94, 95
polyps 100, 102, 236, 307–9
post-nasal drip 233, 235
post-thrombotic syndrome 253
post-traumatic stress disorder (PTSD) 208–9
"postmenopausal zest" 137
postnatal depression (PND) 93, 215
posture 67, 272
pre-eclampsia 30, 128
pregnancy 15, 28, 90
   abdominal pain in 78
   anaemia in 248–9
   asthma in 17, 238
   blood in 247

body changes in 88, 144–5
complications in 28, 30, 59, 124–31
constipation in 303
depression in 17, 214–15
epilepsy in 195
fatty liver in 298
gestational diabetes in 127, 322, 324
hair loss in 369
heartburn in 290
hepatitis B in 118
HIV in 121
hypothyroidism in 327
inflammatory bowel disease in 311
melasma in 361
migraines in 17
perinatal depression in 17, 214, 215
piles in 314–15
rheumatoid arthritis in 17, 268
sinusitis in 235
stress incontinence in 339, 340
uterine prolapse in 105
valvular heart disease in 174
in your 40s 34
see also childbirth; infertility
premature delivery 129
premature ovarian failure (POF) 30
premenstrual dysphoric disorder (PMDD) 92, 93, 211
premenstrual syndrome (PMS) 92–3, 134, 276
progesterone 89, 112, 134
   and the menopause 136, 137, 138
prolapse, uterine 105
pruritus ani 315
psoriasis 63, 72, 356–7
psoriatic arthritis 356
psychological wellbeing 50
psychotherapy, for mental health 224–6
psychotropic medication 226–7
puberty 12–13, 144
pulmonary embolism (PE) 252–3
pyelonephritis (PN) 335, 338

R

radioallergosorbent (RAST) test 355
radiotherapy 255
rashes 72, 74, 77, 81, 83, 84
   eczema 315, 354–5, 359
   food allergies 52
   see also acne
Raynaud's phenomenon 270
relaxation 62–3

renal cell cancer 348
repetitive strain injury (RSI) 280–1
reproductive system 13, 15, 88–141
respiratory system 230–43
retinoids 364, 365
rheumatoid arthritis 17, 266–8, 282
rosacea 364–5

S

salt 54, 172
screening tests 29, 30, 35, 39, 43, 45
seasonal affective disorder (SAD) 213
seizures 194–5
sex
   contraception 132–5
   pain during 109–10, 112–13, 343
sexual disorders 44, 222–3
sexual health
   at different life stages 28, 30, 34, 38
   libido 34–5, 44
sexually transmitted infections (STIs) 38, 114–21, 132–5
shingles 43
shoulder pain 67, 82, 282
sinusitis 233, 235
Sjögren's syndrome 271
skeleton 12, 14
  see also bones
skin 46, 67, 352–67
   acne 72, 134, 353, 362–4, 373
   cancer 28–9, 358–60
   cosmetic dermatology 372–3
   eczema 315, 354–5, 359
   rashes 72, 74, 77, 81, 83, 84
sleep 39, 51, 56, 60–1
slipped discs 272–3, 274
smoking 23, 51, 64
   Alzheimer's disease 47
   bladder cancer 349
   breathing 231
   Crohn's disease 311
   diabetes 322
   emphysema 240–1
   eyes 68
   heart disease 163, 172
   hormonal diseases 319
   incontinence 342
   insomnia 61
   lung cancer 242–3
   osteoporosis 261
   skin 67
social anxiety disorder 206

speech, slurred 75
sperm 112–13
spermicides 134, 135
spinal cord 178
spinal disorders 260, 261, 272–4
spleen 254
spots
see acne; eczema; rashes
squamous cell carcinoma (SCC) 111, 358, 359
statins 16
sterilization 135
steroids 331
stomach disorders
gastroenteritis 300
hiatus hernia 291
stomach ache 78
strength-training exercises 57
stress 172, 208–10
breast pain 149
from modern life 22–3
heart disease 163
inflammatory bowel disease 311
insomnia 61
managing 51, 56, 62–3, 180
migraines 183
sexual disorders 222–3
see also mental health
stress incontinence 339, 340–1
stretches 60
strokes 16, 192, 196
substance abuse 166, 206, 218, 220–1
sun protection 66, 67
syphilis 38, 115

T

teeth care 26, 64, 68–9
and heart conditions 162
in old age 45
telogen effluvium 369
tendinitis, calcific 282
tennis elbow 281
testosterone 13, 95, 364
throat disorders 75, 236–7
thrombocytopenia 250
thrombosis 252–3
thrush
oral 288–9
vaginal 108, 109
thyroid gland 318, 319
disorders 190, 283, 326–9
thyrotoxicosis 328

thyroxine 326–8
tinnitus 188, 193
tiredness 278–9, 319
tongue disorders 75, 288–9
tooth see teeth
toxaemia 128
trichomoniasis 108, 119
tumours
brain 181, 188, 194
pituitary 330–1
see also cancer
Turner's syndrome 327

U

ulcerative colitis 308, 310–11
ulcers 288, 292
unipolar depression 211
ureter 338, 346, 348–9
urethra 119, 335
urinary tract disorders 79, 81, 334–49
urticaria 52
uterine disorders 91, 98–105, 130, 138

V

vaccinations 29, 33, 37, 41, 43, 47
vagina 88
disorders 80, 108–11, 339–40
vaginal intra-epithelial neoplasia (VAIN) 111
vaginal therapy 138–9
valves, heart 160, 161, 174
valvular heart disease 166, 167, 174
varicose veins 175
vascular disease 175
venous thrombosis 252–3
verrucas 366
vertigo 192, 193
vesicovaginal fistula 339–40
vestibular neuritis 193
vision disorders 182, 189
vitiligo 361
vocal cord nodules 237
vulva disorders 108, 112–13, 115–17

W

walking 56
warts 85, 366
genital 29, 38, 117
weight
weight loss 23, 36, 57, 59, 233

weight problems 32, 58–9, 216–17
whiplash 272
von Willebrand's disease 250
wrinkles 353, 372–3

Y

yoga 60

Acknowledgments

Publisher's Acknowledgments

Dorling Kindersley would like to thank the following: Hilary Mandleberg for her unfailing professionalism throughout this project; John Freeman for photography; model Holly Newbury; Dawn Bates and Emma Forge; Dr Naomi Craft; Jane de Burgh; Dr Laszlo Tabar for the information in the graph on p153; Fiona Hunter, Bsc (Hons) Nutrition, Dip Dietetics; Yvonne Bishop-Weston, Foods for Life nutrition clinics, www.optimumnutritionists.com, email: clinic@ foodsforlife.co.uk, tel: 0871 288 4642; Elma Aquino, Will Hicks, and Adam Walker for design assistance; Mary Lambert for proofreading; Vanessa Bird for the index.

All illustrations by Juliet Percival

Picture Credits

The publisher would like to thank the following for their kind permission to reproduce their photographs:

(Key: a-above; b-below/bottom; c-centre; f-far; l-left; r-right; t-top)

Alamy Images: amana images inc. 7tc; Daniel Dempster Photography 172; FogStock 41c; Guy Croft SciTech 197l; Bubbles Photolibrary 305b; Phototake Inc 162, 243; botonics Limited (www.botonics.co.uk): 373; Corbis: Heide Benser 37c; Bettmann 17; Envision 93l; Howard Sochurek 166; DK Images: Stephen Oliver 141cla; Courtesy of the Royal Botanic Gardens, Edinburgh 93r; Getty Images: Alterndo Images 20r; altrendo images 7tr; Cornelia Doerr 62; Michael Goldman 50; Hulton Archive 22; William McCoy-Rainbow 205; Benn Mitchell 47r; Thomas Northcut 140; Marc Romanelli/The Image Bank 47l; Terry Vine 37r; Health and Safety Executive: poster Skin Checks for Dermatitis (c) Crown copyright material is reproduced with the permission of the Controller of HMSO and Queen's Printer for Scotland 354t; iStockphoto.com: Carmen Martínez Banús 20l; Jill Chen 141cl; Martina Ebel 353b; Quavondo Nguygen 353t; Anthony Rosenberg 23; Thomas Stange 32c; Valeria Titova 139; Mediscan: 153; Owen Mumford Ltd: 110; Photolibrary: 133ca; BananaStock 40c; Big Cheese 46l; Blend Images 32l, 33r, 41l, 353ca; Brand X Pictures 237; Corbis 7bc, 353cb; Digital Vision 2, 41r, 46r, 202; image100 168; Juice Images 33l; moodboard 40r, 353c; Photoalto 226; Photodisc 37l, 46c; Photographer's Choice 145; Purestock 36c; Phototake: PDSN 171; PunchStock: Mixa 32r; Rex Features: Garo/ Phanie 138, 195r; RESO 40l; Voisin / Phanie 204; Science Photo Library: 106r, 114, 174, 260l, 260r, 295, 296b, 299, 309; AJ Photo 271; Samuel Ashfield 155;

Biophoto Associates 12; Dee Breger 319; BSIP / Laurent / Laetitia 217; BSIP, Cavallini James 255; BSIP, Ducloux 197r; CDC 296t; Centre for infections/ Health protection agency 366; CNRI 338, 349b, 360fbl; Custom Medical Stock Photo 133cb, 195l, 360r; Michael Donne 372; Du Cane Medical Imaging Ltd 253, 313; Eye of Science 120, 367; Simon Fraser 273, 298; Dr. Robert Friedland 185; Chris Gallagher 169; Adam Gault 161, 344; GJLP 331; Steve Gschmeissner 251, 251cr, 254, 289, 297, 343, 349t; Gusto Images 95, 347; Institut Pasteur/ Unite Des Virus OncongenesF 278; ISM 94, 97, 328; Kwangshin Kim 336; James King-Holmes 123, 252; Mehau Kulyk 148, 264; Dr. Najeeb Layyous 131; Living Art Enterprises 282; Dr. Karl Lounatmaa 115; Dr P. Marazzi 260c, 265, 360l; Dr. P. Marazzi 272, 360c; BSIP 291b; David M. Martin, M.D. 291t; Moredun Animal Health Ltd 119; Don Fawcett 122, 305t; Professors P.M. Motta & F.M. Magliocca 301; Dr.Gopal Murti 232; Susumu Nishinaga 368; D. Phillips 300; Dr Linda Stannard, UCT 116; James Stevenson 360fbr; Saturn Stills 135b, 355b; Andrew Syred 246; Dr E Walker 106l, 249, 288; Dr Keith Wheeler 89; Zephyr 267l; Shutterstock: J.T. Lewis 268; William Stuart: 139r; SuperStock: 47c; age fotostock 135c

All other images © Dorling Kindersley
For further information see: www.dkimages.com